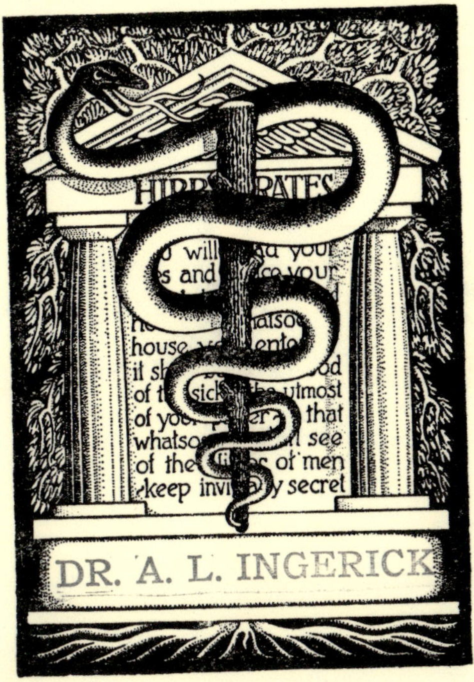
DR. A. L. INGERICK

1993
YEAR BOOK OF
EMERGENCY MEDICINE®

Statement of Purpose

The YEAR BOOK Service

The YEAR BOOK series was devised in 1901 by practicing health professionals who observed that the literature of medicine and related disciplines had become so voluminous that no one individual could read and place in perspective every potential advance in a major specialty. In the final decade of the 20th century, this recognition is more acutely true than it was in 1901.

More than merely a series of books, YEAR BOOK volumes are the tangible results of a unique service designed to accomplish the following:

- to *survey* a wide range of journals of proven value
- to *select* from those journals papers representing significant advances and statements of important clinical principles
- to provide *abstracts* of those articles that are readable, convenient summaries of their key points
- to provide *commentary* about those articles to place them in perspective.

These publications grow out of a unique process that calls on the talents of outstanding authorities in clinical and fundamental disciplines, trained literature specialists, and professional writers, all supported by the resources of Mosby–Year Book, the world's preeminent publisher for the health professions.

The Literature Base

Mosby–Year Book subscribes to nearly 1,000 journals published worldwide, covering the full range of the health professions. On an annual basis, the publisher examines usage patterns and polls its expert authorities to add new journals to the literature base and to delete journals that are no longer useful as potential YEAR BOOK sources.

The Literature Survey

The publisher's team of literature specialists, all of whom are trained and experienced health professionals, examines every original, peer-reviewed article in each journal issue. More than 250,000 articles per year are scanned systematically, including title, text, illustrations, tables, and references. Each scan is compared, article by article, to the search strategies that the publisher has developed in consultation with the 270 outside experts who form the pool of YEAR BOOK editors. A given article may be reviewed by any number of editors, from one to a dozen or more, regardless of the discipline for which the paper was originally published. In turn, each editor who receives the article reviews it to determine whether or not the article should be included in the YEAR BOOK. This decision is based on the article's inherent quality, its probable usefulness to readers of that YEAR BOOK, and the editor's goal to represent a balanced picture of a given field in each volume of the YEAR BOOK. In addition, the editor indicates when to include figures and tables from the article to help the YEAR BOOK reader better understand the information.

Of the quarter million articles scanned each year, only 5% are selected for detailed analysis within the YEAR BOOK series, thereby assuring readers of the high value of every selection.

The Abstract

The publisher's abstracting staff is headed by a physician-writer and includes individuals with training in the life sciences, medicine, and other areas, plus extensive experience in writing for the health professions and related industries. Each selected article is assigned to a specific writer on this abstracting staff. The abstracter, guided in many cases by notations supplied by the expert editor, writes a structured, condensed summary designed so that the reader can rapidly acquire the essential information contained in the article.

The Commentary

The YEAR BOOK editorial boards, sometimes assisted by guest commentators, write comments that place each article in perspective for the reader. This provides the reader with the equivalent of a personal consultation with a leading international authority—an opportunity to better understand the value of the article and to benefit from the authority's thought processes in assessing the article.

Additional Editorial Features

The editorial boards of each YEAR BOOK organize the abstracts and comments to provide a logical and satisfying sequence of information. To enhance the organization, editors also provide introductions to sections or individual chapters, comments linking a number of abstracts, citations to additional literature, and other features.

The published YEAR BOOK contains enhanced bibliographic citations for each selected article, including extended listings of multiple authors and identification of author affiliations. Each YEAR BOOK contains a Table of Contents specific to that year's volume. From year to year, the Table of Contents for a given YEAR BOOK will vary depending on developments within the field.

Every YEAR BOOK contains a list of the journals from which papers have been selected. This list represents a subset of the nearly 1,000 journals surveyed by the publisher, and occasionally reflects a particularly pertinent article from a journal that is not surveyed on a routine basis.

Finally, each volume contains a comprehensive subject index and an index to authors of each selected paper.

The 1993 Year Book Series

Year Book of Anesthesia and Pain Management: Drs. Miller, Abram, Kirby, Ostheimer, Roizen, and Stoelting

Year Book of Cardiology®: Drs. Schlant, Collins, Engle, Gersh, Kaplan, and Waldo

Year Book of Chiropractic: Drs. Phillips and Adams

Year Book of Critical Care Medicine®: Drs. Rogers and Parrillo

Year Book of Dentistry®: Drs. Meskin, Currier, Kennedy, Leinfelder, Berry, Roser, and Zakariasen

Year Book of Dermatologic Surgery: Drs. Swanson, Salasche, and Glogau

Year Book of Dermatology®: Drs. Sober and Fitzpatrick

Year Book of Diagnostic Radiology®: Drs. Federle, Clark, Gross, Madewell, Maynard, Sackett, and Young

Year Book of Digestive Diseases®: Drs. Greenberger and Moody

Year Book of Drug Therapy®: Drs. Lasagna and Weintraub

Year Book of Emergency Medicine®: Drs. Wagner, Burdick, Davidson, Roberts, and Spivey

Year Book of Endocrinology®: Drs. Bagdade, Braverman, Horton, Kannan, Landsberg, Molitch, Morley, Odell, Rogol, Ryan, and Sherwin

Year Book of Family Practice®: Drs. Berg, Bowman, Davidson, Dietrich, and Scherger

Year Book of Geriatrics and Gerontology®: Drs. Beck, Reuben, Burton, Small, Whitehouse, and Goldstein

Year Book of Hand Surgery®: Drs. Amadio and Hentz

Year Book of Health Care Management: Drs. Heyssel, Brock, Moses, and Steinberg, Ms. Avakian, and Messrs. Berman, Kues, and Rosenberg

Year Book of Hematology®: Drs. Spivak, Bell, Ness, Quesenberry, and Wiernik

Year Book of Infectious Diseases®: Drs. Wolff, Barza, Keusch, Klempner, and Snydman

Year Book of Infertility: Drs. Mishell, Paulsen, and Lobo

Year Book of Medicine®: Drs. Rogers, Bone, Cline, O'Rourke, Greenberger, Utiger, Epstein, and Malawista

Year Book of Neonatal and Perinatal Medicine®: Drs. Klaus and Fanaroff

Year Book of Nephrology: Drs. Coe, Favus, Henderson, Kashgarian, Luke, Myers, and Curtis

Year Book of Neurology and Neurosurgery®: Drs. Bradley and Crowell

Year Book of Neuroradiology: Drs. Osborn, Eskridge, Harnsberger, and Grossman

Year Book of Nuclear Medicine®: Drs. Hoffer, Gore, Gottschalk, Zaret, and Zubal

Year Book of Obstetrics and Gynecology®: Drs. Mishell, Kirschbaum, and Morrow

Year Book of Occupational and Environmental Medicine: Drs. Emmett, Brooks, Frank, and Hammad

Year Book of Oncology®: Drs. Young, Longo, Ozols, Simone, Steele, and Glatstein

Year Book of Ophthalmology®: Drs. Laibson, Adams, Augsburger, Benson, Cohen, Eagle, Flanagan, Nelson, Rapuano, Reinecke, Sergott, and Wilson

Year Book of Orthopedics®: Drs. Sledge, Poss, Cofield, Frymoyer, Griffin, Hansen, Johnson, Simmons, and Springfield

Year Book of Otolaryngology–Head and Neck Surgery®: Drs. Holt and Paparella

Year Book of Pathology and Clinical Pathology®: Drs. Gardner, Bennett, Cousar, Garvin, and Worsham

Year Book of Pediatrics®: Dr. Stockman

Year Book of Plastic, Reconstructive, and Aesthetic Surgery: Drs. Miller, Cohen, McKinney, Robson, Ruberg, and Whitaker

Year Book of Podiatric Medicine and Surgery®: Dr. Kominsky

Year Book of Psychiatry and Applied Mental Health®: Drs. Talbott, Frances, Freedman, Meltzer, Perry, Schowalter, and Yudofsky

Year Book of Pulmonary Disease®: Drs. Bone and Petty

Year Book of Sports Medicine®: Drs. Shephard, Eichner, Sutton, and Torg, Col. Anderson, and Mr. George

Year Book of Surgery®: Drs. Copeland, Deitch, Eberlein, Howard, Ritchie, Robson, Souba, and Sugarbaker

Year Book of Transplantation®: Drs. Ascher, Hansen, and Strom

Year Book of Ultrasound: Drs. Merritt, Mittelstaedt, Carroll, Babcock, and Goldstein

Year Book of Urology®: Drs. Gillenwater and Howards

Year Book of Vascular Surgery®: Dr. Porter

Roundsmanship® '93–'94: A Student's Survival Guide to Clinical Medicine Using Current Literature: Drs. Dan, Feigin, Quilligan, Schrock, Stein, and Talbott

1993

The Year Book of EMERGENCY MEDICINE®

Editor

David K. Wagner, M.D.

Professor and Chairman, Department of Emergency Medicine, The Medical College of Pennsylvania, Philadelphia, Pennsylvania

Associate Editors

William P. Burdick, M.D.

Associate Professor, Department of Emergency Medicine; Assistant Professor, Department of Internal Medicine; The Medical College of Pennsylvania, Philadelphia, Pennsylvania

Steven J. Davidson, M.D.

Professor, Department of Emergency Medicine, The Medical College of Pennsylvania, Philadelphia, Pennsylvania

James R. Roberts, M.D.

Professor, Department of Emergency Medicine, The Medical College of Pennsylvania; Chairman, Department of Emergency Medicine, Mercy Catholic Medical Center, Philadelphia, Pennsylvania

William H. Spivey, M.D.

Assistant Professor, Department of Emergency Medicine, The Medical College of Pennsylvania, Philadelphia, Pennsylvania

Mosby

St. Louis Baltimore Boston Chicago London Philadelphia Sydney Toronto

Editor-in-Chief, Year Book Publishing: Kenneth H. Killion
Sponsoring Editor: Katherine Gill
Manager, Literature Services: Edith M. Podrazik
Senior Information Specialist: Terri Santo
Senior Medical Writer: David A. Cramer, M.D.
Assistant Director, Manuscript Services: Frances M. Perveiler
Associate Managing Editor, Year Book Editing Services: Connie Murray
Senior Production/Desktop Publishing Manager: Max F. Perez
Proofroom Manager: Barbara M. Kelly

Mosby, Inc.
11830 Westline Industrial Drive
St. Louis, MO 63146

Editorial Office:
Mosby, Inc.
200 North LaSalle St.
Chicago, IL 60601

International Standard Serial Number: 0271-7964
International Standard Book Number: 0-8151-9064-6

Dedication

The entire emergency medicine community was recently shocked and saddened by the unexpected and untimely death of Bill Spivey. As readers of *Year Book* know, Bill has been a regular contributor as Associate Editor since 1989. With clarity of perception and comments of pertinence, his critiques were welcomed and treasured by all of us. His ability to cut to the heart of the matter, objectively view the data, and succinctly deliver a focused commentary were characteristics of his approach to *Year Book*, as well as to life's situations in general. He was a person of character, integrity, intellect, and honor. His accomplishments were prodigious. He leaves a legacy which will serve both as a model and a stimulus for individuals committed to the growth and development of the discipline of emergency medicine.

D.K. Wagner, M.D.

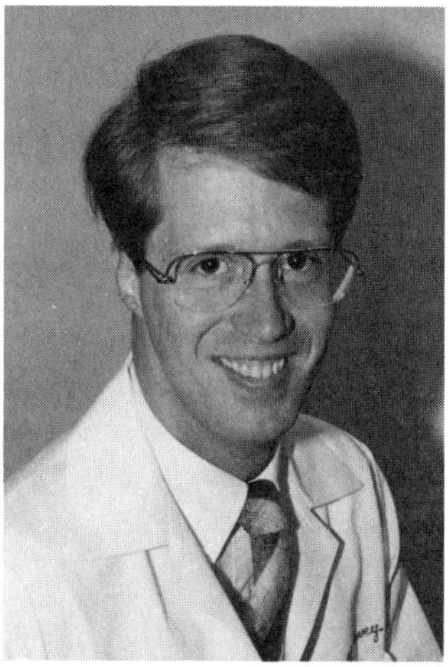

Contributing Editors

James T. Amsterdam, M.D., D.M.D., F.A.C.E.P.
Associate Professor of Emergency Medicine, Northeastern Ohio University College of Medicine; Chairman, Department of Emergency Medicine, Western Reserve Care System, Youngstown, Ohio

Gail V. Anderson, M.D.
Professor and Chairman, Department of Emergency Medicine, University of Southern California School of Medicine, Los Angeles, California

Michael J. Bresler, M.D.
Clinical Professor of Surgery, Division of Emergency Medicine, Stanford University School of Medicine, Stanford, California

David J. Cionni, M.D.
Assistant Professor of Surgery; Director, Prehospital Care, University of Colorado Health Sciences Center; State of Colorado EMS Medical Director, Denver, Colorado

Joseph E. Clinton, M.D.
Clinical Associate Professor of Emergency Medicine, Hennepin County Medical Center, Minneapolis, Minnesota

Jerris R. Hedges, M.D.
Professor of Emergency Medicine, Oregon Health Sciences University, Portland, Oregon

Frederick M. Henretig, M.D.
Associate Professor and Chief, Division of Pediatric Emergency Medicine, The Medical College of Pennsylvania, Philadelphia, Pennsylvania

Jerome R. Hoffman, M.D.
Associate Professor of Medicine, Emergency Medicine Center, UCLA School of Medicine, Los Angeles, California

Mark Joffe, M.D.
Director of Emergency Medicine, St. Christopher's Hospital for Children, Philadelphia, Pennsylvania

John J. Kelly, D.O., F.A.C.E.P.
Assistant Professor, Department of Emergency Medicine, The Medical College of Pennsylvania, Philadelphia, Pennsylvania

William J. Koenig, M.D.
Medical Director, Los Angeles County Emergency Medical Services Agency; Assistant Director, Emergency Department, Long Beach Memorial Medical Center, Long Beach, California

Emily Jean Lucid, M.D.
Associate Professor and Chairman, Department of Emergency Medicine, Medical College of Pennsylvania, Allegheny Campus, Allegheny General Hospital, Pittsburgh, Pennsylvania

Stephen Ludwig, M.D.
Professor of Pediatrics, University of Pennsylvania School of Medicine; Division Chief, General Pediatrics, The Children's Hospital of Philadelphia, Philadelphia, Pennsylvania

Robert N. McNamara, M.D.
Associate Professor of Emergency Medicine, The Medical College of Pennsylvania, Philadelphia, Pennsylvania

Joyce M. Mitchell-Savinsky, M.D.
Clinical Instructor, Department of Internal Medicine, Case Western Reserve University School of Medicine; Department of Emergency Medicine, Mt. Sinai Medical Center, Cleveland, Ohio

James Niemann, M.D.
Director of Research, Department of Emergency Medicine, UCLA School of Medicine; Harbor-UCLA Medical Center, Torrance, California

Gary J. Ordog, M.D.
Assistant Professor of Emergency Medicine, University of California at Los Angeles; MLK/Drew Medical Center, Saugus, California

Edward J. Otten, M.D.
Director, Division of Toxicology, Department of Emergency Medicine, University of Cincinnati Medical Center, Cincinnati, Ohio

Earl J. Reisdorff, M.D., F.A.C.E.P.
Associate Professor, College of Human Medicine, Michigan State University; Assistant Director-Education, Emergency Medicine Residency-Lansing Ingham Medical Center Corporation; Sparrow Hospital, Lansing, Michigan

Suzanne B. Repasky, D.O.
Assistant Professor of Emergency Medicine, The Medical College of Pennsylvania, Philadelphia, Pennsylvania

Ernest Ruiz, M.D.
Chief, Emergency Medicine, Department of Emergency Medicine, Hennepin County Medical Center, Minneapolis, Minnesota

Richard Rutstein, M.D.
Assistant Professor of Pediatrics and Medical Director, Special Immunology Service Division of General Pediatrics, The Children's Hospital of Philadelphia, Philadelphia, Pennsylvania

Robert W. Schafermeyer, M.D., F.A.C.E.P., F.A.A.P.
Associate Chairman, Director, Division of Education, Department of Emergency Medicine, Carolinas Medical Center, Charlotte, North Carolina

John Schoffstall, M.D.
Assistant Professor, Department of Emergency Medicine, The Medical College of Pennsylvania, Philadelphia, Pennsylvania

Kathy N. Shaw, M.D.
Attending Physician, Emergency Department, The Children's Hospital of Philadelphia, Philadelphia, Pennsylvania

Thomas Stair, M.D.
Associate Professor of Emergency Medicine, Georgetown University School of Medicine, Washington, D.C.
Ellen H. Taliaferro, M.D.
Associate Clinical Professor, Department of Surgery, Department of Emergency Services, San Francisco General Hospital, San Francisco, California
Henry D. Unger, M.D.
Director, Division of Emergency Medicine, Assistant Professor, Department of Surgery, Hahnemann University Hospital, Philadelphia, Pennsylvania
Suman Wason, M.D.
Adjunct Associate Professor of Pediatrics and Emergency Medicine, University of Cincinnati; Toxicologist-in-Chief, Cincinnati Drug and Poison Information Center, Children's Hospital Medical Center, Cincinnati, Ohio
Jonathan Wasserberger, M.D.
Associate Professor of Emergency Medicine, Martin Luther King, Jr. General Hospital, Los Angeles, California

Table of Contents

Journals Represented

Mosby-Year Book subscribes to and surveys nearly 1,000 U.S. and foreign medical and allied health journals. From these journals, the Editors select the articles to be abstracted. Journals represented in this YEAR BOOK are listed below.

Acta Neurologica Scandinavica
Americal Heart Journal
American Journal of Cardiology
American Journal of Diseases of Children
American Journal of Emergency Medicine
American Journal of Epidemiology
American Journal of Gastroenterology
American Journal of Hypertension
American Journal of Medicine
American Journal of Obstetrics and Gynecology
American Journal of Physiology
American Journal of Preventive Medicine
American Journal of Public Health
American Journal of Roentgenology
American Journal of Surgery
American Journal of the Medical Sciences
American Surgeon
Anaesthesia and Intensive Care
Anesthesia and Analgesia
Annals of Emergency Medicine
Annals of Internal Medicine
Annals of the Royal College of Surgeons of England
Archives of Disease in Childhood
Archives of Internal Medicine
Archives of Pathology and Laboratory Medicine
Archives of Physical Medicine and Rehabilitation
Archives of Surgery
British Heart Journal
British Journal of Dermatology
British Journal of Surgery
British Medical Journal
Burns
Canadian Journal of Psychiatry
Cardiovascular and Interventional Radiology
Cephalalgia
Chest
Circulation
Circulatory Shock
Clinical Orthopaedics and Related Research
Clinical Pediatrics
Critical Care Medicine
Dysphagia
European Heart Journal
European Journal of Clinical Pharmacology
European Respiratory Journal
Gastroenterology
General Hospital Psychiatry
Human Pathology
Human and Experimental Toxicology
Injury

Intensive Care Medicine
Journal of Allergy and Clinical Immunology
Journal of Applied Physiology: Respiratory, Environmental and Exercise Physiology
Journal of Bone and Joint Surgery (American Volume)
Journal of Bone and Joint Surgery (British Volume)
Journal of Emergency Medicine
Journal of Emergency Nursing
Journal of Family Practice
Journal of Internal Medicine
Journal of Laboratory and Clinical Medicine
Journal of Neuropsychiatry and Clinical Neurosciences
Journal of Neurosurgery
Journal of Otolaryngology
Journal of Pediatric Orthopedics
Journal of Pediatrics
Journal of Trauma
Journal of Urology
Journal of the American College of Cardiology
Journal of the American Geriatrics Society
Journal of the American Medical Association
Lancet
Law, Medicine and Health Care
Medical Care
Neuropediatrics
New England Journal of Medicine
Ophthalmology
Otolaryngology - Head and Neck Surgery
PACE - Pacing and Clinical Electrophysiology
Pediatric Emergency Care
Pediatric Infectious Disease Journal
Pediatrics
Radiology
Respiratory Medicine
Southern Medical Journal
Stroke
Surgery, Gynecology and Obstetrics
Surgical Neurology
Western Journal of Medicine

Standard Abbreviations

The following terms are abbreviated in this edition: acquired immunodeficiency syndrome (AIDS), the central nervous system (CNS), cardiopulmonary resuscitation (CPR), cerebrospinal fluid (CSF), computed tomography (CT), electrocardiography (ECG), human immunodeficiency virus (HIV), and magnetic resonance (MR) imaging (MRI) red blood cell (RBC), white blood cell (WBC).

Publisher's Preface

As publishers, we feel challenged to seek ways of presenting complex information in a clear and readable manner. To this end, the 1993 YEAR BOOK OF EMERGENCY MEDICINE now provides structured abstracts in which the various components of a study can easily be identified through headings. These headings are not the same in all abstracts but, rather, are those that most accurately designate the content of each particular journal article. We are confident that our readers will find the information contained in our abstracts to be more accessible than ever before. We welcome your comments.

Introduction

For the first time in 12 years, the YEAR BOOK OF EMERGENCY MEDICINE has changed the organization of the Table of Contents. This occurred in response to the changing literature base represented by further development of subspecialization within emergency medicine. A portion of the book is now specifically devoted to the developing and recognized areas of special competency available to the emergency physician. Pediatric emergency medicine, emergency medical systems, toxicology, and sports medicine have their own sections. Not far behind may be geriatric emergency medicine, occupational/industrial emergency care, observation/critical emergency care, and hyperbaric medicine. The availability of focused literature, development of training activities, and prospects for formal certification will determine the final format.

The YEAR BOOK continues to focus on the trends in emergency medicine, both clinical and investigative. It attempts to emphasize those conditions that enhance the skill of the practicing physician. To provide practical and pertinent comments with a focus toward clinical practice, a group of associate editors and commentators has been assembled who well represent the breadth and depth of general emergency medicine and the noted areas of subspecialization. Their combined skills, wisdom, and experience are truly outstanding.

As usual and with continued equanimity in the face of hostile deadlines, one person has assembled this manuscript. With patience and persistence, using the carrot without the stick, she brings the material to final form. That's Rose, mom to our favorite teenager, Kelly Schulberger. Thanks, Rose, from all of us!

D.K. Wagner, M.D.

GENERAL EMERGENCY MEDICINE

1 Acute Systems Pathophysiology

Cardiopulmonary, Cerebral Resuscitation

High-Dose Epinephrine Improves the Return of Spontaneous Circulation Rates in Human Victims of Cardiac Arrest

Barton C, Callaham M (Univ of California, San Francisco)

Ann Emerg Med 20:722–725, 1991

1–1

Background.—Recent studies have shown that a standard dose of epinephrine (SDE) as recommended for resuscitating patients in cardiac arrest produces suboptimal myocardial blood flow and resuscitation rates in animals and that a high dose of epinephrine (HDE) improves these parameters in an animal model of prolonged cardiac arrest. Whether HDE similarly improves initial resuscitation rates in human victims of cardiac arrest was studied in 49 victims of nontraumatic prehospital cardiac arrest.

Methods.—The patients were treated in the emergency department (ED) with bolus epinephrine doses ranging from 1 to 15 mg. Epinephrine doses were left to the discretion of the treating physician. High-dose epinephrine was defined as a dose of at least .2 mg/kg, whereas any lower dose was defined as SDE. Patients were divided according to whether they had a return of spontaneous circulation (+RSC) or never regained circulation (−RSC). Patients were further grouped according to their cardiac rhythm on arrival at the ED. A potentially perfusing cardiac rhythm was defined as ventricular tachycardia or electromechanical dissociation and a nonperfusing cardiac rhythm, as asystole or ventricular fibrillation.

Results.—Of the 49 cardiac arrest victims, 12 had a return of circulation and 37 did not. Thirty-nine patients received SDE and 10 were given HDE. Six of the 39 patients (15.4%) who received SDE and 6 of the 10 patients (60%) who received HDE had a return of circulation. The difference was statistically significant. The mean total epinephrine dose given during the entire resuscitation attempt including prehospital epinephrine administration was 7.1 mg in the SDE group and 28.5 mg in the HDE group. Among patients arriving with nonperfusing cardiac rhythms, HDE yielded significantly higher +RSC rates than did SDE, whereas there was no significant difference in +RSC rates among patients arriving with perfusing cardiac rhythms.

Conclusions.—High-dose epinephrine improves the return of spontaneous circulation rates in human victims of cardiac arrest. Its greatest benefit is observed in patients with a nonperfusing cardiac rhythm.

▶ The authors present one of the earlier clinical studies on the use of HDE on human victims of cardiac arrest. While admittedly not all the variables were controlled, there did appear to be some improvement in return to spontaneous circulation in individuals with presumably the lowest coronary perfusion pressures. Other ongoing studies will attempt to sort out the effect of mega epi-infusion early in the course of arrested patients. When all the results are known, the answer to this critical question will have been clarified, and national protocols may need adjustment. Of interest is the fact that patients with potentially low-flow states, i.e., those with an ECG complex without demonstrable pulse, were the least affected by HDE. Whether the low-flow state exists in these patients is a perennial question for which a satisfactory answer is not currently available.—D.K. Wagner, M.D.

Cardiac Resuscitation by Extracorporeal Circulation After Failure of Conventional CPR

Gazmuri RJ, Weil MH, von Planta M, Gazmuri RR, Shah DM, Rackow EC (The Chicago Med School, North Chicago, Ill)

J Lab Clin Med 118:65–73, 1991 1–2

Introduction.—Conventional closed-chest CPR has resulted in disappointingly low survival rates in the past 15 years. Open chest direct cardiac massage presents practical problems and has not been shown in controlled clinical trials to yield superior results. To find an alternative method for cardiac resuscitation, the ability of venoarterial extracorporeal circulation (ECC), with and without the concomitant administration of epinephrine to resuscitate pigs, was compared with that of conventional, closed-chest CPR.

Methods.—The pigs were subjected to alternating current delivered to the endocardium of the right ventricle to induce ventricular fibrillation. After 10 minutes, conventional closed-chest CPR with external defibrillation was initiated. If conventional CPR failed after 15 minutes, ECC was initiated, with or without continuous infusion of epinephrine sufficient to maintain a mean aortic pressure of 60 to 100 mm Hg. Some pigs were indentically instrumented with perfusion cannulas, but were treated with continued precordial compression, with or without the administration of epinephrine (sham ECC). The left external jugular veins and both femoral arteries were used for peripheral vascular access.

Results.—None of 26 animals were successfully resuscitated by conventional CPR. In all 8 pigs subsequently treated by ECC at an average flow rate of 183 mL/kg/min without epinephrine, sinus rhythm was restored. In 6 of these animals, spontaneous circulation was restored after an average of 152 minutes of ECC. When 8 animals were treated with infusions of epinephrine in conjunction with ECC, sinus rhythm was reestablished in all by 4 minutes, and spontaneous circulation occurred after an average of only 23 minutes of ECC. In contrast, none of 5 animals treated with infusions of epinephrine but receiving sham ECC were resuscitated.

Conclusion.—Pigs can be successfully resuscitated, even after failure of conventional chest compression, by ECC in conjunction with epinephrine. Human studies are justified to test the role of ECC in advanced cardiac life support when conventional techniques have failed.

▶ Extracorporeal circulation rapidly restores normal perfusion pressure and in so doing improves cardiac resuscitation. However, in the human model, the question still remains as to the appropriate therapeutic window. Prolonged downtime is associated with morbid neurologic outcome. Initially, this has prehospital implications if the patient does not respond to early defibrillation (if appropriate). Rapid transport is then needed to a center that could perform ECC rapidly, which takes a well-trained team. Animals that have been instrumented and set up prior to initiating the arrest are quite a different model from a patient thrown on the stretcher who was resuscitated in the field 40 minutes before. Extracorporeal circulation may prove promising in patients in the midst of myocardial infarct in cardiogenic shock pending transfer to the catheterization laboratory or operating room in order to maintain organ function (see Abstract 5–31).—J.T. Amsterdam, M.D.

Prevention of Oral Bacterial Flora Transmission by Using Mouth-To-Mask Ventilation During CPR

Cydulka RK, Connor PJ, Myers TF, Pavza G, Parker M (Case Western Reserve Univ, Cleveland, Ohio; Northwestern Univ Med School, Chicago, Ill; Loyola Univ, Chicago)

J Emerg Med 9:317–321, 1991 1–3

Background.—Bystanders are reluctant to perform mouth-to-mouth ventilation on people suffering from cardiac arrest, which may have a significant impact on survival. The use of protective barrier precautions during CPR has been recommended. Seventeen ventilation devices were assessed to determine the adequacy of barrier protection provided against oral aerobic flora transmission.

Methods.—Eight of the devices tested were face shields, 8 were mask devices, and 1 was neither. All the mask devices and 3 face shield devices contained 1-way valves. The devices that contained such a valve were hypothesized to offer better barrier protection against the transmission of oral aerobic bacterial flora than devices not containing such a valve. The valves allowed air in from the rescuer side but did not let air out from the victim's side.

Results.—Forty-one percent of the 17 devices cultured after testing were found to be contaminated with oral aerobic bacterial flora. None of the mask devices was contaminated with oral aerobic bacterial flora as compared with 6 faceshields.

Conclusions.—All ventilation devices with a 1-way valve, except the Sealeasy device, have adequate barrier-type protection from oral aerobic bacterial flora during mouth-to-mouth ventilation simulation. These conclusions are limited because the transmission of anaerobic oral bacterial flora or viruses was not tested and because barrier protection was tested for only 60 seconds, not over the normal course of CPR. Victim barrier protection from an infected rescuer also needs to be addressed in future rescarch.

▶ Transmissibility of infectious disease to emergency personnel is of major concern. The study offers useful information on protection from bacterial transmission. Unfortunately, viral transmission is the real concern that is not addressed.

The article is appropriate and does not overstate conclusions.

A resident in the pre-icteric stage of hepatitis B attended a basic cardiac life support instructor course at our institution several years ago. He became jaundiced 1 week after the course. His fellow students, who shared mannequins with him, were followed for 1 year with serial testing. None of them developed the disease.—J.E. Clinton, M.D.

Comparison of Standard External CPR, Open-Chest CPR, and Cardiopulmonary Bypass in a Canine Myocardial Infarct Model

DeBehnke DJ, Angelos MG, Leasure JE (Wright State Univ, Dayton, Ohio)

Ann Emerg Med 20:754–760, 1991 1–4

Purpose.—In patients with cardiac arrest, the rate of successful resuscitation by standard external CPR (SECPR) is low. Individual comparisons have shown higher rates of resuscitation with open-chest CPR (OCCPR) and cardiopulmonary bypass. A model of myocardial infarct ventricular fibrillation compared all 3 of these techniques.

Methods.—Of 26 mongrel dogs, 9 were randomized to receive SECPR and advanced life support, 9 were randomized to receive cardiopulmonary bypass, and 8 were randomized to receive OCCPR. Each animal had occlusion of the left anterior descending coronary artery. This was followed by 4 minutes of ventricular fibrillation without CPR and then 8 minutes of mechanical chest compression and ventilation. Then, the animals received 1 of the 3 resuscitation techniques, followed by 4 hours of intensive care. Histochemical techniques were used to identify ischemic and necrotic myocardial areas in all resuscitated animals.

Results.—Resuscitation was achieved in all of the cardiopulmonary bypass group, 6 of the OCCPR group, and 2 of the SECPR group. A few of the animals in each group survived to 4 hours. After 2 minutes of attempted resuscitation, the coronary perfusion pressure was 75 mm Hg in the cardiopulmonary bypass group and 56 mm Hg in the OCCPR group vs. 16 mm Hg in the SECPR group. Epinephrine requirements were .10 with cardiopulmonary bypass vs. .28 for SECPR. The ratio of necrotic to ischemic myocardium at 4 hours was .15 with cardiopulmonary bypass and .39 with OCCPR vs. 1.16 with SECPR.

Conclusions.—A study of ventricular fibrillation and myocardial infarct cardiac arrest in dogs shows higher coronary perfusion pressure and resuscitation rates in dogs receiving cardiopulmonary bypass and OCCPR than in those receiving SECPR. Results are similar with cardiopulmonary bypass and OCCPR, although the former requires less epinephrine use. The clinical use of these 2 techniques needs further investigation.

▶ It has been known for a number of years that OCCPR and cardiopulmonary bypass (CPB) are more effective in resuscitating animals from cardiac arrest than standard CPR as taught in the basic and advanced cardiac life support curricula (1). Human case series have also been published. Despite this, no controlled studies of OCCPR or CPB in humans with medical causes of cardiac arrest have been published.

This paper hints at why these invasive resuscitative techniques have not achieved their apparent potential. Although OCCPR and CPB were more effective in resuscitating dogs from cardiac arrest, neither produced better survival at 4 hours. Clearly, it is unrewarding merely to achieve a return of spontaneous circulation (ROSC) in a patient if that patient dies hours or days later. These postresuscitation deaths are usually due to the failure of multiple organs, especially the brain, caused by damage during the no-flow and low-flow states of early arrest and CPR. Human case series have been published that suggest the same thing (2). Until we have better methods of treating so-called postresuscitation disease (see Abstract 3–64 for one possible approach), even these very effective methods of producing ROSC may avail us little.—J. Schoffstall, M.D.

References

1. Safar P, et al: *Am J Emerg Med* 8:55, 1990.
2. Hartz R, et al: *Ann Thorac Surg* 50:437, 1990.

Limitations of Open-Chest Cardiac Massage After Prolonged, Untreated Cardiac Arrest in Dogs

Kern KB, Sanders AB, Janas W, Nelson JR, Badylak SF, et al (Univ of Arizona, Tucson; Purdue Univ, West Lafayette, Ind)

Ann Emerg Med 20:761–767, 1991 1–5

Background.—Open-chest cardiac massage has provided better circulatory support than other forms of CPR both in experimental models and in the hospital setting. It is especially effective when begun within 15 to 20 minutes of circulatory collapse, but the efficacy of later intervention is uncertain.

Objective and Methods.—Open-chest cardiac massage was used to resuscitate dogs from normothermic cardiac arrest after different periods of untreated ventricular fibrillation. Initially it was compared with closed-chest compression after 20 minutes of fibrillation. Open-chest massage was then performed after 10, 20, and 40 minutes of fibrillation.

Observations.—Open-chest massage was significantly more effective than closed-chest compression after 20 minutes of ventricular fibrillation, both in enhancing coronary perfusion pressure and promoting survival. All 10 animals given open-chest massage after 10 or 20 minutes of fibrillation recovered, but none of 5 treated after 40 minutes of fibrillation survived. Open-chest cardiac massage ensured recovery after 20 minutes of fibrillation, but long-term survival was poor.

Implication.—Open-chest cardiac resuscitation can provide a good long-term outcome even if begun after 10 minutes of untreated ventricular fibrillation, but not much more time can elapse without compromising the outcome.

▶ The clinical usefulness of open-chest cardiac massage remains uncertain. As this study points out, it is most useful early in the resuscitation, but the same is so for other measures such as defibrillation. Most long-term survivors come from the group of patients who respond quickly to resuscitation. The questions remaining of open-chest massage are just when to apply it and who will benefit with improved long-term outcomes. The group of patients that this would be used on, those not quickly responding, are likely to have serious underlying pathology, and despite the "improved hemodynamics," benefit will be difficult to demonstrate.—R.M. McNamara, M.D.

Ionized Hypocalcemia During Prolonged Cardiac Arrest and Closed-Chest CPR in a Canine Model

Cairns CB, Niemann JT, Pelikan PCD, Sharma J (Univ of California, Los Angeles)

Ann Emerg Med 20:1178–1182, 1991 1–6

Background.—Free or ionized calcium (Ca^{+2}) plays a vital part in normal cardiovascular function. However, its administration to patients in cardiac arrest is controversial. Research on the levels of Ca^{+2} in cardiac arrest and resuscitation has been inadequate, and exogenous calcium may even worsen ischemic cellular injury. Free calcium was measured during prolonged cardiac arrest and CPR in dogs.

Methods.—After placing central arterial and venous catheters in 9 dogs, ventricular fibrillation was induced by electric means. Countershocks were administered after 7.5 minutes of ventricular fibrillation, and CPR was begun and continued for 20 minutes. Every 5 minutes during resuscitation, arterial pH, ionized Ca^{+2}, lactate, and aortic pressure were measured.

Results.—Systolic arterial pressure averaged 50 mm Hg during resuscitation. A significant decrease in ionized Ca^{+2} occurred within 5 minutes of the initiation of CPR, with a further decrease at 20 minutes—from 5.1 at control to 3.2 mg/dL at 20 minutes. Total Ca^{+2} showed no change during arrest. However, arterial lactate levels increased substantially throughout arrest and resuscitation. Ionized Ca^{+2} was significantly correlated with lactate but not with pH.

Conclusions.—Ionized hypocalcemia appears to occur during prolonged cardiac arrest and resuscitation, possibly because of binding by lactate. Other mechanisms may also contribute, and more research is needed concerning the importance of this phenomenon in cardiac resuscitation.

▶ This study confirms that ionized hypocalcemia occurs in prolonged cardiac arrest and resuscitation. However, the value of calcium administration remains unclear except when wide QRS complexes are present on the ECG before its administration.—G.V. Anderson, M.D.

The Effect of Bicarbonate on Resuscitation From Cardiac Arrest

Federiuk CS, Sanders AB, Kern KB, Nelson J, Ewy GA (Univ of Arizona Health Sciences Ctr, Tucson)

Ann Emerg Med 20:1173–1177, 1991 1–7

Introduction.—The importance of acid-base balance in resuscitation from cardiac arrest remains unclear. The efficacy of treatment of acid-base imbalance during cardiac arrest and the accuracy of measuring acid-base status during arrest through the use of arterial blood gases remains controversial.

Methods.—To determine the effect of administration on resuscitation in a porcine model of prolonged cardiac arrest, 26 swine were instrumented and subjected to ventricular fibrillation for either 15 or 20 minutes without resuscitation attempts. This initial period was followed by open-chest cardiac massage and the administration of epinephrine plus either sodium bicarbonate, 3 mEq/kg, or 3% saline. The 2 groups were compared for rates of resuscitation, hemodynamics, and arterial and mixed venous gases.

Results.—No difference was seen in resuscitation rates between animals in the 2 groups that underwent 15 minutes of fibrillation. No animals in either group survived 20 minutes of fibrillation. Among animals subjected to 15 minutes of fibrillation, those treated with bicarbonate had a mean arterial pH during resuscitation attempts at 18 minutes of arrest of 7.51, significantly greater than the 7.09 mean arterial pH of animals in the control group. After 18 minutes, the bicarbonate-treated animals had a mixed venous pH of 7.31, significantly greater than that of 7 for the control group. The 2 groups of animals that underwent 15 minutes of fibrillation did not differ in systolic or diastolic blood pressures or in myocardial perfusion pressure. The 2 groups of animals that underwent 20 minutes of fibrillation also had similar hemodynamics. Resuscitated and nonresuscitated animals did not differ significantly in arterial or mixed venous pH or in systolic blood pressure. The resuscitated animals had significantly higher diastolic blood pressure and myocardial perfusion pressure than did the nonresuscitated animals.

Conclusion.—Administration of bicarbonate does not improve the rate of resuscitation of pigs after 15 minutes of ventricular fibrillation. Bicarbonate did result in increased arterial and venous pH, but this did not correlate with increased success of resuscitation attempts. The mechanisms leading to irreversibility of arrest after 20 minutes are unclear.

▶ This is another study that demonstrates that administration of sodium bicarbonate has no efficacy in improving outcome in cardiac resuscitation. At the recent AHA meeting, it was given a class IIa recommendation: no proven efficacy and potentially harmful. Certainly, airway maintenance, hyperventilation, reasonable compression, and efforts to maximize end-diastolic pressure to improve cardiac perfusion are all more beneficial than the "amp of bicarb."—J.T. Amsterdam, M.D.

Experimental Models of Ventricular Tachycardia and Fibrillation Caused by Ischemia and Infarction

Wit AL, Janse MJ (Columbia Univ, New York; Univ of Amsterdam, The Netherlands)

Circulation 85 (Suppl 1):32–42, 1992 1–8

Background.—Ventricular tachycardia and fibrillation are important causes of sudden death. It is often not possible to elucidate the mechanisms of potentially lethal ventricular arrhythmias in clinical studies involving patients. A number of animal models have been used to study the causes and mechanisms of ventricular tachycardia and fibrillation.

Experimental Models.—Animal models of ischemic ventricular arrhythmias are studied with the goal of understanding the mechanisms to provide new ways for clinicians to intervene and prevent fatal attacks in human beings. In experiments designed to reproduce the acute arrhythmias caused by transient ischemia or acute myocardial infarction and to illuminate electrophysiologic mechanisms, a variety of techniques are used to induce complete sudden occlusion of a coronary artery or occlusion followed by reperfusion. The animals most often used are dogs. Pigs, cats, rabbits, ferrets, guinea pigs, and rats have also been studied. The results of studies that use different species are sometimes difficult to compare because of the differences in electrophysiologic properties of the heart and in cardiac and coronary artery anatomy. The severity of acute ventricular arrhythmias occurring after a coronary artery has been occluded is related to the particular artery occluded and the distance of the occlusion from the origin of the artery. Experimental models have also been established for subacute arrhythmias and arrhythmias in healing and healed infarcts.

Conclusions.—Animal studies have enabled the vulnerable period of the ventricles to be discovered and characterized and should eventually result in improved defibrillation methods. Animal models of ischemic heart disease and myocardial infarction have helped researchers define the mechanisms of arrhythmias that occur at each stage of infarct development and healing. The findings from such studies have been shown to apply to clinical situations.

Cerebral Dysfunction

Effects of Levemopamil on Neurologic and Histologic Outcome After Cardiac Arrest in Cats

Fleischer JE, Nakakimura K, Drummond JC, Scheller MS, Zornow MH, Grafe MR, Shapiro HM (Univ of California, San Diego; VA Med Ctr, San Diego)

Crit Care Med 20:126–134, 1992 1–9

Background.—Levemopamil is a newly developed calcium channel blocker of the phenylalkylamine class that readily crosses the blood-brain barrier. It was hypothesized that the drug would improve neurologic outcome and neuropathology after complete global cerebral ischemia. The hypothesis was tested in the clinically relevant model of ventricular fibrillation in cats.

Methods.—The study used 54 cats aged 3 to 8 months. After the initiation of cardiac arrest, resuscitation was performed on the animals. Forty-six animals received levemopamil, 1 mg/kg over a 15-minute period followed by 10 μg/kg·min for 16 hours, or saline in a blinded manner. Eight additional animals were pretreated with levemopamil in a nonblinded manner, beginning 45 minutes before cardiac arrest. After resuscitation, the agent was infused at 10 μg/kg·min for 16 hours. The animals in all 3 groups remained sedated, paralyzed, and mechanically ventilated for 24 to 30 hours after resuscitation. Observers graded the animals at 2, 4, and 7 days after resuscitation to generate a neurologic deficit score.

Results.—The 3 groups did not differ in their neurologic deficit scores and overall neuropathologic scores. In the pretreated animals, however, the occipital cortex and CA1 regions showed less severe damage than did those of animals in the other 2 groups.

Conclusion.—Postresuscitation administration of levemopamil improved neither neurologic outcome nor neuropathology in cats. But when given before cardiac arrest, the agent was associated with regionally selective improvement in neuropathology.

▶ Another calcium channel blocker administered after cardiac arrest and resuscitation fails to improve neurologic recovery. Even the results in this small pretreated group are not very promising.—J.M. Mitchell-Savinsky, M.D.

Effects of U74006F on Multifocal Cerebral Blood Flow and Metabolism After Cardiac Arrest in Dogs

Sterz F, Safar P, Johnson DW, Oku K-I, Tisherman SA (Univ of Pittsburgh, Pa)

Stroke 22:889–895, 1991 1–10

Rationale.—Lipid peroxidation reactions taking place during reperfusion after cardiac arrest may contribute to postischemic cerebral hypoperfusion. This in turn could have a role in neurologic dysfunction. A study was designed to show whether the aminosteroid U74006F, which inhibits lipid peroxidation in vitro, protects against cerebral hypoperfusion after cardiac arrest.

Methods.—Cardiac arrest was produced by ventricular fibrillation for 12.5 minutes in dogs, followed by reperfusion for 5 minutes or less. Cerebral blood flow was monitored by the stable xenon CT technique, and cerebral oxygen consumption was estimated from mean blood flow in coronal slices and the cerebral arteriovenous oxygen content difference. Treated animals received U74006F starting at the time of reperfusion and 3 further doses over a period of 4 hours; the total dose ranged from 4.5 to 14.5 mg/kg.

Findings.—Treatment with U74006F did not alter the postarrest hyperemia or prolonged hypoperfusion seen in control animals. In addition, the local blood flow values and the pattern of global cerebral oxygen consumption were the same in treated and control animals. Oxygen consumption was mismatched in both groups 1 to 4 hours after cardiac arrest.

Conclusions.—In a canine model of cardiac arrest and reperfusion, treatment with U74006F does not appear to alter cerebral blood flow or oxygen consumption. If the outcome is improved, mechanisms other than an improved relationship between oxygen need and demand may be responsible.

▶ One theory to explain brain tissue damage and death after cardiac arrest is that oxidation of lipids takes place due to the presence of oxygen free radicals. Inhibiting this oxidation should theoretically reduce breakdown of cell membranes. While this oxidation inhibitor has shown promising results in other animal models, there was no effect on brain metabolism in dogs.—W.P. Burdick, M.D.

Acute Carbon Monoxide Exposure and Cerebral Blood Flow in Rabbits

Meyer-Witting M, Helps S, Gorman DF (Univ of Adelaide, South Australia; Royal New Zealand Naval Hosp)

Anaesth Intensive Care 19:373–377, 1991 1–11

Introduction.—The toxic mechanisms of carbon monoxide (CO) poisoning are not established. Impaired neurologic function can occur, which is usually reversible, but delayed neurologic deterioration is sometimes seen. In several animal species, cerebrovascular dilatation and increased cerebral blood flow and cerebrovascular volume result from CO exposure.

Methods.—To determine the vascular effects of CO exposure and the relationship between pial vascular changes and the carboxyhemoglobin (COHb) concentration, 8 male New Zealand White rabbits were anesthetized and fitted with devices for measuring cerebral blood flow and intracranial pressure. They were administered 1% CO for 15 minutes, after which measurements were taken at 15-minute intervals for 3 hours.

Results.—Although the mean arterial blood pressure decreased 28% during exposure to CO, cerebral blood flow to the left cortex increased by 236%, and to the right cortex it increased by 287%. There were concurrent decreases in cerebrovascular resistance, 71% in the left cortex and 76% in the right. Other changes during CO exposure included increased intracranial pressure, decreased body temperature and ventilation requirement, and metabolic acidosis. When CO was withdrawn, all these changes were rapidly reversed. Changes in cerebral blood flow and cerebrovascular resistance highly correlated with the level of COHb.

Conclusion.—The natural history of CO intoxication in rabbits is similar to that of human beings. The effects of CO correlated with the COHb concentration and were reversible. Cerebrovascular autoregulation is disrupted during CO exposure, which may contribute to CO toxicity in the brain.

▶ This paper provides evidence of yet another aspect of the neurotoxicity that may be attributable to CO poisoning. Frequently cited causes include the effects of cellular hypoxia secondary to COHb in formation along with decreased oxygen-carrying capacity, changes in the oxyhemoglobin dissociation curve, inhibition of mitochondrial heme-containing enzymes, lipid peroxidation of neuronal membranes, and surface adsorption and receptor poisoning. These authors describe, in a rabbit model, significant loss of autoregulation with massive increases in cerebral blood flow and concomitant intracranial pressure. It is quite likely that these effects, either from a direct CO-mediated action on cerebral vessels or in conjunction with the resulting metabolic acidosis and cellular hypoxia, contribute to the significant and often irreversible neuronal pathology that is seen in severe CO poisoning.—F.M. Henretig, M.D.

κ-Opioid Antagonist Improves Cellular Bioenergetics and Recovery After Traumatic Brain Injury

Vink R, Portoghese PS, Faden AI (James Cook Univ of North Queensland, Townsville, Australia; Univ of California, San Francisco; Univ of Minnesota, Minneapolis)

Am J Physiol 261:R1527–R1532, 1991 1–12

Background.—Various agents have been examined in an attempt to limit delayed tissue damage after traumatic injury to the brain. Experimental models of neurotrauma suggest that treatment with opioid-receptor antagonists may be beneficial in improving neurologic outcome. In an attempt to explain the mechanisms underlying the protective actions of these compounds, the effects of nor-binaltorphimine (nor-BNI) and saline treatment after fluid percussion–induced traumatic brain injury in rats were compared.

Methods.—Thirty minutes after trauma, the animals were randomly assigned in groups of 8 to treatment with nor-BNI at intravenous doses of 10 or 20 mg/kg by bolus injection or an equal volume of saline. Metabolic changes were evaluated by ^{31}P MR spectroscopy. In addition, the animals were assessed weekly for neurologic outcome by using a battery of motor function tests.

Results.—Control animals showed a moderately severe neurologic deficit 2 weeks after the injury. Both doses of nor-BNI significantly improved neurologic outcome at 2 weeks post-trauma as compared with controls. During the first 4 hours after injury, treated animals showed significantly greater recovery of intracellular free magnesium concentrations and cytosolic phosphorylation potentials than did controls.

Conclusion.—The hypothesis that κ-opiod receptors such as nor-BNI help to limit delayed tissue damage after traumatic brain injury is supported. This beneficial effect may result from improvement of cellular bioenergetics.

► The development of irreversible neuronal damage after traumatic injury is probably multifactorial. Postulated mechanisms include lactic acidosis, membrane disruption, ionic imbalance, altered bioenergetics, and release of neuronal poisons such as opioids and excitatory amino acids (e.g., glutamate). A number of pharmacologic interventions, some specific and some nonspecific, have been tested in different models of neuronal injury to limit the extent of irreversible injury. In the study by Vink et al, nor-BNI, a highly selective κ-receptor opioid antagonist, was administered to rats after a standard fluid percussion CNS insult. Magnetic resonance spectroscopic and neurologic outcomes were compared between treated rats and a placebo group. Magnetic resonance spectroscopic results at 4 hours indicated greater intracellular magnesium and higher concentrations of high-energy phosphates in the treatment group. Gross overall neurologic funcion was also better 2 weeks postinjury. Neurologic outcome was correlated with enhanced bioenergetics, but not intracellular magnesium. The effects of nor-BNI may well be due to its ability to attenuate phospholipid hydrolysis and release of excitatory amino acids.—J.T. Niemann, M.D.

Shock

Hypertonic Saline Treatment of Uncontrolled Hemorrhagic Shock at Different Periods From Bleeding

Krausz MM, Landau EH, Klin B, Gross D (Hadassah Univ, Jerusalem, Israel)
Arch Surg 127:93–96, 1992 1–13

Background.—Recently, hypertonic saline (HTS) infusion has been recommended in the treatment of hemorrhagic shock. In all previous studies, HTS was administered 5 minutes after the hemorrhagic injury; in this study the physicians examined the effects of giving HTS at several different periods during the first 2 hours.

Methods.—Six groups of rats were studied. Group 1 animals had uncontrolled hemorrhagic shock induced by tail resection and no HTS. Group 2 had HTS administered 5 minutes after shock was induced, group 3 had HTS given after 15 minutes, group 4 had HTS administered after 30 minutes, group 5 had HTS given after 60 minutes, and group 6 had HTS given after 120 minutes. Blood loss was measured during a 4-hour observation period.

Results.—Group 1 animals lost a mean of 2.7 mL of blood in 5 minutes. When HTS was given at 5 and 15 minutes, additional bleeding of 6.3 and 3.8 mL occurred, respectively, and mean arterial pressure decreased to 36 and 56 mm Hg, respectively. Eighty percent of animals in group 2 and 53% of those in group 3 died during the observation period. In groups 4 and 5, HTS infusion increased bleeding only minimally and did not affect mean arterial pressure or survival.

Conclusions.—Animal experiments suggest that HTS infusion within 15 minutes after hemorrhagic insult results in increased bleeding, hypotension, and early death, whereas infusion after 30 or 60 minutes does not alter bleeding, mean arterial pressure, or survival. Early HTS infusion may be dangerous in trauma patients. Ongoing clinical studies are needed to critically evaluate the timing of HTS infusion.

▶ Previously studied HTS administration at 5 minutes in *controlled* hemorrhage improved survival (see Abstract 1–15). In this study, *uncontrolled* bleeding was treated with HTS, and it was found that if given within 15 minutes, mortality was increased and, indeed, was worse than in untreated rats.

The authors point out the implications of these data on prehospital care of trauma victims. It would appear that unless the hemorrhage creating shock can be controlled at the scene, which is not usually the case, HTS should not be utilized in the prehospital volume resuscitation. A better option might be to minimize time away from definitive care and control of hemorrhage. How many of us have received patients with gunshot wounds to the chest who are in arrest and were only 5 minutes away but took 20 minutes to arrive because of intubation, establishing intravenous lines, and ineffective CPR?—J.M. Mitchell-Savinsky, M.D.

Cardiac Contractility and Blood Flow Distribution Following Resuscitation With 7.5% Hypertonic Saline in Anesthetized Dogs

Kien ND, Reitan JA, White DA, Wu C-H, Eisele JH (Univ of California, Davis)

Circ Shock 35:109–116, 1991 1–14

Introduction.—In animals, 7.5% hypertonic saline (HTS) restores cardiovascular function after hypovolemic shock. It is known that HTS has a variety of systemic effects, but it may also increase cardiac contractility.

Methods.—To test this hypothesis, 15 adult mongrel dogs were anesthetized and subjected to rapid hemorrhage to cause a mean decrease in arterial pressure of 50% in 1 hour. Of the dogs, 8 were resuscitated with HTS, 5 ml/kg, and 7 received lactated Ringer's solution (LR), 30mL/kg, the dosage required for comparable restoration of cardiac output. Cardiac contractility was measured by using the slope E_{es} of the linear regression of the left ventricular (LV) end-systolic pressure-diameter relationship. Regional blood flow was assessed by using radioactive microspheres before, during, and after resuscitation. Other hemodynamic measurements were made 10, 30, and 60 minutes after resuscitation.

Results.—With both LR and HTS, the heart rate increased, and similar improvements occurred in mean arterial pressure, cardiac output, and stroke volume. Both LT and HTS resulted in similar changes in vascular resistance of the pulmonary and peripheral beds. Both solutions resulted in similar improvements in blood flow to the heart, muscle, skin, and jejunum 10 minutes after resuscitation, but the administration of HTS resulted in superior improvement in splenic and hepatic perfusion than in the case of LR. Although LR had no effect on cardiac contractility, the administration of HTS increased the slope E_{es} of the LV end-systolic pressure-diameter relationship to 19.4 mm Hg/mm, significantly more than the baseline value of 13.4 mm Hg/mm or the value during hemorrhage of 14.8 mm Hg/mm. Some of this increase was sustained over the 60 minute period.

Conclusion.—Resuscitation of dogs after hemorrhage by using HTS can significantly increase cardiac contractility and result in restoration of blood flow to vital organs by inducing both vascular dilation and increased perfusion pressure. These transient effects may improve survival by limiting ischemic injury.

▶ The use of HTS in dogs after hemorrhage resulted in significant increases in cardiac contractility. There was a gradual fall in cardiac output and arterial pressure over a 60-minute period with either type of fluid, so the effect was transient. The proposed mechanism of action of HTS is rapid immobilization of endogenous fluid, reduction of vascular resistance, and an increase in cardiac contractility. Its low cost, especially the low volumes required, would make this an ideal fluid in the prehospital setting and also have advantages in further resuscitation of a patient, especially with a head injury. Although the effects are transient, tissue damage might be limited during the "golden hour."—J.T. Amsterdam, M.D.

Acute Hypotension Caused by Rapid Hypertonic Saline Infusion in Anesthetized Dogs

Kien ND, Kramer GC, White DA (Univ of California, Davis)

Anesth Analg 73:597–602, 1991 1–15

Introduction.—Animal studies show that resuscitation from severe hemorrhagic shock is possible with a small bolus infusion of 7.5% hypertonic saline solution (HTS). The infusion rapidly improves cardiovascular and metabolic function by increasing plasma volume, inducing vasodilation, and augmenting myocardial performance. Concerns over the safety of rapid infusions of HTS were addressed.

Methods.—Experiments performed on 10 mongrel dogs were designed to evaluate the immediate cardiovascular effects of HTS. Left ventricular pressure and wall motion were measured simultaneously in anesthetized animals for the assessment of cardiac contractility.

Results.—Mean arterial blood pressure was significantly decreased (from 95 to 51 mm Hg) at 45 seconds after the onset of an infusion of HTS (3 mL/kg in 1 minute). This decrease was, however, abrupt and transient. At the same time, there were significant increases in cardiac output (from 2.8 to 3.9 L/min) and coronary blood flow (from 23.7 to 49.8 mL/min). The heart rate remained constant, but increases in systolic shortening of left ventricular diameter and wall thickening occurred and suggested an improvement in cardiac contractility. Decreases in systemic and pulmonary vascular resistance were 60% and 27%, respectively.

Conclusion.—The acute hypotension after a rapid infusion of HTS is secondary to a decrease in systemic vascular resistance. Whereas a brief period of hypotension is well tolerated when circulatory function is normal, adverse consequences may occur in some patients. Hypertonic saline solution should be given slowly to avoid or minimize an acute hypotensive response.

▶ The duration of the hypotensive response in the normovolemic study dogs was 106 ± 9 seconds. Although brief, the marked drop in pressure observed in this study could be disastrous in a very unstable patient. I found the sophisticated techniques used by the authors to measure myocardial contractility and the discussion thereof to be fascinating.—E. Ruiz, M.D.

Experience With Phenylephrine as a Component of the Pharmacologic Support of Septic Shock

Gregory JS, Bonfiglio MF, Dasta JF, Reilley TE, Townsend MC, Flancbaum L (Ohio State Univ, Columbus)

Crit Care Med 19:1395–1400, 1991 1–16

Background.—Patients with septic shock are at risk of multisystem organ failure. The goal of hemodynamic support in these patients is to maintain effective tissue perfusion. Vasopressor agents may improve perfusion and preserve organ function, but the role of such agents in hemodynamic support is a matter of some controversy. The safety and effectiveness of phenylephrine, a selective α_1-adrenergic receptor agonist, was evaluated in patients with septic shock.

Methods.—The study group included 13 surgical intensive care unit patients. Their mean age was 67 years. All were treated with phenylephrine, in addition to standard therapy for septic shock, and underwent invasive hemodynamic monitoring. Phenylephrine was administered at intravenous infusion rates of 0.5 to 9 μg/kg·min in order to maintain a mean arterial pressure (MAP) greater than 70 mm Hg.

Results.—Significant increases in MAP, systemic vascular resistance index, left ventricular stroke work index, and stroke volume index occurred following phenylephrine administration and at the time of highest oxygen consumption. Although the cardiac index was unchanged initially, it increased at the time of highest oxygen consumption. No changes were observed in pulmonary artery occlusion pressure and heart rate. During phenylephrine therapy, average baseline oxygen consumption increased from 145 to 200 $mL/min \cdot m^2$ and oxygen delivery from 447 to 597 $mL/min \cdot m^2$. Serum creatinine concentrations remained unchanged, blood lactate concentrations decreased, and urine output increased significantly.

Conclusion.—Phenylephrine rapidly stabilized MAP at greater than 70 mm Hg with no detrimental effects on cardiac output. Use of the drug in hemodynamic support contributed to improvement in perfusion while allowing optimization of oxygen delivery and consumption.

▶ It is not often in my emergency practice that I have needed a solely vasoconstrictive agent, and I have to admit that phenylephrine is not one of the drugs I have considered when treating hypotensive patients. Many have been cardiac patients requiring inotropic agents, and my experience with patients in a septic state has been that they generally respond to intravenous fluids and varying doses of dopamine.

However, if further evidence confirms that phenylephrine can be given without deleterious effects on end-organ perfusion, it might be ideal for profound dilatory states, not only sepsis but also severe hypersensitivity reactions.—J.M. Mitchell-Savinsky, M.D.

Effects of Bicarbonate Therapy on Hemodynamics and Tissue Oxygenation in Patients With Lactic Acidosis: A Prospective, Controlled Clinical Study

Mathieu D, Neviere R, Billard V, Fleyfel M, Wattel F (Hôpital Calmette, Lille, France)

Crit Care Med 19:1352–1356, 1991 1–17

Background.—Although sodium bicarbonate therapy has been used for at least 30 years to treat lactic acidosis, growing evidence suggests that bicarbonate may be of no benefit or even harmful in such cases. This prospective, randomized, placebo-controlled trial was designed to test the hypothesis that sodium bicarbonate therapy would have negative hemodynamic effects in patients with lactic acidosis.

Methods.—The 8 men and 2 women included in the study were all medical patients with acute circulatory problems and no severe renal failure. All had metabolic acidosis and increased arterial plasma lactate concentrations. At the beginning of 2 successive 1-hour study periods, the patients randomly received an intravenous injection of sodium bicarbonate (1 mmol/kg body weight) or an equal volume of sodium chloride. Hemodynamics and tissue oxygenation were monitored before and repeatedly during the 1-hour postinjection periods.

Results.—In these 10 critically ill patients, sodium bicarbonate increased arterial and venous pH and the serum bicarbonate concentration. Sodium bicarbonate and sodium chloride produced similar hemodynamic responses. No changes were noted in tissue oxygenation, serum sodium concentration, osmolality, arterial and venous lactate, red cell 2, 3-diphosphoglycerate, or hemoglobin affinity for oxygen.

Conclusion.—Results of previous research on the effects of sodium bicarbonate on lactic acidosis were confirmed. Bicarbonate did not improve hemodynamic variables but, at the dose used here, did not worsen tissue oxygenation.

▶ The question of bicarbonate therapy in metabolic acidosis is once again addressed. In this small study of 10 patients, the authors showed that the administration of bicarbonate, while improving pH and the serum bicarbonate concentration, did not have deleterious effects on hemodynamics, tissue oxygenation, and other serum chemistries. In critically ill patients with metabolic acidosis, there may be a tendency to feel that we have to do something. Correcting pH is something we can do. While I do not necessarily advocate this, it would be nice to know that we "do no harm" while we are doing something. Larger prospective studies are needed to prove this.—J.M. Mitchell-Savinsky, M.D.

Circadian Variation in Vascular Tone and Its Relation to α-Sympathetic Vasoconstrictor Activity

Panza JA, Epstein SE, Quyyumi AA (Natl Heart, Lung, and Blood Inst, Bethesda, Md)

N Engl J Med 325:986–990, 1991 1–18

Background.—Several cardiovascular events, including myocardial infarction, sudden death, and stroke, are more frequent in the early morning hours. Because there is a similar circadian pattern for blood pressure and other physiologic variables, circadian variations in vascular tone may have a role in the onset of acute events.

Study Plan.—Baseline blood flow and vascular resistance in the forearm and responses to phentolamine and nitroprusside were examined in 12 normal subjects of both sexes aged 35 to 53 years at 7 A.M., 2 P.M., and 9 P.M. Drugs were infused into the brachial artery, and responses were measured by strain-gauge plethysmography.

Findings.—Mean forearm vascular resistance was significantly higher in the morning than in the afternoon or evening, and blood flow was significantly lower in the morning. This pattern was evident in 10 of the 12 subjects evaluated. Phentolamine-induced reductions in vascular resistance were most marked in the morning in 11 subjects. The degree of nitroprusside-induced vasodilation did not differ significantly at different times of day.

Conclusions.—Circadian change in the degree of α-sympathetic–mediated vasoconstriction has an important role in varying arterial tone throughout the day. The findings may well relate to the higher blood pressure and increased occurrence of cardiovascular events noted in the early morning.

▶ Do not be put off by the "basic-science tone" of the title of this article. It is well worth reading carefully. Every emergency physician has experienced the arrival of a severely ill patient with an acute myocardial infarction or a massive stroke at 5:30 A.M. This study postulates a relationship between α-sympathetic vasoconstrictor activity in the early morning hours and these cardiovascular events. This relationship could have an enormous impact on the development of future therapeutic regimens.—E.J. Lucid, M.D.

2 Trauma Emergencies

General Trauma Problems

Adult Minor Trauma Patients: Good Outcome in Small Hospitals

Hedges JR, Osterud HR, Mullins RJ (Oregon Health Sciences Univ, Portland)

Ann Emerg Med 21:402–406, 1992 2–1

Background.—Little information is available on the outcomes of patients who have sustained minor trauma and were treated in small, rural hospitals. Whether adult victims of minor trauma admitted to small hospitals have a mean length of stay and fatality rate comparable to those treated in larger hospitals was determined.

Methods.—A cohort of 6,739 trauma victims discharged from Oregon hospitals in 1987 was retrospectively analyzed. All patients included in the study were aged 18 years and older, had an Injury Severity Score (ISS) of less than 10, and left the hospital only with medical approval. The mean length of stay (LOS) among survivors and fatality rates were the outcome measures. Seventy-two hospitals were represented in the study.

Results.—Two of the hospitals were sponsored by the U.S. government and had a longer mean LOS than the other hospitals. Mean LOS was positively correlated with patient age, ISS, and hospital size. One hundred thirty-six deaths occurred in this low-ISS population. Fatality rates were independent of hospital size and trauma facility designation. Patients who died were significantly older than those who survived.

Conclusions.—Minor trauma victims treated at smaller hospitals have a shorter mean LOS and a similar fatality rate when compared with those treated at larger hospitals and level I and II trauma facilities. Elderly patients hospitalized for minor injuries have a higher death rate than younger patients, regardless of hospital size and a low ISS.

▶ This paper underscores the need for further research concerning the outcome of minor trauma patients, not only in small hospitals but also in large non–trauma center hospitals in urban centers. It makes good sense to send minor trauma patients to non–trauma centers for 2 reasons: the minor trauma patients might well fare better, and the focus and impact of the trauma center might well improve if the minor trauma patients are not present to dilute the staff's attention and care.—E.H. Taliaferro, M.D.

Autokabalesis: A study of Intentional Vertical Deceleration Injuries
Isbister ES, Roberts JA (Western Infirmary, Glasgow, Scotland)
Injury 23:119–122, 1992 2–2

Introduction.—Autokabalesis is a new term referring to suicidal jumping from a height. This is a relatively rare form of self-harm, but it has been increasing in incidence, and a marked seasonal variation has been recently noticed. Intentional jumping in the general population was studied epidemiologically.

Patients.—The study included 60 incidents of jumping by 58 individuals over a 5-year period. Thirty-one of these patients survived to make it to the hospital; 11 subsequently died. Another 27 were killed outright, and these were studied through their postmortem records. There were 40 men and 18 women with an average of 37.5 years, 53% being in the 20 to 40-year-old group. The general pattern was of a young, single, unemployed man. Jumps were most common in April, June, November, and December. Most had a psychiatric diagnosis, usually depression or psychosis. Thirty-two percent had alcohol or drug ingestion sufficient to affect mental processes.

Jumps varied from 1 to 27 floors in height; those over 6 floors were fatal except in 1 case where the patient landed in the water. The chance of survival was 70% when jumping from the first floor and 50% when jumping from the third floor. Subjects usually landed feet first in jumps from lower floors and head first in jumps from above 13 floors (Fig 2–1). Injury Severity Score highly discriminated survivors from nonsurvi-

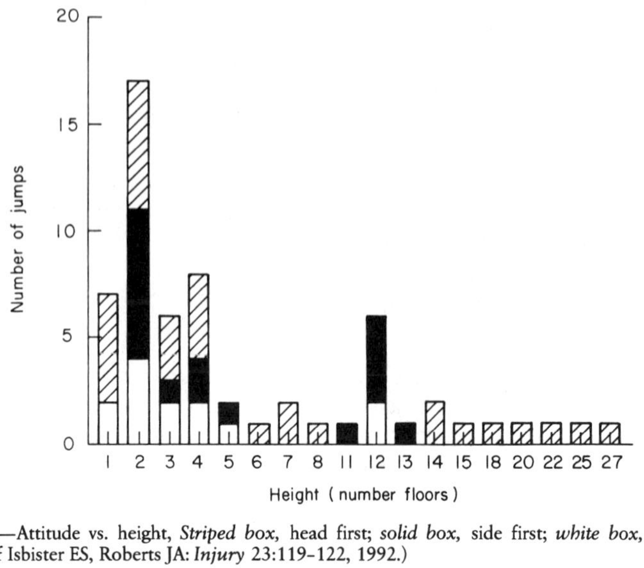

Fig 2–1.—Attitude vs. height, *Striped box,* head first; *solid box,* side first; *white box,* feet first. (Courtesy of Isbister ES, Roberts JA: *Injury* 23:119–122, 1992.)

vors: only 1 with a score more than 29 survived, and only 1 with a score less than 29 died.

Conclusions.—Depression and anxiety appear to be more common in jumpers than psychosis is. Patients will often travel considerable distances to jump from a sufficiently high venue, thus suggesting that these acts may be more premeditated than has been previously suggested.

▶ Study bias: All jumpers landed in Glasgow. Best quote: "The height from which an individual has a 50/50 chance of survival can be approximated to 1 floor for head-first, 3 or 4 floors for side-first, and 4 or 5 floors for feet-first".—T. Stair, M.D.

The Spectrum of Abdominal Injuries Associated With the Use of Seat Belts

Rutledge R, Thomason M, Oller D, Meredith W, Moylan J, Clancy T, Cunningham P, Baker C (Univ of North Carolina; Charlotte Mem Hosp; North Carolina Baptist Hosp; Duke Univ, Durham; New Hanover Mem Hosp; et al)

J Trauma 31:820–826, 1991 2–3

Background.—Recently, there have been reports of abdominal injuries associated with seat belt use (i.e. "seat belt syndrome"). From a sample population from the North Carolina Trauma Registry, the distribution of abdominal injuries after motor vehicle crashes was compared in belted and unbelted patients.

Patients.—A total of 3,901 patients involved in motor vehicle crashes were admitted to trauma centers. When compared with unbelted patients, belted patients had fewer head injuries, lower mean scores on the Injury Severity Score and Abbreviated Injury Scale, shorter length of hospital stay, and a lower mortality rate. Abdominal injuries occurred in 531 (13.6%) patients. The incidence of abdominal injuries was similar in belted (13.9%) and unbelted (13.4%) patients, but the spectrum of organs injured was different. Gastrointestinal tract injuries involving the stomach, small bowel, colon, and rectum were significantly more frequent in belted (3.4%) than in unbelted (1.8%) patients. Liver and spleen injuries occurred with similar frequency in the 2 groups. Patients with abdominal injuries had a significantly higher frequency of chest injuries, a higher overall severity of injury, and more than twice the frequency of deaths than did patients without abdominal injuries.

Conclusions.—Although the incidence of abdominal injury after motor vehicle crashes is similar in belted and unbelted patients, the spectrum of injuries is different in the 2 groups, with hollow viscus injuries more common in belted patients.

▶ This study points out a number of interesting statistics. In the study group of patients admitted to the hospital for injuries sustained in motor vehicle accidents, only 40% of males vs. 50% of females wore seat restraints. Additionally, although it is not noted to be statistically significant, the average age of unbelted patients was 29 years, and it was 37 years for those who were restrained. Perhaps young motor vehicle riders (males especially) should consider this a type of Darwinian selection pressure.

This paper complements a study I reviewed in a previous YEAR BOOK describing the "seat belt syndrome." Both papers point out that there are significant gastrointestinal injuries associated with lap belt use. The physician must be cognizant of this and have a high degree of suspicion that an abdominal injury exists when cutaneous signs of lap belt trauma are present. Perhaps this study cannot answer the question of whether or not restraints decrease injuries (since it looked only at admitted patients), but it certainly should point out that injuries to the head and neck, which can result in more morbidity and mortality, are limited with seat belt use.—H.D. Unger, M.D.

Falls and Ejections From Pickup Trucks

Bucklew PA, Osler TM, Edison JJ, Clevenger FW, Olson SE, et al (Univ of New Mexico, Albuquerque)

J Trauma 32:468–472, 1992 2–4

Introduction.—Falls and ejections from pickup truck beds are especially common in the southwest United States (Fig 2–2). An analysis of 50 such injuries was conducted.

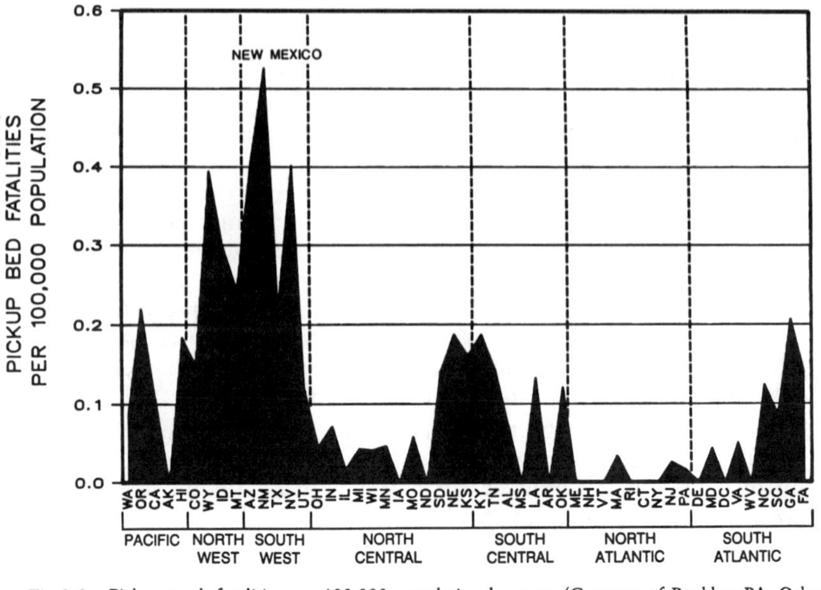

Fig 2–2.—Pickup truck fatalities per 100,000 population by state. (Courtesy of Bucklew PA, Osler TM, Eidson JJ, et al: *J Trauma* 32:468–472, 1992.)

Patients.—The patients were admitted to a level I trauma center during a 5-year period. Sixty-four percent were male, and the mean age was 18 years. Most of the accidents occurred in the summer during the afternoon or evening. Seventy percent of the adults had detectable serum ethanol levels. Twenty-three patients were ejected from the pickup truck bed in a collision, and 27 simply fell out. The average Injury Severity Score was 15.4 for those ejected and 17.4 for those who fell. Three patients in each group died. The average Injury Severity Score was 16.5 in the patients studied vs. 14.5 for those in simple motor vehicle collisions. The head was injured in 68% of the cases, the extremities were injured in 46%, the face was injured in 28%, the thorax was injured in 22%, and the abdomen was injured in 10%. All of the deaths resulted from head injury. In an additional examination of state medical examiner records, 16 more fatalities were discovered. The average age of this group was 24 years; all but 1 of the deaths resulted from a fall rather than an ejection, and 13 resulted from a head injury.

Conclusions.—Falls and ejections from pickup truck beds are infrequent accidents, but the injuries are severe, and many of the victims are children. The authors call for protective legislation—possibly the use of helmets, passenger restraints, and cab covers, but preferably simple prohibition of passengers from cargo spaces.

▶ The authors of this study have done a nice job of pointing out an infrequent but very severe problem. Like motorcycle accidents, it is evident that when falls occur from pickup trucks, they can often be severe. For this reason, I agree with the authors that if people are going to be allowed in the cargo areas of vehicles, they need restraints just as if they were in the front seat. Here, again, is an excellent example of where emergency physicians can make an impact with the state legislators. We have a very real interest in changing behavior that leads to a decrease in accidents. This is clearly a behavior that potentially drains medical resources and increases the price of health care.—W.H. Spivey, M.D.

A Comparison of HIV-1, HBV, and HTLV-I/II Seroprevalence Rates of Injured Patients Admitted Through California Emergency Departments

Rhee KJ, for the California HIV-1 Emergency Department Seroprevalence Study Group (Univ of California, Davis)

Ann Emerg Med 21:397–401, 1992 2–5

Background.—Emergency personnel inevitably come into contact with blood containing hepatitis B virus (HBV) or the human T-lymphotropic virus (HTLV-I/II). The risks of transmission of either or both may therefore be significant. The seroprevalence rates of HBV and HTLV-I/II were studied and compared with HIV-1 seroprevalence in injured patients admitted through 1 of 10 emergency departments in California.

Methods.—All injured adults admitted in consecutive 3-month periods were studied. The 10 participating hospitals reflected geographic and demographic diversity. Prospective blinded testing for serologic markers for HBV, HTLV-I/II, and HIV-1 on routinely collected blood samples was performed.

Results.—The seroprevalence rate of HBV was 2.6%, which was slightly higher than the 1.4% rate for HIV-1.

Conclusions.—In this series, the seroprevalence rate of HBV was slightly greater than that of HIV-1. However, mortality estimates indicate that HBV and HIV-1 pose roughly similar risks to emergency department personnel. Consistent with previous studies, this study suggests that the incidence of HTLV-I/II in the United States is low. The relative health risks from HTLV-I/II to emergency department workers appear minimal at this time.

▶ This study basically supports those previous studies that have demonstrated that there is a low, but very real incidence of HBV and HIV-1 seroprevalence in patients in the emergency department (see Abstracts 4–2 and 4–4). One nice aspect of this study is that it is a large multicenter study with patients from diverse backgrounds. Most of the other studies today have been fairly limited, often with only 1 or 2 institutions participating. It is hoped that the authors will follow this study for 3 to 5 years to see whether this prevalence is increasing.—W.H. Spivey, M.D.

Sexual Violence Against Women: Prevalence, Consequences, Societal Factors, and Prevention

Schwartz IL (Univ of Arizona Health Sciences Ctr, Tucson)

Am J Prev Med 7:363–373, 1991 2–6

Background.—The prevalence of sexual assault among American women may be 25% or more. Most survivors of sexual assault know their assailants. The consequences of such assault can be severe and prolonged. Fear and anxiety, depression, suicide attempts, problems in daily functioning and interpersonal relationships, sexual dysfunction, and a range of somatic complaints can result. The prevalence of rape, its medical and psychological consequences, societal factors identified with it, and the implications these hold for prevention were examined. A model for primary, secondary, and tertiary prevention of rape was studied.

Consequences and Societal Factors.—The "rape trauma syndrome," a constellation of physical and psychological symptoms, includes fear, helplessness, shock and disbelief, guilt, humiliation, embarrassment, anger, and self-blame. Flashblacks and nightmares retraumatize the victim and produce a high level of anxiety. In the long term, rape survivors can have depression, insomnia, sexual dysfunction, difficulties in relationships, fear and phobias, and more nightmares. Functioning at work and family relationships can be greatly impaired. Social isolation, depression, and suicidal ideation are common after rape. Almost 1 in 5 rape victims attempts suicide. Family members often refuse to discuss the rape. Rape victims also rate themselves as significantly less healthy than women who had never been criminally assaulted. Recovery from rape varies in length. Societal factors have recently been implicated in the etiology of sexual violence against women. These include acceptance of rape myths, rigid sex role stereotyping beliefs, and acceptance of violence as a legitimate way to obtain compliance in interpersonal relationships.

Conclusions.—Primary rape prevention involves a program of anticipatory guidance in a developmental framework. Identification of and early intervention in dysfunctional families are part of secondary prevention. Tertiary prevention consists of appropriate treatment for rape victims to prevent or help minimize later physical and psychological difficulties. This preventive model may be incorporated into clinical preventive medicine and primary-care practice.

▶ The author of this article does a nice job reviewing the severe consequences of rape of women. Much of the paper centers on education and recognition of symptoms of rape trauma and the need for follow-up. Although it is difficult for emergency physicians to be active in the education to prevent rape, one group that is certainly at high risk and needs this to be discussed is the battered wife. Women who come to the emergency department after physical abuse are likely to be the victims of sexual abuse also. It is much easier to take care of a laceration and avoid questions about sexual abuse, but we should take a few minutes to discuss it with the patient. Even if they have not been sexually abused, the possibility certainly should be raised to the patient and the appropriate counseling and follow-up arranged.—W.H. Spivey, M.D.

Interpersonal Violence-Related Injuries in an African-American Community in Philadelphia

Wishner AR, Schwarz DF, Grisso JA, Holmes JH, Sutton RL (Philadelphia Dept of Public Health; Children's Hosp of Philadelphia; Univ of Pennsylvania)

Am J Public Health 81:1474–1476, 1991 2–7

Introduction.—Violence is a significant cause of fatal and nonfatal injuries in inner-city communities. In this study, the interpersonal violence-related injuries (IVRIs) in an indigent Philadelphia community were studied.

Methods.—Data on all injuries from a 1-year period were collected from emergency room records, the office of the medical examiner, and death certificate files. The community studied consisted of 68,103 residents, 97.2% African American, with a median family income of $11,810.

Results.—One thousand six hundred ninety persons had IVRIs. Among people aged 15 through 49 years, the rate of IVRIs was higher than that of any other injury type. Among people of all ages, the rate of IVRIs, 28.7 per 1,000 residents, was the second highest of all injury types, less than the rate of 31.7 per 1,000 for falls, and greater than the rate of 22 for motor vehicle accidents. Violence also resulted in a higher death rate than with other injury types. Residents aged 15 through 39 years, who composed 38% of the population, incurred 72.2% of all IVRIs. In this age group, the rate of IVRI was twice as high among males as among females. Even in residents in the 0- to 4-year-old age group, the rate of IVRI was significant at 9.19 injuries per 1,000 residents. The IVRI rate was highest in those aged 15 through 39 years and then fell. Even among residents aged 55 to 59 years, the rate of violence-related injuries was substantial at 12.08 per 1,000. Much information, including the alcohol or drug status of the victim or the assaulter, the relationship between the victim and the perpetrator, the time and place of the injury, and the role of weapons in the injury, was generally unavailable from emergency room records.

Conclusion.—These findings show the staggering extent of violence in this community. Improving the data available would assist in the design of violence prevention programs.

▶ The data presented in this article should be of no surprise to any emergency physician, especially those who work in departments serving inner-city populations. The degree of violence that is obvious is alarming. Now, as requested by the AMA, emergency physicians are asked to probe the events surrounding all injuries to determine the potential for abuse against women, the elderly, and of course, children. This article also underscores the importance of security for emergency department (ED) staff, so often neglected by hospital administrators as "not important" or "bad PR." Perhaps the time has come for OSHA to mandate (1) 24-hr/day armed security in the ED and (2) the use of metal detectors for screening all who enter the ED, backed up by federal statute of mandatory jail sentences for anyone who enters an ED armed with a deadly weapon. This would be similar to standard airport security.—J.T. Amsterdam, M.D.

Injuries in Working Populations: Black-White Differences

Wagener DK, Winn DW (Ctrs for Disease Control, Atlanta, Ga)

Am J Public Health 81:1408–1414, 1991 2–8

Introduction.—Injuries are an important cause of the loss of working years of life and result in significant medical costs. Reports by employers have shown that injury rates and work loss due to injuries have been increasing. Although white employees report more injuries than do black employees, they are less likely than blacks to have fatal injuries. The pattern of injuries in working adults in relation to known important parameters such as race was examined.

Methods.—The incidence of injuries was analyzed by using data from the National Health Interview Survey from 1983 through 1987. Only persons between 18 and 64 years of age were included. Over 200,000 interviews were conducted (with a response rate between 95% and 98%) and dealt with demographic and personal characteristics, illnesses, injuries, current health resource use, and other health topics. Injury rates were determined for adults of different ages, races, gender, occupation, and income.

Results.—The annual weighted estimate for injuries in the U.S. working population was 27,382,000. Eighty-nine percent of injuries were medically attended, and 55% involved at least a half day of restricted activity. Subgroups with higher-than-average injury rates included young males, persons with lower incomes, and whites. Higher injury rates were found among blue-collar and farm workers. Working blacks had lower injury rates than working whites in all family income groups for both genders and for all ages except 45 through 64 years. Men aged 18 to 44 years had a significantly higher reported injury rate than did women the same age. There was little difference between the rates at which older black and white men incurred injuries at work.

Conclusion.—This analysis confirms the high rate of injuries to U.S. working adults and the higher rate for all injuries reported by whites than by blacks. The sociodemographic factors analyzed here, such as occupation and income level, did not explain this racial difference.

▶ This article does point out an alarming number of injuries among the U.S. working population. Certainly, emergency medicine has a role to play in the prevention of such injuries if they are related to unsafe working environments, practices, or the use of drugs and alcohol. In this study, the higher rate of injuries in whites could not be explained by sociodemographic factors. Access to health care was not an issue. Individuals working in service occupations are less likely to have health insurance coverage, sick leave, and work flexibility. In this study, blacks were found to be more likely in these positions. The key to injury management is truly prevention. Education is the key to prevention, which makes studies such as this important so that efforts are directed to appropriate individuals in the right social context.—J.T. Amsterdam, M.D.

Bonfire and Barbecue Burns

Regan PJ, Budny PG, Lavelle JR, Roberts AHN (Stoke Mandeville Hosp, Aylesbury, England)

Burns 17:306–308, 1991 2–9

Introduction.—Over 2 consecutive hot spring and summer seasons, a large number of patients were treated for burns caused by barbecues and bonfires, thus prompting a 10-year review of data on 54 patients with these types of burns.

Patients.—The patients accounted for 2.16% of all burns seen over the study period. There were 10 times as many males as females, the mean patient age was 30.5 years, and 80% of patients were aged 14 to 49 years. Most patients were burned in 1987 to 1989, a time when the summers were hot. Burns were more likely to occur in the months of April, June, July, and November; bonfires are traditional on November 5. In 80% of the episodes, the patient had thrown an inflammable liquid at the fire. The mean total body surface area burned was 10.6%, with most burns covering less than 10%. Excision and grafting was performed in 31 patients with a mean total body surface area burn of 6%. The mean hospital stay was 15.7 days; the face, dorsum of the hands, front of the chest, and anterior aspects of the legs were most often burned. None of the patients died.

Conclusion.—Burns resulting from bonfires and barbecues appear to be increasing. Most of these injuries result from throwing inflammable liquid onto a live fire; patients are often unable to tell whether the fire is lit because of bright sunlight. Children may burn their feet by walking on hot embers.

▶ As this article would indicate, if education could prevent individuals from pouring or throwing inflammable liquids onto hot fires, especially in the sunlight when it is difficult to see whether a fire or hot embers are present, there would be one less problem to see in the emergency department. Emergency physicians should also be aware that many states have a suspicious burn-reporting act that includes respiratory and second- and third-degree burns from incendiary devices or fires such as bonfires. Failure to report such injuries may result in a misdemeanor.—J.T. Amsterdam, M.D.

Snowmobile Trauma: An Eleven-Year Experience

James EC, Lenz JO, Swenson WM, Cooley AM, Gomez YL, et al (Univ of North Dakota, Grand Forks)

Am Surg 57:349–353, 1991 2–10

Background.—The first snowmobile was designed by a Canadian in 1923. Modern machines may weigh as much as 600 lb and may be capable of speeds up to 100 mph. The center of gravity of a snowmobile is low, but it is not a stable machine and can easily turn over on a slope or incline. Because registration is not necessary for snowmobiles used on private property, figures for registered snowmobiles in North Dakota dropped from 14,000 in 1982 to 6,415 in 1987. During the 11 years from 1977 through 1987, 88 patients were treated in 1 hospital for injuries resulting from snowmobiling.

Findings.—Data collected included age, sex, method and degree of injury, use of safety attire, and risk factors. Seventy-seven males and 11 females were treated for a total of 205 injuries that required 760 hospital inpatient days. One hundred percent of the injuries in children younger than 16 years involved extremities caught in the track of the snowmobile. Hitting obstacles led to fractures and even loss of consciousness in the majority of accidents in persons older than 16 years. There were 3 fatalities.

Conclusions.—The leading contributors to accidents in 88 patients seen over an 11-year period in 1 hospital were driver inexperience or carelessness, prior use of alcohol, excessive speed, and poor adherence to the manufacturer's recommendations. Education to promote the safe handling of snowmobiles and requiring safety courses, licensure of drivers, and mandatory use of protective footwear and helmets are recommended.

▶ Snowmobiles and motorcycles have much in common. They are unstable and heavy and afford no protection to the rider(s). While I am not surprised with the frequency and severity of injuries associated with their use, I am amazed at the lack of legislation governing people who use them, especially when it comes to snowmobiles. In most states, motorcyclists are required to wear helmets, and in all states they are required to have an operator's license. Since snowmobiles are often used on private property and off-road sites, there is even less control exerted by state and local officials. As with motorcycles, proper headgear, boots, and training would limit the extent of injuries on the snowmobile. Allowing children who have not reached mental, much less physical puberty run these machines further places the public at risk. The authors strongly support licensure following training for those over 16 years of age. Although substance abuse was documented only in the case of death, I am quite sure that similar to other types of motor vehicle accidents, it would be found in the majority of snowmobiling injuries.—H.D. Unger, M.D.

Head, Neck, Vertebral

Skull Radiography in the Evaluation of Acute Head Trauma: A Survey of Current Practice

Hackney DB (Hosp of the Univ of Pennsylvania, Philadelphia)
Radiology 181:711–714, 1991 2–11

Background.—It has long been reported that skull radiography had a low diagnostic yield when used for mild head trauma, and presently skull radiography is not used in high-yield patients when CT is available. However, despite advances in CT and MRI, there may be suboptimal use of skull radiography and these more advanced technologies. The influence of reports over the last 20 years of the superiority of CT and

MRI over skull radiography on the diagnostic evaluation of trauma patients was investigated.

Methods.—A telephone survey of radiologists was conducted in 53 hospitals with both an emergency room and a CT scanner to determine the use of skull radiography for the evaluation of head trauma. The presence of a CT scanner ensured that if skull radiography was used, it was being used inappropriately.

Findings.—More than half of the 53 hospitals reported that skull radiographs were always or often obtained for head trauma cases, and only 3 reported that radiographs were never a part of the evaluation of acute head injuries. The high usage rates were not related to the teaching or nonteaching status of the hospital, the size of the hospital, or the availability of CT. Skull radiography was frequently used in the evaluation of minor injuries, and CT was always used in cases of severe head trauma. However, MRI was rarely used for evaluating head trauma despite reports of its superiority to CT imaging in many cases of severe brain parenchymal injuries.

Conclusions.—Although the low utility of skull radiographs in evaluating head trauma has been known for many years, radiographs are used in substantial numbers of patients with minor trauma. The overuse of skull radiography increases health care costs, increases the radiation dose to the population, and exacerbates a worsening shortage of radiologic technologists. Additionally, MRI is superior to CT in some trauma cases.

▶ This study is purported to be a study of practice patterns, although the subjects surveyed were radiologists, not the actual practicing physicians who saw the patients and ordered the examinations. Therefore, this paper has little significance to emergency medicine other than to reaffirm a long-standing premise, namely, that skull films have virtually no place in the diagnosis of head trauma in the emergency center (see also Abstract 2–12).—G.J. Ordog, M.D.

Is Routine Computed Tomography Scanning Too Expensive for Mild Head Injury?

Stein SC, O'Malley KF, Ross SE (Robert Wood Johnson Med School, Camden, NJ)

Ann Emerg Med 20:1286–1289, 1991 2–12

Objective.—Routine early CT has become an integral part of the management of moderate to severe head injury, but it has been considered too costly for use in milder injury. Such preventive scanning can, however, provide valuable guidance. An experience with the cost-effectiveness of CT was reviewed.

Methods.—The experience consisted of 658 consecutive patients with mild head injuries, all of whom underwent cranial CT scanning. The patients' records were reviewed, and hypothetical costs based on the actual length of hospitalization, surgical intervention, and other services were calculated. The costs of different treatment protocols were then compared.

Results.—If every patient had been admitted for observation and skull radiographs, the average cost would have been $1,207. If CT were used to find those with intracranial lesions and all others were discharged, these costs would have been reduced by nearly 10%. Using skull radiographs to screen admissions would have reduced costs by 22% as compared with CT scanning; however, skull films would miss intracranial lesions that CT would find.

Conclusions.—Computed tomography was recommended for head injury patients with loss of consciousness or posttraumatic amnesia. Patients with a normal CT scan and no other need for admission can be discharged. This approach optimizes medical care and cost-effectiveness.

▶ The purpose of this study was *not* to determine which patients with minor head injury should be scanned. The message here is simple, namely, patients with minor head injury who have a negative CT scan can be discharged home and are not likely to deteriorate at a later time. This observation is supported by other investigators (1). Indeed, the routine use of CT for all patients with loss of consciousness or posttraumatic amnesia has quietly become the standard of care.—J.T. Niemann, M.D.

Reference

1. Stein SC, Ross SE: *Neurosurgery* 26:638, 1990.

Head-Injured Patients Who Talk and Deteriorate Into Coma: Analysis of 211 Cases Studied With Computerized Tomography

Lobato RD, Rivas JJ, Gomez PA, Castañeda M, Cañizal JM, et al
(Complutense Univ, Madrid, Spain)

J Neurosurg 75:256–261, 1991 2–13

Introduction.—Twelve percent to 32% of patients who go into a coma after head injury speak sometime after the trauma but before their condition deteriorates. Few studies have addressed the mechanisms of deterioration and the avoidable factors leading to unfavorable outcomes in this potentially salvageable group of patients. The clinical and pathologic findings of patients who talked before coma were analyzed and compared with findings in patients who did not speak.

Patients.—The study included 838 patients with severe head injuries who were admitted over a 12-year period since the advent of CT. Of those, 211, or 25.1%, spoke sometime between their injury and subsequent deterioration into coma. In 71% of cases, deterioration occurred sometime during the first day.

Findings.—In the group of patients who talked, the pathologic category was brain contusion/hematoma in 42.2%, epidural hematoma in 21.8%, subdural hematoma in 16.6%, and no focal mass lesion in 19.4%. Thus most patients had a mass lesion potentially requiring surgery; the mass was intracerebral in 52.3% of cases and extracerebral in 47.6%. In patients aged 20 years or younger, the likelihood of having a nonfocal mass lesion was 39%; epidural hematoma, 29%; and intradural mass lesion, 32%. For patients older than 40 years, the chance of having a nonfocal mass lesion was only 3%, and the chance of having epidural hematoma was 18%, but the chance of having an intradural mass lesion was 79%. The patient survived in 67.8% of cases and dies in 32.2%. The most significant independent predictor of outcome was the Glasgow Coma Scale score after deterioration, followed by the highest intracranial pressure, the degree of midline shift, the type of intracranial lesion, and patient age. The result was unaffected by the mechanism of injury, verbal Glasgow Coma Score while the patient was talking, and the time until deterioration or operative intervention.

Conclusions.—Most patients who deteriorate into coma after a seemingly nonserious head injury have a focal mass lesion that usually requires neurosurgical intervention. Intracranial complications need to be recognized and treated earlier; current strategies regarding precautionary admission and CT examination should be modified. Postponing surgery because of a normal initial intracranial pressure can result in severe brain damage.

▶ The authors did not attempt to describe the patient at risk for neurologic deterioration after head injury, but rather looked at management strategies to avoid unfavorable outcome in these patients. I took home a few points. Many of these patients have surgical lesions and should not be lost while in an extensive noncritical workup of other injuries (i.e., orthopedic). Early surgical intervention may prevent a bad outcome. Five patients had normal initial CT scans, which is a reminder that one cannot always utilize normal, early CT results as a screen to clear the patient for discharge.—J.M. Mitchell-Savinsky, M.D.

Transcranial Doppler Ultrasound Following Closed Head Injury: Vasospasm or Vasoparalysis?

Gomez CR, Backer RJ, Bucholz RD (St Louis Univ, Mo)

Surg Neurol 35:30–35, 1991 2–14

Background and Methods.—Transcranial Doppler sonography is a safe and reproducible method for obtaining information on blood flow direction, velocity, and pulsatility in the basal cerebral arteries. In this report, physicians examine the results of transcranial Doppler examinations in patients who incurred and survived closed-head injuries. The 5 women and 4 men, who ranged in age from 16 to 49 years, had Glasgow Coma Scores of ≤8 at admission. Five patients had intracranial pressure elevations to ≥20 mm Hg during the first week of hospitalization and were treated with hyperventilation and osmotic diuresis; 1 patient with elevated intracranial pressure was treated with pentobarbital coma. Two patients underwent craniotomy at admission for subdural hematoma and combined subdural and epidural hematoma, respectively.

Results.—Eight patients had abnormally high mean blood flow velocities (MBFVs) in 1 or more vessels within 2 weeks after trauma. The onset, amplitude, and duration of altered flow velocities differed from those seen with vasospasm after aneurysmal subarachnoid hemorrhage. However, cerebral angiography in 1 patient confirmed the presence of vasospasm. Most patients reached peak MBFVs 3 to 6 days after injury, but 1 patient had maximal MBFVs at admission. These decreased as the patient recovered. In the patient treated with pentobarbital coma. MBFVs began increasing after discontinuation of barbiturate use on day 3. By day 7, they were clearly abnormal, and on days 11 through 13, they reached their peak. Although not statistically significant, there was a relationship between the presence of intracranial hemorrhage and the development of abnormal MBFVs. Multivariate regression analysis showed a definate correlation between velocities—even when abnormally elevated—and concurrent pH and partial pressure of carbon dioxide measurements.

Conclusions.—Cerebral vasculature retains vasoreactivity after head injury a finding that would seem to indicate an absence of vasoparalysis. However, inconsistencies in some patients warrant the theory that both vasospasm and vasoparalysis may occur in the same patient after head trauma. If so, these conditions apparently have different temporal profiles.

▶ The paper has no current applicability to emergency medicine. The observed findings of intracranial blood flow velocities measured in head-injured patients are not readily explained. The observation should serve as the basis for future studies to explain the observed differences. The etiologies of the findings are speculated upon by the authors.—J.E. Clinton, M.D.

Does On-Scene Resuscitation Affect In-Hospital "Do Not Resuscitate" Decisions and Mortality in Patients With Severe Head Injuries?

Buchmann B, Kaufmann MA, Scheidegger D, Gratzl O (Univ of Basel/Kantonsspital, Switzerland)

J Trauma 32:459–463, 1992 2–15

Purpose.—Many patients with severe head injuries who previously would have died at the scene or on the way to the hospital now reach the hospital alive; thus on-scene resuscitation may increase morbidity

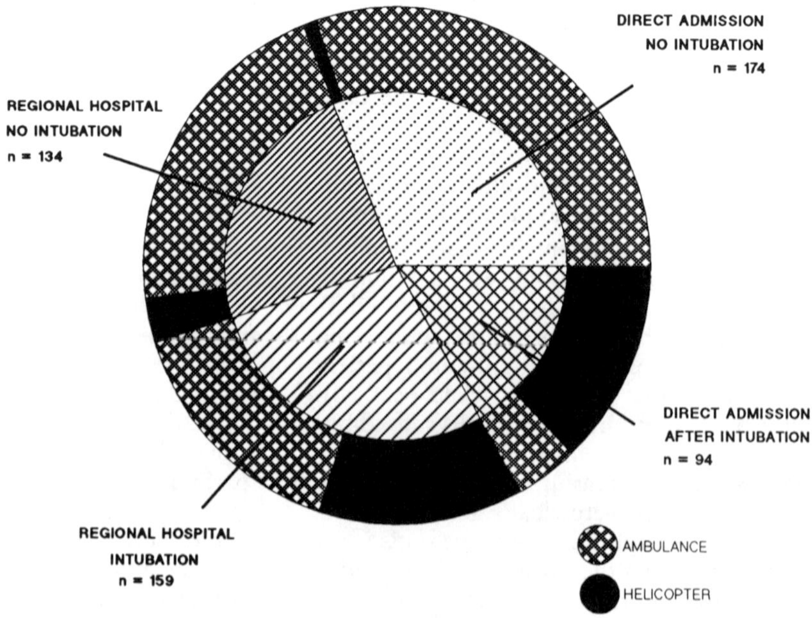

Fig 2–3.—Admission modalities. (Courtesy of Buchmann B, Kaufmann MA, Scheidegger D, et al: *J Trauma* 32:459–463, 1992.)

and in-hospital mortality. On-scene and in-hospital resuscitation of patients with severe head injury was compared with regard to "do not resuscitate" (DNR) orders and mortality rates.

Patients.—The study sample consisted of 561 patients with severe head injuries who were admitted to the surgical intensive care unit (SICU) during a 5-year period. Group 1 consisted of 94 patients resuscitated at the scene of the injury; group 2 included 145 patients resuscitated at a regional hospital before transfer to a neurosurgical center; and group 3 consisted of 130 patients resuscitated after direct admission to a neurosurgical center.

Findings.—Death and DNR rates in the first 48 hours were similar: 13% in group 1, 15% in group 2, and 13% in group 3. Similar results were found for patients intubated within 1 hour of the injury. Seventy percent of patients were transported by ambulance, and 30% were transported by helicopter (Fig 2–3). Of 53 patients who were in the SICU only 1 day, more than 50% died during this day; of 42 patients who stayed in the SICU for more than 3 weeks, all but 3 who died were transferred out.

Conclusions.—In patients with severe head injury, primary aggressive treatment at the scene does not appear to increase DNR and hospital mortality rates or total stay in the SICU. Early management appears to be the best treatment for these patients, although long-term outcome will have to be established.

▶ Prehospital care providers cannot ignore the impact of their efforts on both in-hospital and long-term out-of-hospital health care resources. It is a frequent complaint that survival to hospital discharge is an unfair yardstick because so many variables that may have an impact on outcome are introduced in the hospital and these are not under the control of an emergency medical service system. This compartmentalized approach to health care can lead to faulty judgment when we consider only morbidity or mortality to the emergency department door. Systems are becoming more aggressive in defining the impact of attempting resuscitation on patients whose outcome is inevitably poor and are more and more devoting scarce resources to patients who truly seem to benefit from care. This article attempts to allay some valid concerns regarding the aggressive resuscitation of severely head-injured patients. Despite the aggressive prehospital resuscitation, we do not seem to be "loading" the intensive care units with vegetative patients.—W.J. Koenig, M.D.

Coagulopathy and Catecholamines in Severe Head Injury

Kearney TJ, Bentt L, Grode M, Lee S, Hiatt JR, et al (Cedars Sinai Med Ctr, Los Angeles, Calif)

J Trauma 32:608–612, 1992 2–16

Background.—Between 3% and 13% of all patients who sustain severe head trauma have clinical and laboratory evidence of coagulopathy. It is believed that the damaged brain tissue releases thromboplastain, which activates the extrinsic clotting cascade and initiates disseminated intravascular coagulation (DIC). The catecholamine release seen in severe head injury may stimulate platelets and increase endothelial damage, thus further exacerbating the coagulopathy. The relationship between DIC, catecholamine levels, and outcome was assessed in 36 patients with severe head injury.

Patients.—Ten of the patients sustained penetrating gunshot wounds to the head, and 26 had severe blunt head trauma. All patients had an initial Glasgow Coma Scale score of 9 or less. Blood samples were collected on average 7 hours after admission and analyzed for platelet count, prothrombin time (PT), partial thromboplastin time (PTT), and fibrinogen, D-dimer, antithrombin III, protein C, and protein S levels. A 24-hour urine sample was collected and measured for vanillylmandelic acid (VMA), normetanephrine, and metanephrine levels. Five patients undergoing elective neurosurgery served as controls.

Results.—Eighteen patients (50%) died before hospital discharge. Of the 18 survivors, 4 were in a vegetative state, 6 were severely disabled, 2 were moderately disabled, and 6 had a good outcome. When survivors were compared with nonsurvivors, statistically significant differences were present for platelet count, PT, and fibrinogen activity. There were no significant differences in any of the other coagulation parameters or in urinary catecholamine levels, although many values were abnormal. Significant differences between trauma patients and controls were found for D-dimer and protein C levels, PT, PTT, normetanephrine levels, and DIC scores.

Conclusions.—The coagulopathy that is present in patients with severe head trauma appears to correlate with poor survival and may be related to a catecholamine surge. Interventions to correct the coagulopathy of severe head injury may significantly reduce mortality and morbidity rates.

▶ The authors developed data to support 3 conclusions: (1) that patients with severe head injuries develop a DIC-type coagulopathy not noted in nontraumatic elective surgery; (2) that head-injured, nonsurviving patients have more severe manifestations of DIC than do head-injured survivors; and (3) that a trauma-related catecholamine response may initiate and be responsible for the severe DIC response. The first conclusion has been broadly supported in the literature, while the latter 2 points are less well agreed upon. Whenever emergency physicians or others involved in trauma resuscitation are faced with the "C" condition (coagulopathy), the outcome becomes precarious. Any information that may be utilized to thwart such a development will be welcomed by all individuals involved in the care of traumatized patients.—D.K. Wagner, M.D.

Fractures of the Atlas

Levine AM, Edwards CC (Univ of Maryland, Baltimore)

J Bone Joint Surg (Am) 73:680–691, 1991 2–17

Introduction.—Atlas fractures make up about one fourth of all injuries to the atlantoaxial complex and 10% of all cervical spine injuries. A recent study suggested a relationship between nonunion of atlas fractures and the degree of displacement.

Series.—The outcome of 34 patients with fractures of the atlas who were followed for an average of 4½ years was evaluated. All the injuries resulted from major trauma. The mean age was 37.9 years.

Posterior Arch Fractures.—Seventeen patients had bilateral fractures of the posterior arch of C1 at the junction of the arch with the lateral masses. Associated injuries were frequent, the most common being posteriorly displaced odontoid fractures and spondylolisthesis of the axis. Eight patients were immobilized in a cervical orthosis and had no long-term problems. Two of the 9 patients with other injuries to the atlantoaxial complex died, but no neurologic problems resulted from injury to the posterior arch. With 1 exception, the posterior arch fractures united solidly.

Other Fractures.—Six patients had fractures of the lateral masses, 1 just anterior to or within the anterior part of the lateral mass of C1 and another posterior to the lateral mass of C1 on the same side. Radiographs demonstrated asymmetric displacement of the lateral masses. Eleven patients had a Jefferson, or burst, fracture of C1. They had either 2 fractures in the anterior and 2 in the posterior arch or 1 in the anterior arch and 2 in the posterior arch. If spreading of the lateral masses exceeded 7 mm, they were reduced by axial traction until the arch healed. No patient had atlantoaxial instability at follow-up, but most patients had occasional neck pain. There was 1 nonunion.

▶ This is an excellent review of 34 atlas fractures and describes the three distinct types of atlas fractures, along with the important roentgenographic features of each.

I highly recommend that you pull the original article and review the plentiful and technically excellent cervical spine radiographs that are very educational for every practicing emergency physician. No matter how many (or how few) atlas fractures you have diagnosed and treated in your career, you will learn from this article (see also Abstracts 2–18 and 2–19).—J.J. Kelly, D.O., F.A.C.E.P.

Can Burst Fractures be Predicted From Plain Radiographs?

Ballock RT, Mackersie R, Abitbol J-J, Cervilla V, Resnick D, et al (Univ of California, San Diego)

J Bone Joint Surg [Br] 74:147–150, 1992 2–18

Background.—In acute spinal fractures, it is critical that bursting injuries of the vertebral body be identified because misdiagnosis of these fractures as wedge compression fractures may result in progressive deformity and neurologic damage. Plain radiographs of 67 acute spinal compression fractures in 49 patients were analyzed by subjective and objective criteria.

Methods.—With CT as the diagnostic standard, the sensitivity, specificity, and predictive value of plain radiographs in the diagnosis of burst fractures of the thoracic and lumber spine were determined.

Results.—Twenty-nine (43%) fractures were diagnosed as burst injuries based on disruptions of the posterior cortex on the CT scan. By using the variables of interpedicular widening and loss of height of the posterior vertebral cortex, discriminant analysis correctly identified 88% of the fractures. However, 14% of patients with burst fractures were given incorrect diagnoses of wedge compression fractures, which did not differ significantly from the incorrect diagnoses on 25 fractures analyzed by uninformed readers. The overall sensitivity of the plain radiographs in the diagnosis of burst fractures was 83%. The specificity was 92%, and the predictive value was 89%. When the less severe burst fractures were analyzed alone, the sensitivity was 67%.

Conclusion.—A 25% error in the diagnosis of burst injuries based on plain radiographs alone is unacceptably high. Computed tomography of the spine should be performed routinely on all patients with acute thoracic or lumbar compression fractures to reduce this potential diagnostic error.

▶ This extremely useful article highlights the increasing use of CT in defining orthopedic injuries. It emphasizes the need for tomography if there is any doubt regarding the integrity of the vertebral body in spinal compression fractures. The unfortunate situation can arise when a stable-appearing lumbar compression fracture later becomes displaced and results in spinal cord compression and paralysis. When any doubt exists, CT must be used to define the extent of injury in vertebral body compression fractures.—E.J. Reisdorff, M.D.

Evaluation and Treatment of Atlas Burst Fractures (Jefferson Fractures)

Kesterson L, Benzel E, Orrison W, Coleman J (Univ of New Mexico, Albuquerque; Louisiana State Univ, Shreveport)

J Neurosurg 75:213–220, 1991 2–19

Background.—Several large series of atlas fractures have been recently reviewed, but none has concentrated on atlas burst fractures (Jefferson fractures). To clarify the diagnosis and treatment of these fractures, 17 cases of Jefferson fracture are presented here.

Patients and Clinical Methods.—Patients with the diagnosis of Jefferson fracture treated at Louisiana State University between 1982 and 1989 ranged in age from 4 to 78 years. All complained of cervical or occipital pain (or both) following trauma. Only 1 patient showed a neurologic deficit. Routine radiographic evaluation included plain x-ray films, including open-mouth anteroposterior (AP) views, and CT scans; findings were confirmed by conventional tomography. Stable Jefferson fractures were treated with external immobilization. Unstable injuries occurred in 4 cases. These were treated with early operative fixation with occiput-C2 wiring and fusion, followed by external immobilization with a Minerva jacket.

Results.—All 14 patients followed for at least 1 year had reduced pain, and the single patient with a neurologic deficit returned to normal. Three patients with unstable Jefferson fractures had no complaints of restricted cervical movement 1 year after surgery. The fourth patient had an associated type II odontoid fracture and died after an occiput-C2 fusion due to pulmonary complications related to associated injuries. The most common concurrent upper cervical spine fracture was a type II odontoid fracture, which was seen in all patients with unstable Jefferson fractures, including the sole patient who presented with a neurologic deficit.

Conclusions.—Most of these patients with Jefferson fractures were stable and were effectively treated without complications with Minerva jackets or rigid collar stabilization. Diagnosis of this injury may be difficult or delayed due to an absence of neurologic deficits and concern about associated injuries. An adequate open-mouth AP x-ray film of the atlantoaxial articulations is usually pathognomonic for the diagnosis.

▶ This is a very readable review of atlas burst fractures. It reminds us that a good open-mouth AP view of the atlantoaxial junction is mandatory to exclude the diagnosis and that coexistent type II odontoid fractures should be sought. We often use the lateral and AP views to "clear" the cervical spine. These alone may miss Jefferson fractures. In particular, in a patient with upper neck/occipital pain in whom adequate open-mouth views cannot be obtained, further evaluation such as CT should be done.—J.M. Mitchell-Savinsky, M.D.

The Epidemiology of Fractures and Fracture-Dislocations of the Cervical Spine

Ryan MD, Henderson JJ (Univ of Sydney, St Leonards, Australia; Univ of Manchester, England)

Injury 23:38–40, 1992 2–20

Background.—Studies of injuries to the cervical spine have found a preponderance of such injuries in the young with an increased incidence in the sixth and seventh decades. The frequency of these injuries was assessed at different levels, along with the frequency with which they occurred at more than one level.

Patients.—Over a 13-year period, 717 fractures and dislocations of the cervical spine were seen in 657 patients. The C2 vertebra was the most commonly injured, followed by the C5 and C6 vertebrae. The peak incidence was in the third decade of life and decreased thereafter. The indence of C1 and C2 fractures increased with age, however, primarily because odontoid fractures increased (Fig 2–4). Injuries to C1 and C2 commonly occurred together, and 9% of these patients had injuries involving both the upper and lower segments of the cervical spine. Otherwise, there were few multilevel injuries at lower sites in the neck. Odontoid fractures usually happened alone.

Discussion.—If radiographs show a fracture of the upper part of the cervical spine, the physician should exclude another fracture in the upper or lower portions of the cervical spine. An odontoid fracture should be suspected in patients 70 years or older who have neck pain following

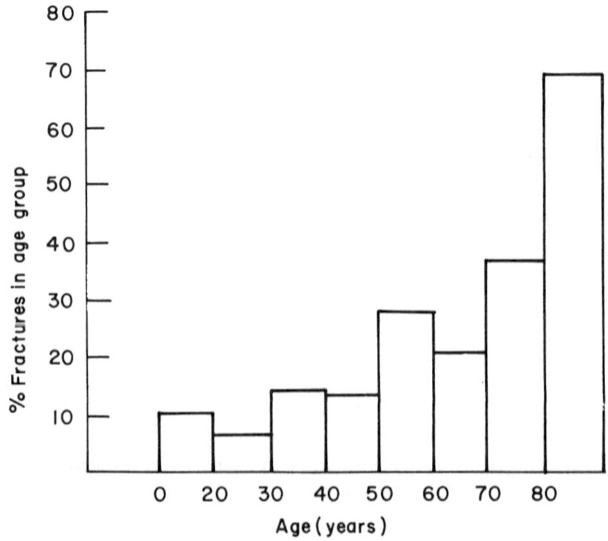

Fig 2-4.—Odontoid fractures (expressed as a percentage of the injuries occurring in each age group). (Courtesy of Ryan MD, Henderson JJ, *Injury* 23:38–40, 1992.)

trauma. All patients with neck injury should have radiographic examination of the entire cervical spine, including the cervicothoracic junction.

▶ This was a retrospective review from 1973 to 1985 at a referral center for acute spinal cord injuries. I doubt that all the fractures were diagnosed on initial emergency department films. It is, however, a good lesson for all of us to look for additional cervical spine fractures.—T. Stair, M.D.

Unstable Occult Cervical-Spine Fracture
Mace SE (St Mary's Hosp, Rochester, NY)
Ann Emerg Med 20:1373–1375, 1991 2–21

Background.—Although physicians have documented occult cervical spine fracture, various studies have recently questioned the occurrence of occult cervical spine fractures in alert patients without neck pain. An alert patient with no symptoms or signs of neck trauma who sustained significant injury to the cervical spine was studied.

Case Study.—A 51-year-old man with a history of seizures and alcohol abuse complained of a sore throat, spitting up saliva, difficulty swallowing, and shortness of breath for 1 day. The patient was taking phenytoin and phenobarbital. Paramedics noted bilateral rales and rhonchi. The patient's blood pressure was 160/98 mm Hg, his pulse was 120, and his respiration was 28. The patient was given 40 mg of furosemide intravenously. The patient was alert and oriented with a class 1 level of consciousness. He was not intoxicated or under the influence of drugs. The patient's tonsils were enlarged and had a white exudate. His neck was supple and nontender; the lungs had scattered bibasilar rales; the abdomen was benign. Neurologic examination was unremarkable. Indirect laryngoscopy detected tonsilar enlargement and tonsillitis but was unable to fully exclude a peritonsillar abscess. A chest radiograph showed a clear lung field. Soft-tissue neck films showed a normal epiglottis with some fullness in the subglottic soft tissues, marked degenerative changes in the cervical spine with large osteophytes, and a type 2 odontoid fracture at its base. There was anterior subluxation of the arch of C1 on C2 of approximately 1 cm. The patient underwent cervical spine immobilization to improve alignment. The patient was treated with 2.4 million units of bicillin and transferred to the neurosurgery spine service, where he was placed in cervical traction. He then underwent fusion of C1-2 and a bone graft. Four months later, he was neurologically intact but still hospitalized.

Conclusions.—Significant cervical spine injury can exist without signs and symptoms of neck injury and even without a history of trauma. Especially in high-risk patients, physicians should maintain high indices of suspicion despite the absence of signs and symptoms.

▶ Other studies have shown that the cervical spine can be "cleared" by an absence of pain and/or tenderness in an awake and alert patient (See Abstract 2–22). This case illustrates the problems with patients who have seizures and alcohol abuse. When documentation exists in the medical literature of this type of problem, it makes us open to liability if we do not clear the cervical spine radiologically in patients who have altered mental status, drug or alcohol abuse, and seizures.—G.J. Ordog, M.D.

Is the Anteroposterior Cervical Spine Radiograph Necessary in Initial Trauma Screening?

Holliman CJ, Mayer JS, Cook RT Jr, Smith JS Jr (The Milton S Hershey Med Ctr, Hershey, Pa)

Am J Emerg Med 9:421–425, 1991 2–22

Background.—In caring for the trauma patient, ruling out a cervical spine fracture or dislocation is important. When a cross-table lateral view alone constitutes the radiographic examination, a relatively low accuracy results. Some researchers therefore advocate the use of a 3-view cervical spine series consisting of lateral, anteroposterior (AP), and odontoid views, although this approach can be time-consuming. A retrospective study was done to examine whether the AP radiograph is useful in diagnosing cervical spine trauma.

Methods.—Sixty cervical spine injuries of which 3 radiographic views were available plus an additional 57 of which original lateral and odontoid, but not AP views existed were reviewed. All radiographs were of patients with cervical spine fractures or dislocations seen at a rehabilitation center over a 10-year period or at a level I trauma center over a 3-year period. A neuroradiologist blinded to the original diagnosis examined the lateral, open-mouth odontoid, and AP radiographs in order so as to make a diagnosis if possible after examining each view and judge whether a final diagnosis was possible.

Findings.—A firm diagnosis was possible from the lateral view alone in 43 of the 60 injuries of which 3 views were available. Four fractures of C2 were confirmed by using the odontoid view. In no case did the AP view show any major injury not previously noted on the lateral or odontoid views. In 15 injuries, the lateral view showed a major vertebral body injury that was absent from or minimally seen on the AP view. In the 57 injuries for which no AP film was available, injuries were evident on the lateral films. In 31 of the 60 injuries with 3 views available, CT was performed. It was judged helpful in 23 of these, and in 4 of them CT showed a fracture at an additional vertebral level from that noted on the plain films.

Conclusions.—An initial AP view was not helpful in diagnosing cervical spine injury. If this finding is confirmed at other trauma centers, the AP view can be dropped without a loss in diagnostic sensitivity. This would result in savings of time, cost, and radiation exposure.

▶ If there is uncertainty about the diagnosis or degree of injury after adequate lateral and open-mouth views, the next procedure should be a CT scan. I agree that the AP view has very little utility. See also Abstracts 2–23 and 8–18.—W.P. Burdick, M.D.

Delayed Presentation of Unstable Cervical Spine Injury With Minimal Symptoms

Cox GR, Barish RA (Univ of Maryland Med System Hosp, Baltimore)
J Emerg Med 9:123–127, 1991 2–23

Introduction.—An emergency physician is more likely to discard the possibility of significant cervical spine trauma if a patient has been ambulatory for some time after a traumatic episode. A patient with multiple cervical fractures did not seek medical care for 6 weeks after falling from a height.

Case Report.—A 65-year-old man walked into the emergency department 6 weeks after falling 10 ft off a garage roof. The accident was not witnessed, and the patient had not sought medical care at the time of the fall. Neck pain developed about 3 days after the fall, and the pain had continued intermittently and gradually worsened. The patient complained of pain in the middle of his neck and numbness of the right upper extremity. He denied having other symptoms. The patient was placed in a Philadelphia collar, and cervical spine radiographs were obtained. The lateral view revealed 75% anterior subluxation of C6 and C7, fractures of the posterior elements of C5 and C6, and a possible fracture of the lamina of C4. Computed tomography at the level of C6 confirmed fractures of the left pedicle and both laminae of C6. The patient was treated with halo immobilization for 6 weeks but later underwent iliac crest bone grafting and Caspar plating.

Comment.—Even significant injury of the cervical spine after a mishap may go unrecognized by the patient. Emergency physicians must not be lulled into complacency because a patient with neck pain has been ambulatory for some time after a traumatic incident.

► Almost all patients with cervical fractures have immediate onset of pain—here is an exception (see Abstract 8–18)—W.P. Burdick, M.D.

Validating the Selective Management of Penetrating Neck Wounds
Mansour MA, Moore EE, Moore FA, Whitehill TA (Denver Gen Hosp; Univ of Colorado)
Am J Surg 162:517–521, 1991 2–24

Background.—Physicians are divided as to the relative merits of mandatory vs. selective management of penetrating neck wounds. On the basis of a 56% negative exploration rate in previous patients, a 12-year prospective study of selective management was conducted.

Methods.—Penetrating anterior neck wounds were selectively managed in 188 patients. The first priority was to achieve airway patency and to tamponade hemorrhage. Patients with expanding hematomas encroaching upon the trachea underwent endotracheal intubation. Neck wounds were examined to determine the level of penetration, but they were not probed. Active bleeding was controlled with direct pressure; vascular structures were not clamped. Patients underwent an anteroposterior chest roentgenogram and anteroposterior and lateral soft tissue neck roentgenograms. Patients with persistent shock, profuse bleeding, or evolving stroke underwent immediate formal neck exploration. Patients with other signs of vascular injury also had early neck exploration if warranted by selective preoperative testing. All stable patients with zone 1 injuries underwent arteriography of the aortic arch and thoracic outlet. Cervical angiography was performed for suspected zone 3 carotid wounds. Patients with suspected zone 1 esophageal injuries underwent flexible endoscopy.

Results.—Sixty-nine patients underwent early neck exploration. Seventy-one specific venous, arterial, digestive tract, airway, and miscellaneous injuries were identified during surgery. Sixty patients in the explored group had significant injuries. The remaining 119 patients were observed in the hospital. These patients underwent ancillary diagnostic tests based on the location of the injury and trajectory. One patient in the observation group required delayed exploration for an occult injury. The average hospital stay for patients who underwent exploration was

8.4 days. When exploration was negative, the hospital stay averaged 4.2 days. Those in the observation group averaged a 1.7-day hospital stay.

Conclusions.—Selective exploration of penetrating neck wounds is efficacious and safe in a level 1 trauma center. The surgeon must have enough clinical experience to be familiar with the physical signs of a benign course. The role of adjunctive tests in patients managed expectantly depends upon the relative expertise available in the institution.

▶ Other studies have shown similar results (1, 2). Selective management of penetrating neck trauma at a trauma center is feasible. This requires the immediate availability of radiographs, angiography, triple endoscopy, CT scanning, and specialists in the various areas of the neck. In other hospitals where immediate workups are not available, then mandatory surgery may still be indicated. See Ordog et al. (1) for a description of what is required to perform selective management.—G.J. Ordog, M.D.

References

1. Ordog GJ, et al: *J Trauma* 25:238, 1985.
2. Ordog GJ, et al: *J Trauma* 28:624, 1988.

The Diagnosis and Initial Management of the Fractured Mandible

Luyk NH, Ferguson JW (Univ of Otago, Dunedin, New Zealand)

Am J Emerg Med 9:352–359, 1991 2–25

Purpose.—Mandibular fractures are the second most common facial fractures and account for 40% to 62% of all facial fractures. The principal causes of mandibular fractures are interpersonal violence and motor vehicle accidents. Other significant causes are falls and sports.

Diagnosis.—Mandibular fractures are frequently associated with other facial and systemic injuries. Following resuscitation and exclusion of

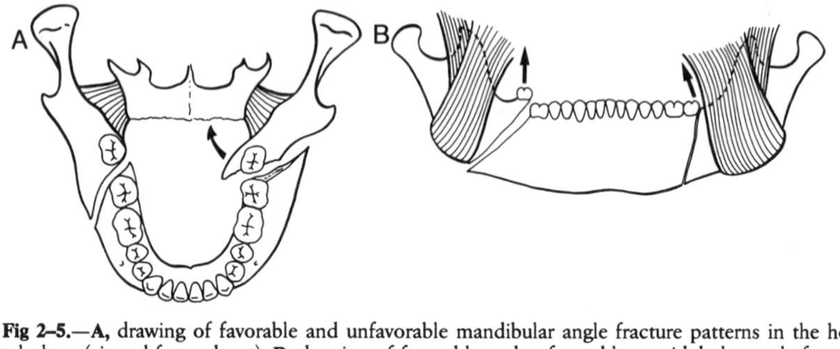

Fig 2–5.—A, drawing of favorable and unfavorable mandibular angle fracture patterns in the horizontal plane (viewed from above). **B,** drawing of favorable and unfavorable manidubular angle fracture patterns in the verticle plane (viewed anteroposteriorly)). (Courtesy of Luyk NH, Ferguson JW: *Am J Emerg Med* 9:352–359, 1991.)

other significant injuries, a detailed examination of the face and jaws should be undertaken. When there is suspicion of a mandibular fracture based on clinical judgement, radiographs consisting of an orthopantomograph, a posteroanterior mandibular view, and a reverse Towne's view of the condylar necks should be obtained. Based on radiographic evaluation, mandibular fractures can be classified as favorable or unfavorable. A favorable fracture occurs when fracture displacement is limited by the disposition of the fracture line; the fracture is unfavorable if otherwise (Fig 2–5).

Management.—Except for the potential for airway obstruction, mandibular fractures are seldom life-threatening and assume a low priority in the initial assessment and management of a severely traumatized patient. Significant bleeding rarely occurs from a ruptured maxillary or inferior alveolar artery. Airway obstruction can occur when tongue support is lost because of bilateral body fracture and fracture of anterior part of the mandible with multiple fractured segments. A pharyngeal airway if often sufficient, but the patient should be intubated if there are other significant injuries. Pain control can be achieved with temporary immobilization of the fragments by passing a bridle wire through the teeth on either side of the fracture site. Tetanus immunization should be evaluated, and antibiotic therapy should be initiated.

▶ Although mandibular fractures are the second most common facial fracture, they are rarely fatal but can cause obstruction of the airway when both rami are fractured. This permits posterior tongue displacement with resultant obstruction. As is the case with head injuries, if shock is present, other causes must be sought.—G.V. Anderson, M.D.

Chest, Cardiac

The Use of Echocardiography in the Emergency Management of Nonpenetrating Traumatic Cardiac Rupture

Schiavone WA, Ghumrawi BK, Catalano DR, Haver DW, Pipitone AJ, et al (Robinson Mem Hosp, Ravenna, Ohio)
Ann Emerg Med 20:1248–1250, 1991 2–26

Background.—The diagnosis of cardiac rupture after blunt trauma may not be immediately apparent because of the absence of the most reliable sign, central venous rupture in the presence of circulatory shock. Echocardiography performed in the emergency department can show pericardial fluid and signs of cardiac tamponade even before increased central venous pressure is clinically evident. Three case reports illustrate situations in which surgical management was facilitated by echocardiography that revealed cardiac tamponade.

Summary of Cases.—Two men aged 35 and 39 years and 1 woman aged 26 years were involved in 3 separate motor vehicle crashes. All sustained blunt, nonpenetrating chest trauma that resulted in right atrial rupture and cardiac tamponade. When they arrived at the emergency department, all patients were hypotensive, and they complained of chest pain. Only 1 patient had jugular venous distension and upper-body cyanosis. All had normal chest radiographs, but 1 had ECG ST elevation. In all 3 patients, echocardiography revealed moderate-sized pericardial effusions and signs of cardiac tamponade. Surgeons attempted emergency thoracotomy and repair of the right atrial rupture in all cases. The 2 men survived the procedures, but the woman died. Both men had uneventful recoveries and left the hospital on days 7 and 12, respectively.

Summary.—The emergency physician should consider cardiac tamponade when a patient is hypotensive and has a history of blunt chest trauma whether or not there are other obvious causes for hypotension. Often the initial chest radiograph and ECG are normal. The patient with multiple trauma can experience hemodynamically significant cardiac tamponade long before the components of Beck's triad—high venous pressure, low arterial pressure, and a small, quiet heart—can be clinically identified. The use of echocardiography in the emergency department can document this process quickly and noninvasively.

▶ As these cases demonstrate, patients with blunt trauma to the chest are candidates for cardiac rupture and tamponade without the classic signs. Echocardiography makes it possible to diagnose the condition at an earlier stage so that definitive surgical treatment is facilitated (see also Abstract 3–32).—G.V. Anderson, M.D.

The Value of SPECT-Thallium Scanning in Screening for Myocardial Contusion

McCarthy MC, Pavlina PM, Evans DK, Broadie TA, Park HM, et al (Wright State Univ, Dayton Ohio; Indiana Univ, Indianapolis)

Cardiovasc Intervent Radiol 14:238–240, 1991 2–27

Background.—Various screening studies are used to detect myocardial contusion in patients who have sustained blunt chest trauma. Single-photon-emission CT (SPECT) can provide early and accurate identification of patients at risk for morbidity resulting from cardiac contusion. The role of SPECT was assessed in a prospective study of 40 patients.

Methods.—Those included in the study had been involved in high-speed motor vehicle accidents and had a high likelihood of myocardial contusion. The group included 28 males and 12 females; their mean age was 38.1 years. All were hemodynamically stable upon admission. In addition to continuous cardiac monitoring and other indicated studies, all underwent SPECT scans within 48 hours of admission.

Results.—Twelve of the 40 patients had evidence of cardiac-related morbidity. Twenty-four of 37 evaluable SPECT-thallium scans were considered abnormal. The sensitivity of SPECT-thallium scanning in predicting myocardial contusion was 55.6%, its specificity was 32.1%, and its overall accuracy was 37.8%. Single-photon-emission CT had a positive predictive value of 20.8% and a negative predictive value of 69.2%. The initial ECG was a superior predictor of patient outcome, however, with a sensitivity of 91.7%, a specificity of 82.1%, and an accuracy of 85%. The positive predictive value of initial ECG was 68.8%, and the negative predictive value was 95.8%.

Conclusion.—The diagnosis of myocardial contusion is difficult in patients who have sustained blunt chest trauma. Single-photon-emission Ct-thallium scanning is not a useful screening tool for this injury. But a normal initial ECG nearly always rules out cardiac complications.

▶ Consideration of myocardial contusion is important in patients sustaining blunt chest trauma.

The SPECT scan is a waste of time and money in patients suspected of having myocardial contusion. The clinical course and ECG remain the best determinants of the condition.—J.E. Clinton, M.D.

Ruptures of the Heart in Seatbelt Wearers

Santavirta S, Arajärvi E (Koskela Hosp; Orthopaedic Hosp of the Invalid Found, Helsinki, Finland)

J Trauma 32:275–279, 1992 2–28

Objective.—There is little question that seat belt use decreases deaths caused by traffic accidents. However, the relationship between seat belt

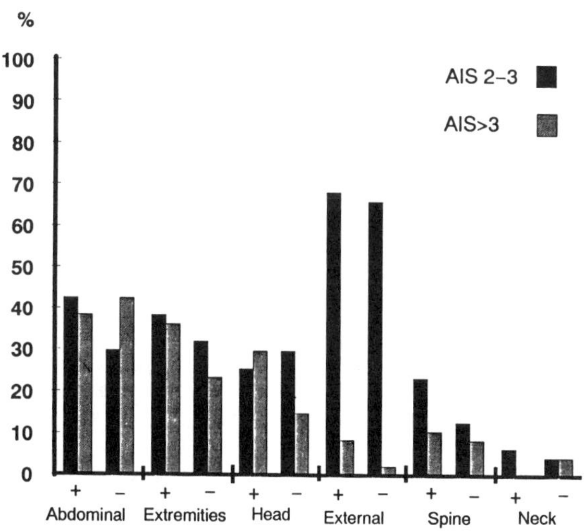

Fig 2–6.—Associated injuries in different body regions in seatbelt wearers (+) and unbelted victims (–) with heart rupture, according to Abbreviated Injury Scale (AIS). (AIS 2–3 = milder injuries; AIS > 3 = severe injuries.) (Courtesy of Santavirta S, Arajärvi E: *J Trauma* 32:275–279, 1992.)

use and rupture of the heart, one of the important causes of such deaths, is unknown. Fatal rupture of the heart in traffic accident victims who were wearing seat belts was studied.

Methods.—The study included 4,169 deaths in 3,468 traffic accidents from 1972 to 1985. Chest injuries were the main cause of death in 1,121 individuals, 207 of whom had been wearing a seat belt. Of these, 75 had rupture of the heart. Complete information on the location and size of the rupture was available for 47 subjects, and these were compared with 47 randomly selected controls with fatal rupture of the heart who had not been wearing a seat belt.

Findings.—Left ventricular rupture was more common in the seat belt wearers, particularly right-front passengers. Some interior part of the car most commonly caused the injury in seat belt wearers, whereas the steering wheel most commonly caused the injury in non–seat belt wearers. Non–seat belt wearers more often had fractures of the left side of the chest and more than 6 rib fractures. In terms of nonthoracic associated injuries, unbelted individuals had only slightly more severe abdominal injuries, most commonly hepatic and splenic rupture (Fig 2–6). According to the Injury Severity Scale, injuries were more severe in victims with rupture of the aorta and in drivers.

Discussion.—In severe traffic accidents, there is a significant incidence of traumatic rupture of the heart, even in seat belt wearers. The mechanism of this injury is usually crushing against the steering wheel, regardless of seat belt use. Almost all patients with fatal heart rupture have multiple injuries. This injury appears to occur only in serious collisions, most often with a heavier vehicle.

► All but 5 of the 75 victims with heart rupture died at the scene of the accident. The 5 immediate survivors all died within 24 hours. One of these made it to the operating room. Emergency ultrasound examination for cardiac tamponade is becoming widely available in our emergency departments, and we should be using it in blunt chest trauma as well as penetrating trauma.—E. Ruiz, M.D.

Recognition, Resuscitation and Management of Patients With Penetrating Cardiac Injuries

Buchman TG, Phillips J, Menker JB (Johns Hopkins Univ, Baltimore, Md)
Surg Gynecol Obstet 174:205–210, 1992 2–29

Background.—Without prompt identification and definitive management, penetrating cardiac injuries are commonly lethal. Diagnosis, resuscitation, and definitive treatment of all patients brought to the emergency department with possible penetrating cardiac wounds must be swift. A retrospective study was done to evaluate clinical performance and identify evolving management strategies.

Methods.—The Adult Trauma Service registry at Johns Hopkins Hospital was searched to identify all victims of penetrating cardiac injury in the 59-month period between 1985 and 1990. Such injury was defined as a perforation of the pericardium associated with a visible wound of the pericardial contents. Twenty-three patients seen with at least 1 sign of life and who subsequently underwent repair of an intrapericardial injury were identified. Their medical records were examined, and their surgeons were interviewed for additional data.

Outcomes.—Twenty-two of the patients survived. Patients with hemodynamically stable presentations and those with unstable presentations did not differ significantly in Injury Severity Score, anatomic complexity, early fluid requirements, or the length of hospital stay. This suggests that the appearance at presentation does not predict injury severity. Rapid volume infusion and prompt drug-assisted endotracheal intubation expedited resuscitation of unstable patients and obviated the need for thoracotomy in the emergency department in 13 of 15 cases.

Conclusions.—In this series, 1 of 3 patients with penetrating cardiac injuries and a sign of life were seen with hemodynamic stability. Patients who were initially stable had injuries as severe as those who were initially unstable. Pressure-driven infusion of warmed fluids can stabilize 85% of those initially unstable and permit transport to the operating room for definitive treatment. Rapid infusion of 2 L of crystalloid into stable patients may serve as a provocative test by increasing central venous pressure to 20 cm water or more in all patients with occult cardiac injuries.

▶ This paper supports what we basically already know, i.e., that early specific diagnosis and aggressive resuscitation will improve survival. Unfortunately, the design is such that it really does not compare patients who survive vs. those who do not survive. Only 1 patient did not survive; therefore, it is difficult to compare what treatment modalities are most effective in resuscitation. This paper, like most retrospective studies, is limited by the data that are available. We have been recording all of our trauma resuscitations on videotape in the emergency department. This provides not only a very useful educational tool but also a very valuable research tool. It is much easier to review tapes retrospectively and collect the necessary data. Videotaping for research purposes is a whole new area that needs to be explored in emergency medicine.—W.H. Spivey, M.D.

"Directed" Emergency Room Thoracotomy: A Prognostic Prerequisite for Survival

Ivatury RR, Kazigo J, Rohman M, Gaudino J, Simon R, Stahl WM (New York Med College, Bronx, NY)

J Trauma 31:1076–1081, 1991 2–30

Background.—Physicians continue to debate the value of resuscitative thoracotomy in the emergency room. A recent study of emergency room thoracotomy (ERT) was evaluated to define appropriate patient selection.

Methods.—The outcomes of 163 patients undergoing ERT were examined. Forty-nine had stab wounds, 85 had gunshot wounds, and 29 had blunt trauma. Four patients had Revised Trauma Scores (RTSs) exceeding 8, 21 had RTSs from 4 to 8, and 138 had RTSs from 0 to 3.

Outcomes.—None of the blunt trauma victims survived. Twelve stab wound victims and 4 gunshot victims were eventually discharged for an overall survival rate of 9.8%. Eight survivors had no vital signs when they arrived in the emergency department, and 1 had signs of life only at the scene. The best survival rate was achieved in patients with thoracic penetration in whom ERT was directed at potential cardiac injury. Fifty-six of these 84 patients had cardiac wounds with tamponade; 21.4% of this subgroup survived. Two of the remaining 28 patients survived, both of whom had pulmonary injuries. When ERT was nondirected, the survival rate was significantly lower.

Conclusions.—In patients with no vital signs, ERT directed at potential cardiac injury based on thoracic penetration has an important impact on survival. However, ERT in blunt trauma victims appears ineffective, and its role in the treatment of patients with penetrating abdominal injuries has yet to be established.

▶ This represents one more example underscoring the futility of emergency room (sic) thoracotomy (see also Abstracts 2–31 and 2–32). As such, it adds weight to guidelines calling for no thoracotomy during the resuscitation of blunt trauma victims who arrive without vital signs.

On a lighter note, won't it be nice when our friends, the operating room doctors, become politically correct and refer to the emergency room as the emergency *department*? When will they "get it"?—E.H. Taliaferro, M.D.

Reappraisal of Emergency Room Thoracotomy in a Changing Environment

Esposito TJ, Jurkovich GJ, Rice CL, Maier RV, Copass MK, et al (Univ of Washington, Seattle)

J Trauma 31:881–887, 1991 2–31

Background.—Authors have questioned the benefit of resuscitative emergency room thoracotomy (ERT), especially in victims of blunt trauma. The wide use of this technique may not be cost-effective, and the risk of exposure and lethal infection to medical personnel during ERT is great. The policy of performing ERT on all moribund patients with penetrating torso injuries and all those with blunt injuries with any evidence of cardiac electric activity was assessed to determine whether such a liberal policy is justified.

Methods.—The charts of all patients who underwent ERT in a 4-year period were analyzed. Of the 112 patients who underwent ERT, 24 had penetrating injuries, and 88 had blunt injuries.

Outcomes.—The overall survival rate was 1.8%. Patients with penetrating injuries had a 4.2% survival rate, and those with blunt injuries had a 1.1% survival rate. None of the patients in whom CPR was started at the scene and required throughout transport survived. Patients with blood pressure and spontaneous respirations in the field had a survival rate of 11.8%. Patients with sinus rhythm or ventricular fibrillation on arrival at the emergency department had a 6.4% survival rate. There were no survivors among the patients coming to the hospital with an idioventricular rhythm or asystole. Total hospital charges for patients having ERT were $59,565 more than reimbursement. Human immunodeficiency virus and hepatitis screening could be documented in only 2 patients, both of whom were negative.

Conclusions.—This liberal policy for performing ERT had dismal results: monetary losses were incurred and the risk of exposure to lethal infection was increased in hospital personnel. Emergency room thoracotomy is warranted only when vital signs or a resuscitatible cardiac rhythm exists in the field or emergency department and deteriorates shortly before the procedure. Such a policy would maximize survival while reducing inappropriate expenditures and risks.

▶ While the success rate for emergency department thoracotomy (EDT) remains low, the attendant risks to the health care worker continue to rise. Human immunodeficiency virus seropositivity has been reported to be as high as 24% in selected populations of trauma patients. In addition, as if this were not risk enough, a recent study from Michael Reese Hospital (1) revealed 20% seropositivity for hepatitis B in a group of trauma patients. Significantly more health care workers die of hepatitis (200 to 300 annually) than of HIV disease acquired from occupational exposures. It is of interest to note that no reports of needlesticks or cutaneous exposures were documented over the 4-year study period in this report. A clinical review at Jackson Memorial Hospital revealed only 16% compliance with universal precautions among housestaff (even with patients strongly suspected of being at high risk for HIV infections!) (2). These data support my theory that there are numerous exposures that remain unreported, thus increasing the risk to health care personnel even more than this study suggests. In view of these risks, EDTs should be limited to those patients who statistically have a chance for meaningful recovery. Employing the procedure as a teaching tool in cases when chances of patient recovery are nil places the health care worker at unnecessary and dangerous risk of contracting a deadly disease.—H.D. Unger, M.D.

References

1. Hammond JS, et al: *J Trauma* 30:555, 1990.

2. Levine EA, et al: *Am Surg* 57:385, 1991.

Resuscitative Thoracotomy Performed in the Operating Room

Jurkovich GJ, Esposito TJ, Maier RV (Univ of Washington, Seattle)
Am J Surg 163:463–468, 1992 2–32

Background.—Investigators have questioned the effectiveness of resuscitative thoracotomy in trauma victims. Survival rates vary, with some being quite low. Patients initially having signs of life who can be transported directly to the operating room before the need for resuscitative thoracotomy may be expected to have higher survival rates.

Methods.—The clinical course of all injured patients undergoing urgent or exigent thoracotomy in the operating room from 1983 to 1989 was studied. Thirty-four patients underwent exigent/resuscitative thoracotomy. Eight had penetrating injuries, 25 had blunt trauma to multiple systems, and 1 had isolated blunt chest trauma. There were 8 median sternotomies and 26 left or bilateral thoractomies. Concurrent exploratory celiotomy was done in 26 patients.

Findings.—Three patients survived for an overall survival rate of 9%. Patients with penetrating injuries had a survival rate of 37.5%. None of the 26 patients with blunt trauma survived. Seventy-four percent of the 54 patients undergoing urgent nonresuscitative thoracotomy survived. Combined group survival rates were 49% overall, 77% for those with penetrating injuries and 22% for those with blunt injuries (table).

Conclusions.—Resuscitative thoracotomy in patients with blunt trauma who have deteriorated to the point of being in extremis is futile. The salvage rates among patients with penetrating injuries were relatively high in this series, thus supporting the continued use of resuscitative tho-

Survival Rates for Exigent/Resuscitative Thoracotomy and Urgent/Nonresuscitative Thoracotomy Performed in the Operating Room and Emergency Department

Indications and Location	Total No. of Patients	No. of Patients Surviving (%)
Total, operating room	88	43 (49)
Operating room exigent/resuscitative thoracotomy	34	3 (9)
Operating room urgent/nonresuscitative thoracotomy	54	40 (74)
Emergency department resuscitative thoracotomy*	112	2 (1.8)
Total	200	45 (22.5)

(Courtesy of Jurkovich GJ, Esposito TJ, Maier RV: *Am J Surg* 163:463–468, 1992.)

racotomy when vital signs are lost, especially if the injury is to the thorax. Variability in previously reported survival rates may be the result of a mix of patients with blunt trauma and penetrating injuries and of disagreement about what constitutes a resuscitative thoracotomy.

▶ There are logical reasons for better survival rates in operating room (OR) thoracotomies than in emergency department thoracotomies. The main reason is supported in this study: the Injury Severity Score was lower (29 vs 47) in the group that underwent OR thoracotomy. Plain and simple, these patients were less severely injured (and more stable) and could tolerate transfer to the OR for definitive surgical care.

Key concepts on this topic of resuscitative thoracotomy are touched upon in this paper. First, victims of blunt trauma who undergo thoracotomy *anywhere* do not do well *anywhere* (1). Second, patients with thoracic stab wounds do better than those with thoracic gunshot wounds. Third, patients with isolated chest injuries do better than those with concomitant chest and abdominal injuries. Finally, in victims of penetrating thoracic trauma, a resuscitative thoracotomy should be done in the emergency center whenever the patient is too unstable to be transported to the OR. The procedure should be done by emergency physicians or trauma surgeons, whoever is right there and ready to perform the procedure at the time it is acutely needed.—J.J. Kelly, D.O., F.A.C.E.P.

Reference

1. Esposito TJ, et al: *J Trauma* 32:881, 1991.

Antibiotic Prophylaxis in Penetrating Injuries of the Chest

Demetriades D, Breckon V, Breckon C, Kakoyiannis S, Psaras G, et al (Baragwanath Hosp, Univ of the Witwatersrand, South Africa)

Ann R Coll Surg Engl 73:348–351, 1991 2–33

Background.—About 85% of patients with penetrating chest injuries can be safely managed by placement of a thoracostomy tube. The value of routine antibiotic prophylaxis in these patients is unclear. Most prospective studies recommend antibiotic prophylaxis while the tube is in place or longer. However, very few randomized studies have been done. A randomized study was performed to compare single-dose prophylaxis with long-term prophylaxis for as long as the drain was in place in patients with penetrating injuries of the chest.

Methods.—One hundred eighty-eight patients with chest injuries requiring a chest drain were enrolled in the 10-month study. Ninety-five received a single dose of ampicillin before the chest tube was inserted, and 93 were given additional antibiotic prophylaxis for as long as the drain was in place.

Findings.—The overall incidence of intrathoracic sepsis—pneumonia and empyema—was 3.2%. The single-dose group had an incidence of 3.1%, and the long-term group had an incidence of 3.2%. Minor sepsis at the thoracostomy tube site occurred in 7.4% and 5.4%, respectively. A residual hemothorax after tube removal was seen in 7.4% in the single-dose group and in 9.7% in the long-term group. The length of hospital stay was increased by the development of intrathoracic sepsis. The overall incidence of sepsis in patients with bullet injuries was 7.1% as compared with 9.2% in patients with knife wounds.

Conclusions.—Single-dose prophylaxis is as effective as prolonged prophylaxis in patients with penetrating chest injuries. Chest physiotherapy immediately after drain insertion is important, as is early removal of the drain.

▶ Patients were randomly assigned to the single-dose or prolonged-coverage groups. The study yields good information and will influence my practice, but ampicillin may not be the antibiotic of choice everywhere.—E. Ruiz, M.D.

Abdominal

Computed Tomography and Diagnostic Peritoneal Lavage: Complementary Roles in Blunt Trauma

Meredith JW, Ditesheim JA, Stonehouse S, Wolfman N (Wake Forest Univ, Winston-Salem, NC)

Am Surg 58:44–48, 1992 2–34

Background.—Authors disagree on the use of CT and diagnostic peritoneal lavage (DPL) in assessing stable patients with blunt abdominal trauma. A study was done to further clarify their independent and combined value.

Methods.—One hundred sixteen patients were enrolled in the prospective study. All were adults satisfying the entry criteria of major blunt torso trauma, hemodynamic stability, equivocal and unreliable abdominal examination, and the absence of prior abdominal surgery and unstable pelvic fractures. The patients were admitted during an 11-month period and underwent CT scanning with a 9800 series GE scanner. The surgeon then examined the results with a CT radiologist and determined whether laparotomy was needed. Patients then underwent DPL. Recommendations for laparotomy after this procedure were based on finding gross blood on the initial aspiration, $>100{,}000$ RBC/mm^3, >500 WBC/mm^3, or the presence of bile or food fibers. A final decision was made on the basis of data from both studies.

Findings.—Twenty-two patients underwent initial laparotomy; yet only 17 had injuries needing repair. Unnecessary laparotomy resulted from DPL findings in 15.5% of the patients as compared with .8% from CT findings. Inappropriate observation was recommended because of DPL findings in 1.7% of the patients and because of CT in 6.9%. Computed tomography failed to identify 5 bowel injuries. Half of the patients with positive DPL findings did not need surgery.

Conclusions.—These findings underscore the complimentary nature of CT and DPL. These modalities are not equivalent tests or substitutes for one another. Further research should focus not on establishing the superiority of 1 test over the other, but on identifying which patients need which tests.

▶ The methods of this study were not well described, but it appears that the physicians first obtained a CT scan and decided whether or not to take a patient to surgery. Patients then had DPL, and the findings were prepared. I question the ethics of performing DPL of the patient's indication for surgery has already been established. Nevertheless, this study does again demonstrate the value of good diagnostic imaging. Other studies have demonstrated that DPL is more effective at diagnosing intra-abdominal pathology than CT scanning is. I suspect that most of these studies report findings that are more of a reflection of the ability of radiologists to interpret the CT scans correctly. As CT scans are improved, no doubt CT scanning will become the best means for diagnosing intra-abdominal pathology.—W.H. Spivey, M.D.

A Prospective, Randomized Comparison of Computed Tomography With Conventional Diagnostic Methods in the Evaluation of Penetrating Injuries to the Back and Flank

Easter DW, Shackford SR, Mattrey RF (Univ of California, San Diego; Univ of Vermont, Burlington)

Arch Surg 126:1115–1119, 1991 2–35

Introduction.—Penetrating injuries to the back and flank remain difficult to assess and manage, but recent reports suggest that CT is an accurate means of evaluating such injuries.

Study Design.—Computed tomography was compared with conventional diagnostic methods in a prospective series of 85 patients at least 18 years old who had penetrating injuries to the back or the posterior aspect of the abdomen. Twenty-four patients underwent immediate laparotomy and were not randomized. Thirty-one of the remaining patients had CT assessment using intragastric contrast medium, while 30 patients were conventionally evaluated.

Outcome.—Nine of the 24 immediate operations proved to be unnecessary. Hospital costs were significantly higher for these patients than for those in either randomized group. In the randomized group there were 3 true-positive and 3 false-positive findings. Both CT assessment and conventional evaluation proved to be highly accurate and specific in patients whose injuries necessitated surgery (table). It took longer to make a hos-

Accuracy of Evaluation Methods*

Result	Immediate Operation*	CT Evaluation	Conventional Evaluation
True-positive	15	2	1
False-positive	9	1	2
True-negative	58 †	28	27
False-negative	3 †	0	0
Total	**85**	**31**	**30**
Predictive value, %			
Positive	65	67	33
Negative	95	97	100
Sensitivity, %	83	97	100
Specificity, %	86	96	93
Accuracy, %	86	97	93

* CT = computed tomographic. Values are number of patients.
† By design, those with "negative" immediate assessment findings were randomized into conventional or CT evaluation.
(Courtesy of Easter DW, Shackford SR, Mattrey RF: *Arch Surg* 126:1115–1119, 1991.)

pital disposition in the CT group, but these patients required fewer diagnostic tests.

Conclusions.—When severe visceral injury is present in a patient with a penetrating injury of the back or flank, it probably will be recognized by either conventional assessment or CT examination. In this study after either CT assessment or conventional evaluation, patients whose findings were normal could have been safely discharged.

▶ Stab wounds to the back and flank remain problematic. Most wounds will miss the colon, renal hilum, and other vital areas. However, delayed recognition of injury to these structures can be disastrous. The authors have shown good reason to take those patients with significant physical findings directly to laparotomy. The increased hospital cost seen with the immediate-laparotomy group was due to the patients' underlying injuries and not the mode of evaluation or therapy.

"Conventional diagnostic methods" in this study refers to workup without CT assessment and includes serial clinical evaluation and selective use of diagnostic peritoneal lavage, urography, cystography, and angiography. The study size is too small to choose between CT assessment or "conventional diagnostic methods" in patients without immediate indications for surgery.

Hence, both approaches seem appropriate at this time for patients without evisceration, a high-velocity missile wound, hemodynamic instability, or signs of peritonitis.—J.R. Hedges, M.D.

Contributions of Peritoneal Lavage Enzyme Determinations to the Management of Isolated Hollow Visceral Abdominal Injuries

McAnena OJ, Marx JA, Moore EE (Denver Gen Hosp; Univ of Colorado Health Sciences Ctr, Denver)

Ann Emerg Med 20:834–837, 1991 2–36

Background.—Counting cells in diagnostic peritoneal lavage (DPL) specimens has improved the sensitivity of the test, but early identification of isolated hollow viscus injury remains a problem. Injured viscera may bleed minimally, and at least 3 hours may elapse before peritoneal inflammation is evident.

Objective.—Markers in DPL effluent that could make it easier to identify injuries to hollow viscera at an early stage were sought in 51 patients with injury limited to one or more hollow visceral structures. Levels of amylase (LAM) and alkaline phosphatase (LAP) in lavage fluid were estimated.

Findings.—Twenty-eight patients had positive DPL findings based on the RBC or WBC count in lavage fluid. Among the 23 patients with conventionally negative lavage findings, all 11 with isolated small-bowel injury had an LAM of 20 IU/L or higher, and 6 of those patients had an LAP of 3 IU/L or higher. All 6 patients with colon injury and 2 with gallbladder injury had an LAM below 20 IU/L and an LAP below 3 IU/L. A patient with a stomach injury had an increased LAP but a normal LAM.

Conclusion.—The finding of increased amylase or alkaline phosphatase in DPL fluid is an accurate predictor of isolated small-bowel injury at a stage when cellular markers of injury are not helpful.

▶ DPL has made a significant impact on the triage and management of blunt and penetrating (nonmissile) abdominal trauma. Depending on the clinical scenario, availability of CT scanning, level of expertise of the radiologist reviewing the CT, and level of experience of the trauma surgeon, DPL still plays a significant role. Interpreting the values of the DPL is the key to improving the sensitivity of this test; however, a major limitation remains early identification of isolated hollow viscus injury (1). The authors nicely (albeit retrospectively) highlight the usefulness of LAM and LAP levels in patients with isolated small-bowel injuries. Interestingly, these lavage enzymes were not helpful in the detection of colonic injuries.—J.J. Kelly, D.O., F.A.C.E.P.

Reference

1. Fischer RD, et al: *Am J Surg* 136:701, 1978.

Evaluation of Diagnostic Peritoneal Lavage in Suspected Penetrating Abdominal Stab Wounds Using a Dipstick Technique

Muckart DJJ, McDonald MA (Univ of Natal, Durban, South Africa)

Br J Surg 78:696–698, 1991 2–37

Background.—The value of diagnostic peritoneal lavage for investigating patients with blunt abdominal trauma is well documented, but its reliability for diagnosing penetrating abdominal trauma is less well established. Furthermore, the diagnostic parameters for this indication are not as clearly defined. The efficacy of measuring the albumin content to estimate the WBC count in lavage effluent by using a dipstick technique for identification of intra-abdominal injury in patients with abdominal stab wounds was investigated.

Patients.—During a 6-month period, 157 patients who sustained stab wounds to the abdomen were divided into 3 groups on the basis of the findings at physical examination. Sixty-six patients underwent immediate laparotomy, and 41 patients underwent observation and repeat examination. The remaining 50 patients had equivocal findings at physical examination because an intra-abdominal injury could not be confirmed or excluded. The latter group consisted of 46 men and 4 women aged 16 to 35 years with a mean age of 23.6 years. Diagnostic peritoneal lavage using the closed guidewire technique was performed in those 50 patients, and the lavage effluent was tested with a urine dipstick. Lavage fluid was considered positive if the protein concentration was l g/L or higher and WBC count was greater than 500 cells/mm^3 as indicated by color changes on the dipstick. Patients with positive lavage findings by those criteria underwent laparotomy, whereas those with negative lavage results underwent observation and repeat physical examination. The results in 46 patients were assessable.

Results.—The lavage effluent was positive in 26 patients, negative in 18 patients, and equivocal in 2 patients. Twenty-three of the 26 patients with positive lavage findings had significant injuries confirmed at laparotomy. Seventeen of the 18 patients with negative lavage results were managed successfully without laparotomy. One patient died of complications attributable to central venous catheterization. Of the 2 patients with equivocal lavage results, one underwent laparotomy, which was negative, and the other recovered uneventfully. The dipstick technique had an overall sensitivity of 100%, a specificity of 86%, a positive predictive value of 88%, and a negative predictive value of 100%.

Conclusions.—Using a urinary dipstick to evaluate peritoneal lavage fluid obtained from patients with stab wounds to the abdomen is an accurate, inexpensive, and rapid means for identifying penetrating intra-abdominal injury.

► Diagnostic peritoneal lavage, in the face of blunt abdominal trauma, has had a high degree of both sensitivity and specificity since its introduction in

1965 by Harlan Root. Its reliability in the face of penetrating trauma has been somewhat more dicey. This is particularly true when injuries are isolated to the diaphragm or in penetration of the small bowel. In such situations, evaluation of the WBC count, protein content, and fiber fragments have been recommended. The authors suggest that a simple and consistent way to evaluate protein and WBC counts resides in the omnipresent urine dipstick. Their results are impressive and appear worthy of serious consideration.—D.K. Wagner, M.D.

Peritoneal Lavage Enzyme Determinations Following Blunt and Penetrating Abdominal Trauma

McAnena OJ, Marx JA, Moore EE (Denver Gen Hosp; Univ of Colorado Health Sciences Ctr, Denver)

J Trauma 31:1161–1164, 1991 2–38

Introduction.—Diagnostic peritoneal lavage is limited in its ability to identify isolated injury to a hollow viscus at an early stage. These structures tend not to bleed much, and at least 3 hours are needed to provoke an inflammatory peritoneal reaction.

Objective and Methods.—The value of estimating lavage amylase (LAM) and lavage alkaline phosphatase (LAP) was examined in a series of 1,969 diagnostic peritoneal lavage studies carried out in injured patients in a 4-year period. Lavage amylase was determined in 96% of studies, and LAP in 88%. The series included 1,536 patients with blunt injury and 433 with penetrating trauma.

Findings.—Sixty-seven patients (3.6%) had negative lavage findings when RBCs were counted but an LAM of 10 IU/L or higher. Fifty-five of those patients had blunt injuries. The mean LAM was 122 IU/L. Thirteen of the 67 patients had an LAP of 3 IU/L or above; 7 of them had significant intra-abdominal injuries. Ten of 13 patients with an LAM of at least 20 IU/L and an LAP of at least 3 IU/L had small-bowel injuries, and the other 3 had pancreaticonduodenal injuries.

Recommendations.—It makes sense to estimate enzyme levels in lavage fluid. An LAM of 20 IU/L or above and an LAP of at least 3 IU/L call for laparotomy if the history is consistent with small-bowel injury. An increase in either enzyme warrants close observation.

▶ See also Abstract 2–37.—J. Wasserberger, M.D.

Diagnostic Peritoneal Lavage: Integration With Clinical Information to Improve Diagnostic Performance

Day AC, Rankin N, Charlesworth P (Middlemore Hosp, Otahuhu, Auckland, New Zealand)

J Trauma 32:52–57, 1992 2–39

Background.—To manage abdominal trauma, physicians must be able to detect the injuries and distinguish patients needing surgery from those who do not. A prospective study was performed to see whether the diagnostic value of diagnostic peritoneal lavage (DPL) after blunt trauma could be enhanced by combining the DPL results with clinical assessment to establish the need for laparotomy.

Methods.—Two hundred patients receiving DPL after blunt trauma were studied prospectively. Relationships among the DPL results, clinical features seen during initial patient evaluation, and laparotomy outcome were determined.

Findings.—The results of DPL alone predicted the need for laparotomy with an accuracy of 93%, a specificity of 96%, a sensitivity of 85%, a positive predictive value of 87%, and a negative predictive value of 95%. Combining clinical features with DPL results increased the positive predictive value and specificity, reduced the number of unnecessary laparotomies performed, but decreased the negative predictive value and sensitivity, thereby increasing the number of needed laparotomies missed. The best diagnostic performance was achieved by combining DPL findings with circulatory status. In this series, the combination predicted necessary laparotomy with an accuracy of 95%, a specificity of 99%, a sensitivity of 81%, and a positive and negative predictive value of 98% and 94%, respectively.

Conclusions.—Diagnostic peritoneal lavage provides rapid, useful information for guiding the decision to perform laparotomy not only in patients with hemodynamic instability despite resuscitation but also in those who have temporary hypotension in the hospital. However, no single investigation can completely differentiate patients needing surgery from those who do not. Clinical decision making is still needed and should consider information obtained by clinical assessment and the results of specialized investigations.

▶ Until the 100% foolproof test comes along, clinical decision making will still be the cornerstone of practice. In this study, interestingly enough, the combination of DPL results and hemodynamic status (defined as a systolic blood pressure of < 100) was the best predictor of necessary laparotomy.

Once again, we see how much and mighty is the information gained from the simple and repetitive measurements of blood pressure, pulse, respiration, and temperature. Apparently, they are called *vital* signs for a reason.—E.H. Taliaferro, M.D.

Unreliability of Standard Quantitative Criteria in Diagnostic Peritoneal Lavage Performed for Suspected Penetrating Abdominal Stab Wounds

Muckart DJJ, McDonald MA (Univ of Natal, Republic of South Africa)

Am J Surg 162:223–227, 1991 2–40

Background.—Diagnostic peritoneal lavage (DPL) is the preferred investigation in patients with equivocal findings in blunt abdominal trauma, and it is also becoming popular in patients with penetrating trauma. However, the standard criteria for blunt abdominal trauma are not reliable for penetrating trauma, particularly in regard to the cell count that should be used to indicate a positive lavage. A prospective study was conducted to determine the role of cell counting in DPL performed for suspected penetrating abdominal stab wounds in patients with equivocal clinical findings.

Methods.—Diagnostic peritoneal lavage was performed before laparotomy on 35 patients with abdominal stab wounds and equivocal clinical findings on 2 separate occasions. Operative findings were compared with the RBC and WBC counts in the lavage effluent. Thirty-two patients were male.

Results.—Twenty-six laparotomies were positive, and 9 were unnecessary. Four of the latter were negative, and 5 were nontherapeutic. Standard quantitative criteria for RBCs in DPL failed to identify significant injury in 8 patients. The standard WBC count missed 6 injuries. Use of both still missed 3 injuries. With the RBC count alone, there were 2 false-positive findings; with the WBC count alone, there were 4 false-positive results. Combined, there were false-positive results in 4 patients.

Conclusions.—The standard quantitative criteria for DPL are superior to clinical evaluation in patients with equivocal findings, but their use in penetrating trauma does not achieve comparable diagnostic accuracy with that in blunt abdominal trauma. The use of standard cell counts in isolation is even less reliable than their combined usage. Because of the much wider range of penetrating injuries and varying degrees of hemorrhage and peritoneal soiling, it is unlikely that any 1 set of standard criteria could be developed for cell counts in DPL performed for penetrating trauma.

▶ Computed tomography scans are the preferred, initial investigation of stable abdominal trauma and not DPL as stated in this article. The results on this study indicate part of the reason why.

With the new ultrafast CT scans, the time factor in doing either investigation is brought down to less than 1 minute, so in actual practice, DPL is rarely performed any more (see Abstract 2–37).—G.J. Ordog, M.D.

Randomized, Prospective Comparison of Open and Closed Peritoneal Lavage for Abdominal Trauma

Troop B, Fabian T, Alsup B, Kudsk K (Univ of Tennessee, Memphis)
Ann Emerg Med 20:1290–1292, 1991 2–41

Introduction.—Blunt abdominal trauma can lead to intra-abdominal bleeding, a diagnosis often made by the procedure of peritoneal lavage. This comparative study investigated the diagnostic results made by using either closed or open peritoneal lavage in individuals who had experienced acute blunt abdominal trauma.

Methods.—Study subjects were selected from patients attending the trauma center who appeared to be candidates for peritoneal lavage. The 2 trauma teams assessing these patients were composed of residents in surgery with 1 to 5 years of training. The lavage procedure received a positive rating if more than 10 mL of blood was removed or if the RBC count netted greater than 100,000 μL^{-1}. Catheter insertion time and fluid removal were also recorded.

Results.—A total of 220 patients with an average age of 31 years entered the study during the 8-month study period. Nineteen patients had positive peritoneal lavage findings in the open procedure group, and 18 had positive results in the closed group. Lavage volume was 538 mL for the open group and 574 mL for the closed group. Catheter insertion times differed significantly between groups, with the open procedure group requiring 6.9 minutes and the closed group requiring 3.6 minutes. One false-positive result occurred in the closed peritoneal lavage group. One patient in the closed lavage group experienced a urinary bladder perforation that responded quickly to treatment. The closed lavage procedure cost about $27 less per patient than did the open lavage procedure. Most of the peritoneal lavage procedures were performed by a third-year resident.

Conclusions.—The open peritoneal lavage procedure posed greater technical difficulties than did the closed procedure. The closed peritoneal procedure has the advantages of requiring less time for insertion of the catheter, being easier to perform, and having lower expense. The safety record was demonstrably similar for both procedures because the complication rates were approximately the same.

▶ In this study, closed lavage differed from open lavage in only the time required to perform the procedure. The importance of a $27 cost savings is arguable. It would seem that the best lavage technique is the one with which the trauma team is most familiar. In addition, the role of peritoneal lavage in the management of blunt abdominal trauma appears to be declining with the increasing use of abdominal CT scanning. The reader is reminded that the closed technique should not be used in patients with prior abdominal surgery (particularly a pelvic procedure) or in a pregnant trauma victim.—J.T. Niemann, M.D.

Autotransfusion of Potentially Culture-Positive Blood (CPB) in Abdominal Trauma: Preliminary Data From a Prospective Study

Ozmen V, McSwain NE Jr, Nichols RL, Smith J, Flint LM (Tulane Univ, New Orleans, La)

J Trauma 32:36–39, 1992 2–42

Background.—The increased use of autotransfusion for trauma-induced bleeding may decrease the amounts of banked blood needed for severe injuries. Although autotransfusion is standard for traumatic hemothorax, its use has been limited in patients with abdominal injuries. A prospective study was done on autotransfusion of potentially culture-positive blood (CPB) in patients with abdominal injuries.

Methods.—Microbiologic data on 152 patients with intestinal trauma were used. When blood loss was anticipated to be greater than 1,000 mL, blood from the peritoneal cavity was cultured, washed, concentrated, and recultured for reinfusion. The Penetrating Abdominal Trauma Index (PATI) was used to stratify infection rates. Fifty patients with PATI values exceeding 20 who received a mean of 1,800 mL of banked blood were compared with 20 patients who received a mean of 3,900 mL of autotransfused, potentially CPB.

Outcomes.—Wound infection occurred in 25% of patients in both groups. When the severity of injury was stratified according to PATI, there were no significant increases in site-specific infection risk. Bacteria cultured from autotransfused blood did not cause bacteremias, pulmonary infections, or urinary infections.

Conclusions.—Autotransfusion of blood aspirated from the peritoneal cavity is feasible and can reduce the need for banked blood in trauma victims. Blood washing removes bacteria from most of the units. Infusion of CPB does not increase the risk of subsequent infection in seriously injured patients. Further research is needed to assess the use of this technique in a larger group of patients.

▶ This technique shows great promise for the resuscitation of seriously injured trauma patients suffering from massive hemorrhage. The authors conclude that further research is needed to assess the use of this technique in a larger group of patients. Such research will, we hope, validate the feasibility and safety of this procedure for trauma victims and will also address the possibility of harvesting HIV, hepatitis-negative blood for blood bank use when the blood is not utilized by the patient.—E.H. Taliaferro, M.D.

Base Deficit as an Indicator of Significant Abdominal Injury

Davis JW, Mackersie RC, Holbrook TL, Hoyt DB (Univ of California, San Diego)

Ann Emerg Med 20:842–844, 1991 2–43

Introduction.—Intra-abdominal injury (AI) after blunt trauma is not always evident on physical examination, and patients with suspected AI often undergo unnecessary diagnostic peritoneal lavage or CT for confirmation. Thus there is a need for more specific indicators of AI to help physicians decide which patients should undergo diagnostic peritoneal lavage or CT. Intra-abdominal injury is often associated with hemorrhage and therefore with an increased serum lactate and arterial base deficit (BD). Whether BD is a reliable indicator of AI was determined in a review of the records of 3,011 patients admitted because of blunt trauma during a 3½-year period.

Methods.—The BD was calculated from admission femoral arterial blood gas values determined by using the Sigaard-Anderson nomogram. Four other indicators of injury, specifically, chest injury, pelvic fracture, hypotension in the field, and admission hypotension, were included in the analysis.

Results.—Significant AI was present in 240 (7.9%) patients. A normal BD of −2 or less was present in 1,901 patients, a mild BD of −3 to −5 was present in 838 patients, a moderate BD of −6 to −14 was present in 227 patients, and a severe BD of −15 or greater was present in 45 patients. Field hypotension was present in 773 patients (25.7%) and admission hypotension in 288 patients (9.6%). Chest injuries occurred in 567 patients (18.8%) and pelvic injuries in 314 patients (10.4%). No indicators of AI were present in 1,647 patients. The case-control analysis for the association of BD category with AI showed that a BD of −6 or less was the single most important indicator of AI and that the odds ratio for AI increased with each category of increasing severity of BD. Admission hypotension, major chest injury, pelvic fracture, and field hypotension were also significantly associated with AI. However, hypotension was not as good a predictor of AI as was a BD of −6 or less.

Conclusion.—Arterial BD is a powerful indicator of AI. Although a normal BD does not exclude AI, the presence of a BD of −6 or less in a patient who has suffered blunt trauma should be considered a strong indication for performing diagnostic peritoneal lavage or CT.

► An unexplained BD, or metabolic acidosis, in a trauma patient means persistent lactic acid production and therefore persistent shock. This usually correlates with persistent hypotension and tachycardia, although occasionally hemodynamic compensatory mechanisms may raise the blood pressure to the normal range while shock at the cellular level persists. With unexplained hypotension, the patient clearly requires diagnostic peritoneal lavage or CT scan of the abdomen. If these tests are negative, a blood gas study may be useful to determine whether this "low" blood pressure is, in fact, "normal" for the patient or whether the patient's body is perceiving an inadequate cardiac output as minifested by lactic acidosis. Similarly, in patients who are not doing well despite a "normal" blood pressure, an arterial blood gas value indicating metabolic acidosis may lead the physician to further investigation of the abdomen.—W.P. Burdick, M.D.

Diagnosis of Pelvic Fractures in Patients With Acute Pelvic Trauma: Efficacy of Plain Radiographs

Resnik CS, Stackhouse DJ, Shanmuganathan K, Young JWR (Univ of Maryland, Baltimore)

AJR 158:109–112, 1992 2–44

Background.—Computed tomography has been a valuable addition to the evaluation of acute pelvic trauma. However, in serious injuries, surgeons may rely heavily on plain films in deciding whether immediate external fixation is necessary. The efficacy of plain radiographs in detecting pelvic fractures and dislocations was investigated with CT used as the gold standard.

Methods.—The radiographs and CT scans of 50 patients with acute pelvic injuries were reviewed independently in a blinded fashion. An anteroposterior radiograph and CT scan were obtained for all patients within 24 hours of admission. Most patients had other radiographic studies as well.

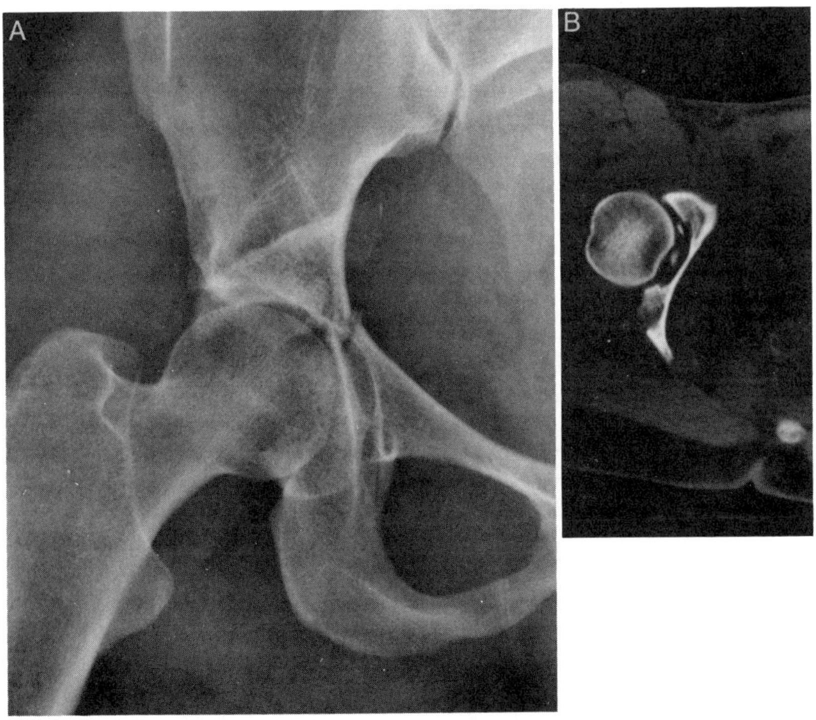

Fig 2–7.—Misdiagnosed intra-articular fragment. **A,** radiograph shows fracture of the right acetabulum, but intra-articular fragments are not visible. **B,** CT scan shows fracture of posterior aspect of right acetabulum with 2 intra-articular bone fragments. (Courtesy of Resnik CS, Stackhouse DJ, Shanmuganathan K, et al: *AJR* 158:109–112, 1992.)

Findings.—There were a total of 162 fractures and dislocations, only 9% of which were misdiagnosed on plain films (Fig 2–7). In none of these subtle injuries was the patient's management altered by the misdiagnosis. Eighty percent of intra-articular fractures were not noted on plain films.

Conclusions.—Almost all clinically important pelvic fractures and dislocations can be adequately detected by plain radiography. After the patient's condition is stabilized, CT can be used to detect fractures within the joint. These findings disagree with the high rates of misdiagnosis reported in previous studies.

▶ I, too, have seen subtle fractures of the acetabulum visible only on CT, but this study reassures me that plain films are still adequate for secondary assessment of the multiple-trauma patient.—T. Stair, M.D.

Penetrating Injury to the Gluteal Region

Gilroy D, Saadia R, Hide G, Demetriades D (Univ of Witwatersrand, Johannesburg, Republic of South Africa)

J Trauma 32:294–297, 1992 2–45

Background.—Most reports of traumatic damage to the gluteal or internal pudendal arteries have concentrated on the late presentation of posttraumatic false aneurysms. However, the same problems can apply to injuries seen acutely, in which case damage to the pelvic and abdominal viscera or vessels can also occur. Eight patients had lesions of the gluteal or internal pudendal arteries after relatively minor penetrating trauma.

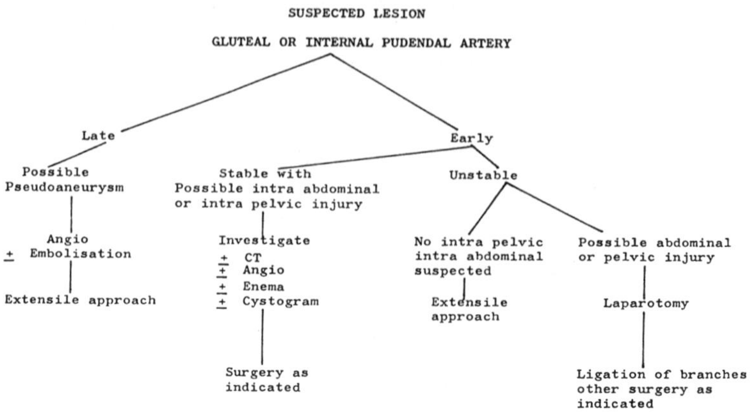

Fig 2–8.—Algorithm for management of suspected gluteal or pudendal artery injury. (Courtesy of Gilroy D, Saadia R, Hide G, et al: *J Trauma* 32:294–297, 1992.)

Patients.—Over a 6-year period, 7 men and 1 woman ranging in age from 22 to 45 years were seen with gunshot or stab wounds to a buttock. Three patients presented early after the injury, 2 with profuse external hemorrhage and 1 with acute false aneurysms. The other 5 were seen late with chronic false aneurysms, with infection in 1 case. The problem was at first wrongly assessed in 7 of the 8 cases, and the lesions were inappropriately excised or explored. One patient died of acute hemorrhage and another of generalized sepsis. Four patients were definitively managed by a direct approach through the gluteal muscle, with great difficulty in 1 case. This approach failed in another patient, who required transperitoneal ligation of the gluteal and internal pudendal arteries. Ligation of the internal iliac was tried in 3 cases but only successful in 1. The other patient was managed by formal extensile exposure.

Discussion.—For patients with penetrating trauma to the gluteal region, direct incision of suspected abscesses is dangerous because the lesion may turn out to be a false aneurysm. The physician should suspect problems with these vessels, even if the injury seems minor. Each patient must undergo sufficient investigation and planning before surgery (Fig 2–8).

▶ One gluteal/internal pudendal arterial injury was immediately obvious and fatal. One hematoma was digitally explored 1 hour postinjury and 4 swellings incised at 6 to 90 days, all under local anesthesia and all with profuse bleeding and hypotension. The only patient who did not bleed into shock died of sepsis. The U.S. practice of early suspicion and evaluation with CT provides better results than these late, blind incisions and drainage in South Africa.—T. Stair, M.D.

Guaiac Testing in the Diagnosis of Rectal Trauma: What Is Its Value?

Levine H, Simon RJ, Smith TR, Ivatury R, Stahl W (New York Med College, Bronx, NY)

J Trauma 32:210–212, 1992 2–46

Background.—Acutely traumatized patients in the emergency department routinely undergo rectal examination with guaiac testing. The value of guaiac testing in detecting occult rectal injury has been questioned. This question was addressed in a retrospective review of 19 patients with suspected rectal injury.

Patients.—The seventeen men and 2 women with a mean age of 26 years sustained acute trauma, including 10 abdominal injuries, 9 injuries to the buttock, and 3 to the thigh.

Findings.—Guaiac testing proved to have a sensitivity of 69% and a specificity of 33%. By contrast, rigid sigmoidoscopy had a sensitivity of 100% and a specificity of 67%. When guaiac testing and rigid sigmoidoscopy were combined, the sensitivity was 100%.

Conclusions.—Guaiac testing alone is not sufficient to confirm or exclude the presence of occult rectal injury in acutely traumatized patients in the emergency department. Even when guaiac test results are negative, physicians must aggressively pursue the diagnosis in patients with highly probable occult rectal injury.

Vascular, Urogenital, Musculoskeletal

Duplex Scanning for Arterial Trauma

Meissner M, Paun M, Johansen K (Harborview Med Ctr, Seattle, Wash)
Am J Surg 161:552–555, 1991 2–47

Introduction.—Blunt or penetrating trauma without overt hemorrhage or distal ischemia is commonly investigated by arteriography to exclude occult arterial trauma. However, the utility of arteriography in this setting has been questioned lately since most arteriograms are either normal or show minor abnormalities that do not require surgical intervention. The utility of noninvasive duplex sonography as a screening tool for arterial injuries was assessed.

Patients.—During a 4-year period, 89 patients with a mean age of 29.5 years underwent duplex sonography scanning for 93 known or suspected arterial injuries to the extremities or the cervicothoracic region. Sixty scans were done solely for wound proximity to nearby vascular structures, 19 scans were obtained because of suspected vascular injuries, and 12 scans were done for postoperative follow-up. One patient underwent duplex scanning for serial evaluation of an unoperated lesion.

Results.—Four of the 60 scans (6.7%) performed for wound proximity alone showed abnormalities, but each of those 4 arterial injuries remained stable during follow-up. Thirteen of the 19 (68%) scans done for clinical indications were positive. Six of the 12 (50%) scans performed for postoperative follow-up also showed abnormalities, but no new injuries were discovered. Four patients (4.3%) with normal duplex studies had abnormal angiograms, but none of those patients had major arterial injuries. There were no false-positive studies.

Conclusion.—Duplex sonography is a rapid, noninvasive, inexpensive, and portable diagnostic modality that reliably aids diagnosis and localization of sites of arterial disruption. A noninvasive vascular diagnostic algorithm for evaluating patients who may harbor a potential traumatic vascular injury is proposed. The algorithm limits contrast arteriography to patients who have abnormal findings on physical examination or an abnormal Doppler arterial pressure index.

▶ The authors conclude that duplex scanning represents a reliable alternative to angiography in the evaluation of occult arterial injuries. This is supported by others who have found an overall accuracy of 98% when utilizing this modality (1). Angiography is not without its morbidity, and the amount that often transpires when attempting to get angiographic studies accomplished in the middle of the night might be reason enough to look for alternative dianostic choices! As with most ultrasonographic studies, however, accuracy is operator dependent, and this factor must be considered when choosing between the two tests.—H.D. Unger, M.D.

Reference

1. Bynoe RP, et al: *J Vasc Surg* 14:346, 1991.

Evaluation and Treatment of Blunt Renal Trauma

Herschorn S, Radomski SB, Shoskes DA, Mahoney J, Hirschberg E, et al (Univ of Toronto, Canada)

J Urol 146:274–277, 1991 2–48

Background.—In the United States and Canada, blunt trauma to the kidneys is far more common than penetrating trauma. A retrospective study was done of patients with blunt renal trauma treated at 1 trauma unit over a period of 13 years.

Patients.—Of 3,993 patients admitted to this regional trauma unit, 126 (3.1%) had blunt renal trauma. Patients ranged in age from 13 to 87 years, with a mean of 32. The male-to-female ratio was 3:1. The patients were followed for a mean of 7 months. Renal injury was minor in 72%, moderate in 17%, and major in 11%. Nine patients had genitourinary surgery; 114 were treated conservatively.

Outcomes.—Results were excellent in 87% and good in 8%. In 5% of the patients, treatment failed. All those with microscopic hematuria without shock had minor injuries. Excretory urograms were normal in 74% of those with minor injuries and in 39% of those with moderate injuries. All those undergoing CT scanning had abnormal results. Computed tomography was more sensitive and specific than intravenous pyelography.

Conclusions.—Most patients with blunt renal trauma can be managed conservatively with an excellent outcome. Patients with microscopic hematuria and no shock need not undergo radiologic assessment. When radiologic study is indicated, the imaging modality of choice is CT scanning.

▶ This retrospective study confirms previous studies that even more convincingly demonstrate that microscopic hematuria without shock is a benign finding rarely associated with any significant renal pathology. A prospective study in 1987 (1) followed 506 patients with blunt trauma and hematuria who were all studied by intravenous pyelography (IVP). They found that of the 365 patients with microscopic hematuria without shock, 3 injuries were found—2 renal contusions and 1 minor renal laceration. Microscopic hematuria is clearly a benign finding and unless complicated by shock, does not require evaluation with IVP and should simply be rechecked in 48 hours for persistence.—W.P. Burdick, M.D.

Reference

1. Hardeman SW, et al: *J Urol* 138:99, 1987.

Blunt Traumatic Bladder Rupture: The Role of Retrograde Cystogram

Rehm CG, Mure AJ, O'Malley KF, Ross SE (UMDNJ/Robert Wood Johnson Med School; Cooper Hosp/Univ Med Ctr, Camden, NJ)

Ann Emerg Med 20:845–847, 1991 2–49

Purpose.—Blunt traumatic bladder rupture is most often seen in acute blunt abdominal trauma, particularly when associated with a pelvic fracture. A delay in the diagnosis and treatment of a bladder rupture may significantly increase mortality. The importance of microscopic and gross hematuria and the role of retrograde cystography and CT in the diagnosis of blunt traumatic bladder rupture were examined.

Methods.—Trauma victims with blunt abdominal injury who had a suspected bladder injury underwent complete urinalysis with microscopic examination and anteroposterior radiography of the pelvis. A retrograde cystogram was obtained in the anteroposterior projection only because of the risk associated with moving multiply injured patients. A postvoid or washout film was also obtained. Patients suspected of having a pelvic fracture underwent CT of the abdomen and pelvis with intravenous contrast medium.

Patients.—During a 39-month period, 719 patients admitted with blunt abdominal trauma were considered to be at risk for bladder rupture. Eleven men and 10 women aged 14 to 87 years had a bladder rupture, and all had associated major injuries. Eighteen (86%) patients also had pelvic fractures. Eight patients died and 13 survived. All 21 patients had RBCs in their urine. Seventeen of them had gross hematuria, and 4 had microhematuria. All 3 patients with bladder rupture but no pelvic fracture had gross hematuria. Retrograde cystography accurately identified the bladder rupture in all 20 patients who underwent this procedure. One bladder rupture was found at emergency laparotomy for other injuries. Seven patients underwent CT of the abdomen and pelvis, which failed to demonstrate the bladder rupture. None of the patients with bladder rupture had associated urethral injuries.

Conclusions.—Hematuria is the principal indication for evaluating bladder injury in patients with blunt abdominal trauma, particularly when associated with pelvic fracture. Retrograde cystography is the diagnostic procedure of choice, whereas CT is of no use in diagnosing bladder ruptures.

▶ The authors review the diagnosis of traumatic bladder rupture in light of the availability of new diagnostic modalities. Interestingly enough, basic bedside and emergency center evaluation remains the most sensitive way to identify this condition. While not all individuals with traumatic microscopic hematuria require retrograde cystography, it is to be remembered that when a rupture is suspected, cystographic evaluation is the diagnostic modality of choice. This is particularly important to bear in mind since current practice in a hemodynamically stable patient with microscopic hematuria and blunt abdominal trauma is to obtain CAT scan evaluation of the abdomen. Such evaluation alone, even with the addition of double contrast, may not provide the diagnosis of bladder disruption. Additional application to the bladder of contrast material in the amount of 300 cc or more is necessary to fully delineate traumatic rupture in adult patients.—D.K. Wagner, M.D.

Isolated Clavicle Fracture With Associated Pneumothorax: A Case Report

Meeks RJ, Riebel GD (State Univ of New York, Syracuse)

Am J Emerg Med 9:555–556, 1991 2–50

Background.—Isolated fractures of the clavicular shaft typically heal uneventfully after routine treatment, but when acute complications occur, they can be serious. A case of pneumothorax caused by an isolated midshaft clavicle fracture is reported.

Case Study.—A 35-year-old man developed left-sided pleuritic chest pain after a vehicular collision. Physical examination indicated respiratory distress and extensive subcutaneous emphysema. The patient had decreased breath sounds on the left side and tenderness with deformity over the left clavicle. He had no neurovascular compromise of the arm, was hemodynamically stable, and had no other injuries. A chest radiograph confirmed the pneumothorax. The patient had a displaced transverse midshaft clavicle fracture along with thoracic scoliosis and a 30% left pneumothorax. Respiratory status improved after placement of a thorocostomy tube. Further imaging investigations revealed no other problems except for pulmonary contusions found on a subsequent radiograph. The patient required chest-tube draining for 4 days for a persistent air leak. He was discharged with a figure-of-8 clavicular strap.

Conclusions.—Although rare, complications occasionally occur with isolated clavicular fractures. The emergency physician should be aware of these complications and obtain a thorough history and physical examination, particularly of the chest. Careful reading of the radiograph will confirm the diagnosis of pneumothorax.

▶ This case reinforces the important clinical point that just because a given type of injury has a low associated complication rate, the possibility of those complications must be considered at the time of evaluation.—G.V. Anderson, M.D.

A Flexion Adduction Method for the Reduction of Posterior Dislocation of the Hip

Bassi JL, Ahuja SC, Singh H (Dayanand Med College and Hosp, Ludhiana, Punjab, India)

J Bone Joint Surg [Br] 74:157–158, 1992 2–51

Background.—The Bigelow method for reduction of posterior dislocations of the hip requires forcible traction. A new, simpler method that is less likely to produce complications is described.

Method.—The procedure is performed with the patient under general anesthesia and supine on the operating table. The surgeon stands on the unaffected side of the patient, lifts the dislocated leg to a position of 90 degrees of flexion and maximum adduction, and applies traction in the long axis of the femur. An assistant stands on the other side of the table, stabilizes the pelvis with one hand, and pushes the head of the femur into the acetabulum with the other hand (Fig 2–9).

Results.—Twenty consecutive type I or type II dislocations were reduced by this method. Five hips had a significant associated acetabular fractures and were reduced even more easily. Eighteen cases were fol-

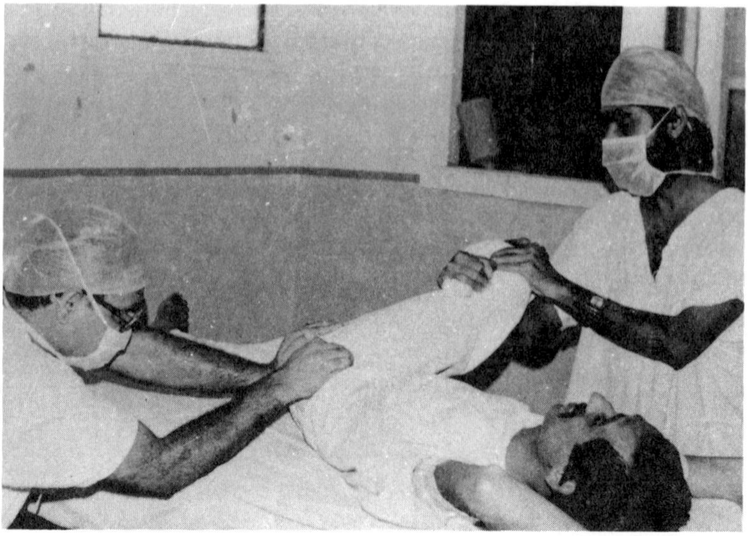

Fig 2–9.—Method for reduction of posterior dislocation of the hip. The dislocated leg is lifted to a position of 90 degrees of flexion and maximum adduction from the unaffected side. Traction is applied in the long axis of the femur while the pelvis is stabilized and the head of the femur pushed into the acetabulum. (Courtesy of Bassi JL, Ahuja SC, Singh H: *J Bone Joint Surg* 74 (Br): 157–158, 1992.)

lowed for at least 5 years and showed no evidence of avascular necrosis or myositis ossificans. Some minor degenerative changes were observed in patients with significant fractures of the acetabular rim.

Conclusion.—Application of a corrective force directly to the femoral head allows reduction to be controlled and achieved with minimal trauma. Damage from excessive traction can be avoided, as well as conversion into an anterior dislocation. The method is useful in treating type I and type II traumatic dislocations and dislocation of a hemiarthroplasty or total hip replacement.

▶ Emergency medicine physicians would be eager to embrace an easy technique for reduction of posterior hip dislocations. Although the reported technique offers promise, in this series it was always performed with the patient under general anesthesia. Too often, the emergency physician sedates the patient, struggles to reduce the hip dislocation, and ultimately requests an orthopedist for final reduction.—E.J. Reisdorff, M.D.

3 Organ System Emergencies

Respiratory Emergencies

ASTHMA

Aminophylline Therapy for Acute Bronchospastic Disease in the Emergency Room

Wrenn K, Slovis CM, Murphy F, Greenberg RS (Emory Univ, Atlanta, Ga; Univ of Rochester, NY)

Ann Intern Med 115:241–247, 1991 3–1

Introduction.—Aminophylline is no longer a mainstay in the treatment of acute bronchospastic disease because of the drug's narrow therapeutic index and a lack of convincing evidence of its efficacy. A double-blind, placebo-controlled trial was designed to assess the role of aminophylline as an adjunct to β-agonists and corticosteroids in patients coming to an emergency room with acute bronchospastic disease.

Patients.—Study participants included 133 adults with either asthma or chronic obstructive pulmonary disease. All came to the emergency department with asthma exacerbation or wheezing and were treated with both aerosolized metaproterenol and intravenous methylprednisolone. The patients were randomly assigned to receive either aminophylline or placebo, followed by a routine infusion.

Results.—Spirometric values at 60 and 120 minutes showed no significant difference in improvement between the aminophylline and placebo groups. Side effects were similar for the 2 groups, although nausea was reported more often in the aminophylline group. Time in the emergency department, patient satisfaction, and the investigator's assessment of response to therapy were similar for the 2 groups. Yet, aminophylline was associated with fewer hospital admissions; 6% of the patients in the aminophylline group and 21% of those in the placebo group were hospitalized.

Conclusion.—Because aminophylline treatment reduced the likelihood of hospital admission by 71%, its use in emergency department patients with an acute exacerbation of bronchospastic disease could considerably reduce treatment costs. The mechanism of the agent's favorable effects is not fully understood.

▶ The findings need explanation. An unmeasurable effect of aminophylline should prompt further research to determine the etiology of the effect.

The unexplained decrease in hospital admissions of patients receiving aminophylline is a justified conclusion of the study. Why this occurred cannot be determined from those data. Further study of this phenomenon is needed to include a confirmatory study.

Authors refer to the "asthma room of the emergency department" in the methods section; yet they use the term "emergency room" in the paper title. "Emergency department" in the title would be preferable and a more accurate sobriquet.—J.E. Clinton, M.D.

The Use of β-Agonists and the Risk of Death and Near Death From Asthma

Spitzer WO, Suissa S, Ernst P, Horwitz RI, Habbick B, et al (Montreal Gen Hosp, McGill Univ, Montreal; Yale Univ, New Haven, Conn; Univ of Saskatchewan, Saskatoon; Saskatchewan Health, Regina, Sask; Oregon Health Sciences Univ, Portland; et al)

N Engl J Med 326:501–506, 1992 3–2

Background.—Previous studies have suggested that use of fenoterol is associated with an increased risk of death from asthma, and 1 study showed that regular use of fenoterol, not "as-needed" use, was associated with poor control of asthma symptoms. Whether these observations also apply to other β_2-agonists is not clear. The current case-control investigation asked whether regular, long-term use of β-agonists, especially fenoterol, is associated with an increased risk of death or near death from asthma.

Methods.—From a cohort of 12,301 Canadian patients taking asthma medications between 1978 and 1987, 129 patients who had fatal or near-fatal events were identified. These were matched with 655 control patients who also took asthma medications. Case and control patients were matched for region of residence, age, receipt of social assistance, and previous hospitalization for asthma. Data were available on the number of metered-dose inhalers dispensed per months.

Results.—Case patients were hospitalized more frequently, used the services of physicians more often, and used more classes of medications other than asthma drugs more often than control patients. The use of inhaled β-agonist bronchodilators, especially fenoterol and albuterol, was associated with an increased risk of death from asthma or near-fatal asthma. Use of these drugs was also associated with an increased risk of death alone, with an odds ratio of 2.6 per canister per month. Only when the odds ratio for albuterol was calculated by using a weight-for-weight comparison with fenoterol were comparable, significant risks seen. Increased risks were also associated with the use of nebulized albuterol, other inhaled β-agonists, theophylline, and oral corticosteroids, but not with the combined use of inhaled corticosteroids and cromolyn. The odds ratios for death from asthma were also significantly elevated in patients thought to be at low risk who used both albuterol or fenoterol on a regular, long-term basis.

Conclusions.—The risk of death or near death from asthma is associated with the regular use of inhaled β-agonist bronchodilators. It is unclear whether the use of these agents is responsible for these adverse effects or whether they are a marker for more severe disease. In either case, heavy use of these medications should alert the physician that further evaluation is needed.

▶ The findings of this study are provocative, but the caveat stated by the authors in their conclusion is most important, that is, the increased risk of death may simply mean that the patients using β-agonists are sicker.—E. Ruiz, M.D.

Dose of Nebulized Ipratropium Bromide in Acute Severe Asthma

Whyte KF, Gould GA, Jeffrey AA, Airlie MAA, Flenley DC, et al (City Hosp, Edinburgh, Scotland)

Respir Med 85:517–520, 1991 3–3

Background.—Adding ipratropium bromide to nebulized β_2-agonists can improve peak flow in patients with acute asthma. The current maximum dose of ipratropium is 500 μg, but it is not clear whether this dose is sufficient to produce maximum effectiveness. The effects of .5 mg vs. 1 mg of nebulized ipratropium bromide were compared as to peak expiratory flow (PEF), heart rate, blood pressure, and ear oxygen saturation in 26 patients admitted with acute severe asthma.

Methods.—Variables were measured at baseline and regularly after treatment with nebulized ipratropium bromide in saline. All patients first received 200 mg of hydrocortisone administered intravenously. Thirteen patients were randomized to each group. Two hours after nebulization of ipratropium, patients received 5 mg of terbutaline administered by nebulizer. Variables were measured again 15 and 30 minutes later.

Results.—The peak expiratory flow increased by 51% in the .5-mg ipratropium group and by 37% in the 1-mg group 1 hour after nebulization. There were no significant differences between groups in either the absolute or percent increase in PEF rate. Also, there were no significant differences between groups in heart rate or ear oxygen saturation. In both groups, the pulse rate declined from a mean of 120 beats per minute to 110 beats per minute. Two hours after nebulization, PEF did not differ significantly between groups. The baseline PEF rate increased 86%

overall after the administration of .5 mg of ipratropium plus 5 mg of terbutaline and 65% after 1 mg of ipratropium plus 5 mg of terbutaline. There were no cholinergic side effects in either group.

Conclusions.—The lower dose—.5 mg—of nebulized ipratropium is as effective as 1 mg in the treatment of patients with acute severe asthma. Ipratropium should be combined with a β_2-agonist.

▶ The above article on the issue of ipratropium in acute, severe asthma unfortunately is flawed technically. Each patient was given 200 mg of intravenous hydrocortisone prior to receiving nebulized ipratropium. One hour after the patients received both drugs, measurements of pulmonary function were made. The PEF increased by 37 to 51%. These findings are encouraging, except for the fact that there is no control group to let us see what percent increase in PEF would have occurred with the intravenous administration of 200 mg of hydrocortisone alone.

In asthmatics, ipratropium can augment the response produced by β-adrenergic agents, although when this does occur, it is not often very marked. Inhaled anticholinergics, .5 mg of ipratropium or .5 mg of atropine, may be of benefit in patients not responding to more conventional therapy.—J. Wasserberger, M.D.

Aminophylline in the Emergency Department: Maximizing Safety and Efficacy

Kino R, Day RO, Pearce GA, Fulde GWO (St Vincent's Hosp, Darlinghurst, NSW, Australia)

Chest 100:1572–1577, 1991 3–4

Background.—The use of intravenously administered aminophylline improves pulmonary function in patients with acute asthma, but this drug has a low therapeutic ratio and pronounced intersubject variability in its metabolism. Although theophylline dosages are generally determined from the patient's weight and/or the intuition of the physician, the use of a computer-assisted dosage prediction program might provide superior results. In addition, a new bedside kit for measuring plasma theophylline levels might help determine an appropriate theophylline loading dose. This study tested whether residents of an emergency department could better determine aminophylline loading and maintenance dosages by using the Acculevel assay kit together with the computer-based "theophylline program."

Methods.—This sequential, prospective trial involved 46 patients with acute bronchospasm who received intravenously administered aminophylline according to a standard, empirical emergency department protocol and another 43 dosed according to the "theophylline program." The standard protocol used a loading dose of 5 mg/kg, followed by an infusion of .4 to .8 mg/kg/hr. No loading dose was given if the patient had taken orally administered theophylline within 12 hours of hospital admission. The experimental protocol involved determining baseline theophylline concentrations within 15 to 20 minutes by using the Syva "Acculevel." With this protocol, a "theophylline program" on a personal computer was used to calculate loading and maintenance doses. A standard laboratory technique was used to determine 1- and 6-hour theophylline levels of plasma in all patients.

Results.—After 1 hour, the mean plasma concentration in patients dosed according to the standard protocol was 51.5 μmol/L, which is below the therapeutic range and significantly lower than the range of 68.8 μmol/L of patients in the experimental group. The target plasma concentration was 70 μmol/L. After 6-hours, the mean plasma concentration of patients in the experimental group was 69.8 μmol/L, not significantly different from that of 59.7 μmol/L in the control group. At 1 hour, use of the experimental protocol resulted in 81% of the patients having theophylline concentrations in the accepted therapeutic range, significantly more than the 26% of the patients dosed according to the standard protocol. At 6 hours, 91% of the experimental patients had plasma concentrations in the standard therapeutic range, significantly more than the 37% of patients who received standard dosing. No patients whose doses were determined according to the experimental protocol had levels in the toxic range at either 1 or 6 hours, whereas 7% to 10% of the patients who received standard dosing had plasma levels in the toxic range.

Conclusions.—This quick and easy new protocol for determining intravenously administered aminophylline dosages appears to result in superior accuracy than when the conventional method is used. Without undue strain on busy housestaff, the use of this protocol should maximize both the safety and efficacy of theophylline administration.

▶ Despite my personal aversion to computers, I was intrigued by this article because it truly appears to offer a better way to accurately achieve therapeutic theophylline levels *quickly* in an acute situation. In my opinion, the bedside measurement of plasma theophylline levels is the real key to the solution, and I am personally anxious to try it myself. It would be very interesting to repeat this study by using only the rapid measurement of theophylline levels and not using the computer-assisted pharmacokinetic prediction because most emergency departments do not have a computer readily available.—E.J. Lucid, M.D.

Reversible T-Wave Abnormality in Severe Acute Asthma: An Electrocardiographic Sign of Severity

Efthimiou J, Hassan AB, Ormerod O, Benson MK (John Radcliffe and Churchill Hosps, Oxford, England)

Respir Med 85:195–201, 1991 3–5

Background.—Patients with severe acute asthma may develop reversible ECG abnormalities. Inversion of T-waves in the inferior leads has been reported only rarely, and their frequency and significance are undocumented. Seventy patients with severe acute asthma were studied to investigate inferior-lead T-wave abnormalities and their relationship to the severity of the attack.

Methods.—There were 40 females and 30 males ranging from 16 to 62 years of age. The main reason for admission was severe acute asthma. All had a 12-lead ECG on admission and during recovery. In patients who had inferior-lead T-wave flattening or inversion or any sign of right or left heart disease, follow-up studies were done. Ten patients with and 10 without T-wave abnormalities had 2-dimensional echocardiography in the acute and recovery phases.

Results.—Admission ECGs showed inferior-lead T-wave inversion in 34% of patients. Inversion of T-waves was the most common ECG abnormality after sinus tachycardia. Asthma was more severe in the patients with inferior T-wave inversion, as indicated by the degree of pulsus paradoxus, peak expiratory flow rate, forced expiratory volume in 1 second, and arterial blood oxygen tension. Six of 10 patients with T-wave abnormalities had echocardiographic evidence of right ventricular pressure overload as compared with only 1 of 10 patients without T-wave abnormalities. Voluntary hyperventilation and exercise testing could not reproduce the ECG changes in tests done after recovery.

Conclusions.—Patients with severe acute asthma may have reversible inferior-lead T-wave abnormalities that may be related to the severity of the attack. The ECG change may reflect acute right ventricular strain related to pressure overload and could play an important part in assessing the severity of attacks.

▶ The authors make a strong case for the observed T-wave inversions in multiple inferior leads being the result of right ventricular strain and pressure overload in the setting of acute pulmonary hypotension with hypoxemia. They anecdotally note that similar ECG findings occur with other respiratory disorders associated with severe hypoxemia, including severe pneumonia and severe exacerbations of chronic obstructive lung disease and cystic fibrosis.

While this ECG finding may help stratify the severity of the patient's respiratory status, it also raises the issue of concurrent non–Q-wave myocardial infarction. Such patients will require admission to a monitored hospital bed and further investigation of cardiac status with serial cardiac enzyme levels and ECGs.—J.R. Hedges, M.D.

Decreased Duration of Emergency Department Treatment of Chronic Obstructive Pulmonary Disease Exacerbations With the Addition of Ipratropium Bromide to β-Agonist Therapy

Shrestha M, O'Brien T, Haddox R, Gourlay HS, Reed G (Univ of Texas Southwestern Med Ctr, Dallas; Univ of California, San Diego)

Ann Emerg Med 10:1206–1209, 1991 3–6

Introduction.—Ipratropium bromide is a bronchodilator without the systemic anticholinergic side effects of atropine. In patients with chronic obstructive pulmonary disease (COPD), ipratropium can result in bronchodilatation nearly equal to or greater than that produced by β-agonists. A previous study showed that patients with COPD who were seen in the emergency department had only small improvements in spirometry after treatment with a single dose of fenoterol in combination with ipratropium.

Methods.—The effects of adding ipratropium to repeated doses of nebulized β-agonist during acute exacerbations of COPD were investigated in a double-blind randomized study of 76 patients who were treated in the emergency department of a busy, inner-city hospital. The patients were randomized to receive either the standard regimen of nebulized isoetharine, .5 mL of a 1% solution every hour, or the same regimen plus ipratropium bromide, 54 μg after the first isoetharine treatment and 36 μg after the second and fourth treatments. The trial was blinded by the use of a placebo metered-dose inhaler by patients receiving the standard treatment. The duration of therapy and number of treatments required in the 2 groups were compared.

Results.—After a mean of 226 minutes in the emergency department, 30 patients in the ipratropium group were discharged. This was significantly less time than that of the 25 patients in the control group. The experimental patients required an average of 3.7 treatments, significantly fewer than the average of 4.8 required by the controls. Patients in both groups had similar pulmonary function values as determined both initially and on discharge. No significant difference was seen in relapse rates between the 2 groups.

Conclusion.—Patients with acute exacerbations of COPD spent an average of 91 minutes less in the emergency department and required an average of 1 less treatment when β-agonist therapy was combined with ipratropium bromide. Ipratropium seems to accelerate the improvement of these patients.

► Given that the armamentarium is quite limited for the treatment of exacerbation of COPD and asthma in the emergency department (ED), the addition of ipratropium is welcome and simple to administer in combination with inhaled β-agonists. Certainly, the early use of steroids appears to have helped to shorten the stay in the ED as well as on the floor (admitted or observation status). This study was not controlled for the administration of steroids or aminophylline, and interestingly, 60% of patients in the control group received aminophylline as compared with 37% of the experimental group. A similar percentage of patients received steroids in each group. One would like to see a larger repeat study using albuterol aerosols every 20 to 30 minutes and controlled for the administration of other agents before drawing a firm conclusion about the emergent use of ipratropium in conjunction with β-agonists.—J.T. Amsterdam, M.D.

Rehabilitation of Patients With Quadriparesis After Treatment of Status Asthmaticus With Neuromuscular Blocking Agents and High-Dose Corticosteroids

Apte-Kakade S (Hennepin County Med Ctr, Minneapolis, Minn)

Arch Phys Med Rehabil 72:1024–1028, 1991 3–7

Background.—Patients with severe asthma not responding to maximum medical therapy require mechanical ventilation. Neuromuscular blocking agents are often used in such cases to relax the muscles and reduce airway pressure during anesthesia. However, these agents sometimes have adverse effects. Four patients who had quadriparesis after treatment of status asthmaticus with neuromuscular blocking agents and high-dose corticosteroids were successfully rehabilitated.

Patients and Outcomes.—Twenty-seven of 51 asthmatic patients consecutively treated with mechanical ventilation were given neuromuscular blocking agents. All 27 received high-dose intravenous steroids. Quadriparesis that was more severe distally developed in 4 patients. No cranial nerve or sensory involvement was noted. The 4 patients underwent physical and occupational therapy. Three were transferred to a rehabilitation unit. The patients had steady improvement in muscle strength and by discharge, they had independence in mobility and activities of daily living.

Summary.—Four asthmatic patients receiving neuromuscular blocking agents and high-dose corticosteroids during intubation and mechanical ventilation had quadriparesis, an uncommon complication. These patients had an excellent outcome after treatment in a rehabilitation unit. Early rehabilitation is strongly urged. The cause of this complication is not known, but it may result from steroid-induced acute myopathy facilitated by neuromuscular blocking agents.

▶ It remains unclear whether the myopathies observed in these patients were due to corticosteroids, neuromuscular blocking agents (NMBs), or a combination of the two. Clearly, it is a time- and dose-related phenomenon.

For the unstable asthma patient who fails to improve with conventional therapy (including steroids), the use of NMBs and intubation remains a therapeutic cornerstone. While the physician should be aware of the potential for neurologic sequelae when both these drugs are used, it should not change the course of acute therapy.

For those physicians involved in the continued care of these patients, added emphasis on early extubation and limited use of NMBs may be appropriate.—H.D. Unger, M.D.

Methylprednisolone Does Not Protect the Lung From Inhalation Injury

Nieman GF, Clark WR, Hakim T (State Univ of New York, Syracuse)
Burns 17:384–390, 1991 3–8

Introduction.—Corticosteroids are contraindicated in the treatment of acute smoke inhalation. However, in some critical cases, they are still used in hope of reversing the acute pathophysiologic response. The effects of methylprednisolone in dogs subjected to amoke inhalation were studied.

Methods.—After anesthetization, 30 mongrel dogs were intubated and ventilated with a mixture of smoke and room air. Three experiments were performed: 1 to assess hemodynamics, gas exchange, lung compliance and lung water; 1 to evaluate pulmonary vascular permeability by cannulating the afferent tracheobronchial lymphatic and calculating the osmotic reflection coefficient at high lung lymph flows; and 1 to study pulmonary surfactant function by using a Wilhelmy balance.

Results.—None of the values measured were different in animals that received methylprednisolone as compared with those for control animals. Methylprednisolone pretreatment—30 mg/kg—did not attenuate the adverse responses to smoke inhalation. Lung water was only moderately increased in both groups. Methylprednisolone did not protect minimum surface tension of extractable surfactant.

Conclusions.—Methylprednisolone has no beneficial effect on any of the pathologic responses to smoke inhalation injury, even when adequate tissue levels are seen when the injury occurs. This study and previous clinical studies show no benefit of corticosteroids in patients who should be treated for smoke inhalation.

▶ The benefit of corticosteroids in inhalation injuries continues to be questioned. In fact, their use may be associated with increased risk of infection. The difficulties associated with this type of study relate to the fact that the exact type of inhalation injury cannot be easily standardized or simulated.—G.V. Anderson, M.D.

MAGNESIUM THERAPY

Intravenous Magnesium Sulfate in Acute, Life-Threatening Asthma

Kuitert LM, Kletchko SL (Middlemore Hosp, Auckland, New Zealand)

Ann Emerg Med 20:1243–1245, 1991 3–9

Background.—Magnesium is a physiologic calcium antagonist that has a direct effect on calcium uptake in smooth muscle and results in smooth muscle relaxation. Research on magnesium sulfate infusions in patients with mild or moderate-to-severe acute asthma indicates that it may have a significant bronchodilatory effect, comparable to that of salbutamol. A case was presented.

Case Study.—A 56-year-old woman was brought to the emergency department in cardiorespiratory arrest. She was successfully defibrillated, although manual ventilation was difficult because of high airway pressure. Wheeze was audible through the lung fields. Her history included lifelong mild-to-moderate asthma. In the next 1½ hours, she was given 100% inspired oxygen, 19.5 mg parenteral salbutamol, 250 mg aminophylline followed by an infusion of 45 mg/hr, 200 mmol sodium bicarbonate for severe and persistent mixed metabolic and respiratory acidosis, 200 mg hydrocortisone, and 2 mg adrenaline parenterally for bradycardia and hypotension. Her condition minimally improved. Manual ventilation continued to be difficult because of her severe persistent bronchospasm. She was transferred to the intensive care unit. Three hours after the arrest and despite aggressive treatment, her condition was not improved. Magnesium sulfate infusion was begun, for a total of 100 mmol over a period of 20 minutes. She had a dramatic physiologic and clinical improvement in her asthma. Airway pressure dropped, compliance increased, and $ETCO_2$ increased to 5 kPa. Tidal volumes could be increased to 800 mL without a rise in peak airway pressure. Her condition continued to improve over the next 2 hours. The rest of the patient's hospital stay was uneventful, and she was discharged after 5 days.

Conclusions.—This patient with severe asthma responded to a magnesium sulfate intravenous infusion after failing to respond to aggressive pharmacologic management. Magnesium sulfate may prove to be a valuable addition to treatment options for asthmatic patients. It may be particularly beneficial in patients who do not respond to conventional treatment.

Intravenous Magnesium for Acute Asthma: Failure to Decrease Emergency Treatment Duration or Need for Hospitalization

Green SM, Rothrock SG (Riverside Gen Hosp, Calif; California Emergency Physicians Med Group, Oakland)

Ann Emerg Med 21:260–265, 1992 3–10

Background.—Findings suggest that routine early administration of magnesium to asthmatic patients may add to or synergize with conventional treatment. The addition of magnesium was compared with conventional treatment alone.

Methods.—One hundred twenty patients aged 18 to 65 years were enrolled consecutively in the prospective trial. All patients had acute asthma and were unresponsive to a single albuterol treatment. All were given oxygen, 125 mg of methylprednisolone intravenously, and hourly albuterol inhalations. The study group was also given magnesium sulfate, 2 g intravenously, infused over a 20-minute period.

Results.—The 2 treatment groups were similar in demographic and clinical characteristics. Thirteen of the 58 patients receiving magnesium needed to be hospitalized as compared with 11 of 62 patients given conventional therapy alone. The duration of treatment in the emergency department among those discharged was 224 minutes in the study group and 228 in the control group. Changes in peak expiratory flow were also not significantly different.

Conclusions.—The addition of magnesium to conventional treatment in patients with acute asthma does not significantly affect the rate of hospitalization, peak expiratory flow measures, or emergency department treatment time for discharged patients. The routine use of magnesium in such patients does not therefore alter treatment outcomes.

▶ Anecdotal cases have suggested that intravenous (IV) magnesium may be beneficial for asthmatic patients who fail to respond to β-agonists. According to the authors of Abstracts 3–9 and 3–10, the early administration of IV magnesium offered no advantage in the routine treatment of asthma. However, it is important to note that the above study does not necessarily apply to critically ill asthmatic patients. What is of great concern is that those asthmatics requiring mechanical ventilation at any point during their emergency department visit or subsequent hospitalization were totally excluded in the above study. Thus, the group of asthmatics facing impending intubation (the group of greatest concern to emergency physicians) was not studied at all, and to date, no data on this critical subset of patients are available. The closest data we have to this subset of severe asthmatics come from Skobeloff, who in 1989 found an increased peak expiratory flow rate after the administration of IV magnesium in patients who were refractory to inhaled β-agonists (1).

Of note is that administering large doses of magnesium or administering magnesium too rapidly can cause hypotension and bradycardia. Eight grams of magnesium can cause muscle paralysis and respiratory arrest.

Data on the effects of magnesium on asthma patients who are in extremis are needed to determine whether magnesium is effective in helping to prevent the need for intubation and, if so, at what dose. Likewise, better data are also needed on the use of inhaled atropine or iprapropium in this same group of critically ill patients (see Abstract 3–3).—J. Wasserberger, M.D.

Reference

1. Skobeloff EM, et al: *JAMA* 262:1210, 1989.

Magnesium Deficiency: Recognition and Treatment in the Emergency Medicine Setting

Reinhart RA (Marshfield Clinic, Wis)
Am J Emerg Med 10:78–83, 1992 3–11

Conditions Associated With or Causing Magnesium Deficiency

- Renal loss
  - Diuretic (excluding potassium/magnesium-sparing drugs)
  - Osmotic agents (including hyperglycemia)
  - Antibiotics (carbenicillin, ticarcillin, gentamicin, tobramycin, amphotericin B)
  - Cisplatin
  - Cyclosporine
  - Alcohol
  - Diabetes mellitus and diabetic ketoacidosis
  - Renal tubular acidosis
  - Hyperparathyroidism (and other causes of hypercalcemia)
  - Postobstructive diuresis
  - Hyperaldosteronism
  - Hyperthyroidism
- Redistribution
  - Exchange transfusion
  - Acute pancreatitis
- Reduced intake
  - Starvation
  - Prolonged intravenous therapy without magnesium supplement
- Impaired intestinal absorption
  - Chronic diarrhea
  - Ileal resection
  - Malabsorption syndromes (including familial magnesium-specific)
- Miscellaneous
  - Acute myocardial infarction (intracellular shift)
  - Excessive sweating
  - Digitalis toxicity
  - Congestive heart failure

Data from Reinhart RA: *Arch Intern Med* 148:2415–2420, 1988; Wacker WEC, Parisi AF: *N Engl J Med* 278:658–663, 712–717, 772–776, 1968; Elin RJ: Disease-a-Month 34:161–218, 1988.
(Courtesy of Reinhart RA: *Am J Emerg Med* 10:78–83, 1992.)

Background.—Magnesium deficiency is commonly seen in acutely ill patients. Magnesium must sometimes be given empirically since serum and intracellular magnesium concentrations are not correlated. Conditions associated with magnesium deficiency that respond to supplementation were studied.

Clinical Conditions.—Because of modern food-refining techniques and softening of hard water, much of the population has subclinical magnesium deficiency. This deficiency may only become apparent during acute illnesses (e.g., acute myocardial infarction or congestive heart failure (table). Diuretic use, alcoholism, and starvation may also increase the risk of magnesium deficiency.

Assessment.—Relatively acute magnesium loss may be diagnosed by a low serum magnesium concentration. Deficiency may also be diagnosed by measurement of intracellular magnesium in mononuclear cells or RBCs by calculating the proportion of magnesium retained after infusion, measuring skeletal or cardiac muscle magnesium, or performing magnesium balance studies. Most intracellular magnesium is bound, with the free component being physiologically active at the molecular and cellular levels. The reference range for serum magnesium concentrations is 1.4 to 2 mEq/L, but it may not fall until several hours after the onset of acute illness. Thus, empirical magnesium replacement should be instituted for high-risk patients.

Treatment.—Intravenously administered magnesium may be given for urgent conditions, with chronic oral supplementation used for more chronic depletion. Patients with normal renal function tolerate magnesium well, whereas those with abnormal renal function need periodic serum magnesium determinations. Magnesium-sparing diuretics can be used for patients with magnesium loss caused by diuretics.

Discussion.—The associated conditions, diagnosis, and treatment of magnesium deficiency, including available preparations and recommended doses, were examined. Precautions for patients with renal insufficiency were also studied.

▶ Magnesium is involved in many of the enzymatic reactions in the body. It is essential for the cleavage of phosphate from ATP and release of energy. Clinically, this translates into reactions that regulate smooth muscle tone and neuroexcitatory activity. It is not surprising that if the magnesium content is low, these enzymatic reactions either do not grow as quickly or do not grow at all. Our own work in asthma suggests that some chronic asthmatics may have low magnesium stores. It is unclear whether this is due to medications taken or whether these patients have a baseline magnesium deficiency that increases the resting bronchoconstriction.

The interrelationship between calcium and magnesium is a fascinating one, and one that I think is going to be very important for us to understand in the future (see also Abstract 3–27).—W.H. Spivey, M.D.

Serum Magnesium Levels in Asthmatic Patients During Acute Exacerbations of Asthma

Falkner D, Glauser J, Allen M (Mount Sinai Med Ctr, Cleveland, Ohio)

Am J Emerg Med 10:1–3, 1992 3–12

Background.—There has been increasing interest in the beneficial effects of magnesium sulfate as an adjunct in the treatment of acute exacerbations of asthma. However, it is not clear whether hypomagnesemia plays a role in asthma attacks. Whether serum levels of magnesium in asthmatic patients with acute exacerbation differ from those of a control population was examined in a case-control study.

Patients.—Twenty-three patients with known asthma who were seen in the emergency department in acute exacerbation of asthma and 15 nonasthmatic patients matched for age, sex, race, and socioeconomic status were evaluated. The case patients were aged 18 to 50 years with no history of alcoholism, heart disease, renal disease, or diuretic use.

Findings.—Mean serum levels of magnesium did not differ significantly between the case and control patients. Analysis for β-error showed the true difference of the means to be less than .1 (95% confidence) or less than .13 (99% confidence). Except for 1 patient in each group, serum levels of magnesium were within normal range. Furthermore, serum levels of magnesium did not correlate with the severity of asthma.

Conclusion.—Determination of the serum level of magnesium does not play a useful role in the evaluation and treatment of asthmatics for acute exacerbation of asthma in the emergency setting.

► This article results from a growing interest regarding the use of intravenous magnesium in the treatment of acute bronchospasm. The study tried to define the role hypomagnesemia plays in precipitating an asthmatic attack. The authors' conclusion that "serum levels of magnesium did not correlate with the severity of asthma" has limited implications for the pharmacologic use of magnesium in bronchospasm. If intravenous magnesium proves to be therapeutic in relieving bronchospasm, therapy should be empirical and not guided by the patient's baseline serum magnesium level (see also Abstract 3–11).—E.J. Reisdorff, M.D.

PULMONARY EMBOLISM, PNEUMOTHORAX, PNEUMONIA

Clinical, Laboratory, Roentgenographic, and Electrocardiographic Findings in Patients With Acute Pulmonary Embolism and No Pre-Existing Cardiac or Pulmonary Disease

Stein PD, Terrin ML, Hales CA, Palevsky HI, Saltzman HA, et al (Henry Ford Hosp, Detroit; Maryland Med Research Inst, Baltimore; Massachusetts Gen

Hosp, Boston; Univ of Pennsylvania, Philadelphia; Duke Univ, Durham, NC; et al)
Chest 100:598–603, 1991 3–13

Background.—In patients without preexisting cardiac or pulmonary disease, the history, physical examination, chest radiograph, and ECG are useful in diagnosing acute pulmonary embolism (PE). A study was done to evaluate those clinical characteristics attributable only to PE.

Patients.—The patients were participants in the national Prospective Investigation of Pulmonary Embolism Diagnosis study. Acute PE was confirmed in 117 and excluded in 248 patients. Angiography aided the diagnosis of PE in 98% of the first group and the exclusion of PE in 71% of the second group. Dyspnea or tachypnea was present in 90% of the patients with PE; 91% had dyspnea, hemoptysis, or pleuritic pain. Eighty-four percent had an abnormal chest radiograph showing atelectasis and/or pulmonary parenchymal abnormalities in 79 of the 117 patients.

Results.—The most prevalent predisposing factor (56%) for PE in patients with no preexisting cardiac or pulmonary disease was immobilization, usually because of surgery. There was a history of neoplasia in 23% of the patients and one of thrombophlebitis in 14%. The most prevalent mode of presentation was the syndrome of pleuritic pain or hemoptysis (65%). The ECG was abnormal in 70% of patients with PE.

Conclusion.—The clinical manifestations of PE, considered together, are nonspecific. Only a small proportion of patients, however, did not have these important manifestations of PE. Thus, clinical evaluation is useful in identifying those patients in whom ventilation/perfusion scans and angiography may be necessary.

Clinical Characteristics of Patients With Acute Pulmonary Embolism

Stein PD, Saltzman HA, Weg JG (Henry Ford Heart and Vascular Inst, Detroit; Duke Univ, Durham, NC; Univ of Michigan, Ann Arbor)
Am J Cardiol 68:1723–1724, 1991 3–14

Introduction.—By using data from the National Heart, Lung, and Blood Institute Prospective Investigation of Pulmonary Embolism Diagnosis (PIOPED) study, the characteristics of patients with pulmonary embolism (PE) were evaluated. Symptoms suggestive of PE were required within 24 hours of entry into the study.

Methods.—There were 2 groups in the PIOPED study. The 251 patients in the first group were required to undergo pulmonary angiography if their ventilation/perfusion scans were abnormal. Those in the second group were not required to undergo this diagnostic procedure, although many did. The clinical characteristics of acute PE in the 383 patients with acute PE who were in either arm of the PIOPED study were reviewed and compared with those of 843 others in whom suspected PE was excluded.

Results.—The most common symptoms among the 383 patients with acute PE were dyspnea (78%), pleuritic pain (59%), and cough (43%). Frequent signs included tachypnea (73%), rales (55%), and tachycardia (30%). The 843 patients without PE did not differ significantly in the frequency of their symptoms and signs. Radiography revealed atelectasis or a pulmonary parenchymal abnormality in 69% of patients with PE and in 39% of patients without PE. The partial pressure of oxygen in arterial blood with the patient breathing room air was less than 80 mm Hg in 226 of 280 with and 458 of 624 without PE.

Conclusion.—Among patients in whom PE was confirmed, all but a few had a number of important manifestations. Although these manifestations are not specific for PE, they may be of help in identifying patients who require ventilation/perfusion scans and/or angiography.

▶ This study confirms what we already knew to be true, and that is that there is no single symptom, sign, or test (short of pulmonary angiography) that can definitively diagnose a pulmonary embolus. Thus, it remains for the emergency physician to maintain a high index of suspicion in any patient who presents with any of the signs or symptoms described in this article. To this list should also be added a sudden syncopal episode. I have seen several patients who ultimately were found to have a pulmonary embolus whose only complaint was syncope. However, during further workups they were found to be tachypneic and to have abnormal blood gases.

This diagnosis remains as one of our greatest diagnostic challenges.—E.J. Lucid, M.D.

Usefulness of Noninvasive Diagnostic Tools for Diagnosis of Acute Pulmonary Embolism in Patients With a Normal Chest Radiograph

Stein PD, Alavi A, Gottschalk A, Hales CA, Saltzman HA, et al (Henry Ford Hosp, Detroit; Univ of Pennsylvania, Philadelphia; Michigan State Univ, East Lansing; Massachusetts Gen Hosp, Boston; Duke Univ, Durham, NC; et al)

Am J Cardiol 67:1117–1120, 1991 3–15

Objective.—Clinical experience suggests that patients with severe dyspnea and a normal chest radiograph are likely to have pulmonary embolism (PE) and that, intuitively, ventilation/perfusion scans should work better in patients with a normal chest radiograph. The value of bedside examination and a ventilation/perfusion scan in the diagnosis of acute PE in patients with a normal chest radiograph was evaluated.

Patients.—Clinical characteristics and ventilation/perfusion scans were evaluated in 20 (8%) patients with normal chest radiographs among 260 patients with acute PE and 113 (18%) patients with normal chest radiographs among 642 patients in whom PE was excluded.

Findings.—The occurrence of a partial pressure of oxygen of $\leq$ 70 mm Hg in arterial blood and dyspnea was significantly more frequent

Sensitivity and Specificity of Ventilation/Perfusion Scans in Patients With a Normal Chest Radiograph

Scan Categories	Sensitivity (n = 20)	Specificity (n = 113)
High probability	6 (30%)	110 (97%)
High or intermediate probability	10 (50%)	97 (86%)
High, intermediate or low probability	18 (90%)	79 (70%)

(Courtesy of Stein PD, Alavi A, Gottschalk A, et al: *Am J Cardiol* 67:1117–1120, 1991.)

among patients with PE (53%) than those in whom PE was excluded (19%). However, neither this combination nor any other combination of blood gases, signs, and symptoms was strictly diagnostic. Pulmonary embolism occurred in 67% of the patients with a high-probability ventilation/perfusion scan and 17% of patients with a low-probability ventilation/perfusion scan. The ventilation/perfusion scans were less sensitive and more specific when scan categories (e.g., high or intermediate probability) were considered (table). An advantage of ventilation/perfusion scans in patients with normal chest radiographs appeared to be a reduction in the percentage of patients with intermediate-probability scans.

Conclusion.—Although not diagnostic, the combination of dyspnea and hypoxia in a patient with a normal chest radiograph is a useful clue to the diagnosis of PE. The ventilation/perfusion scan is not more effective in establishing a correct diagnosis in these patients.

► This report from the Prospective Investigation of Pulmonary Embolism Diagnosis (PIOPED) study reinforces the uncertainty that clinicians work under when attempting to diagnose PE. The authors note the association of dyspnea, hypoxia ($Pao_2 \leq$ 70 mm Hg), and a normal chest film with the presence of a pulmonary embolus. Unfortunately, from the authors' data that combination has a positive predictive value of only 33% for PE in a selected subpopulation having a 15% prevalence of emboli. Furthermore, that criteria set identified < 7% of all patients diagnosed with pulmonary emboli in the PIOPED study.—J.R. Hedges, M.D.

Simultaneous Bilateral Spontaneous Pneumothorax: Case Report

Hay E, Sternfeld M, Rashid A, Kunichevsky S, Eliraz A (Kaplan Hosp, Rehovot, Israel)

Am J Emerg Med 10:50–52, 1992 3–16

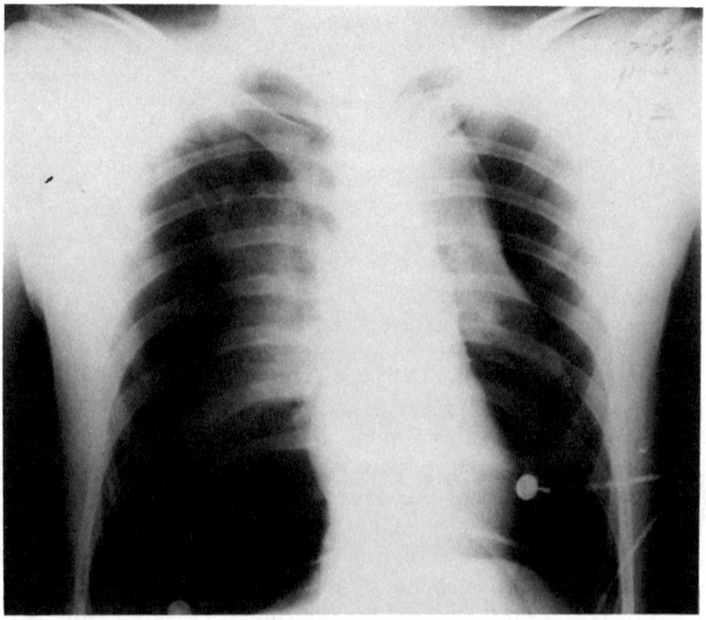

Fig 3–1.—Chest x-ray study showing bilateral pneumothorax with collapsed lungs. Note midline position of mediastinum. (Courtesy of Hay E, Sternfeld M, Rashid A, et al: *Am J Emerg Med* 10:50–52, 1992.)

Introduction.—Simultaneous bilateral spontaneous pneumothorax (SBSP) is a rare condition with diverse clinical manifestations. A patient developed acute respiratory failure necessitating mechanical ventilation.

Case Report.—A 22-year-old man was admitted with severe sudden dyspnea and chest pain. He had no history of health problems but smoked up to 4 packs of cigarettes a day. When the patient became severely agitated and cyanotic within minutes of admission, he was intubated nasotracheally and artificially ventilated with 100% oxygen. Bilateral pneumothorax was diagnosed from a chest x-ray study performed immediately before intubation (Fig 3–1). Chest tube drainage brought about full expansion of the lungs (Fig 3–2). A chest CT scan showed diffuse emphysematous bullae. The patient recovered and was able to be discharged 1 week later (Fig 3–3). He continued smoking and suffered a left spontaneous pneumothorax 4 months later.

Discussion.—Bilateral pneumothorax occurs in association with a variety of conditions, including trauma, lung tumor, and anesthesia. In SBSP, clinical diagnosis is difficult because there is no shift of the trachea. Although the etiology and pathology of SBSP are not fully understood, the risk of pneumothorax appears to be significantly increased by cigarette smoking. Symptoms in the present case resembled those of an acute

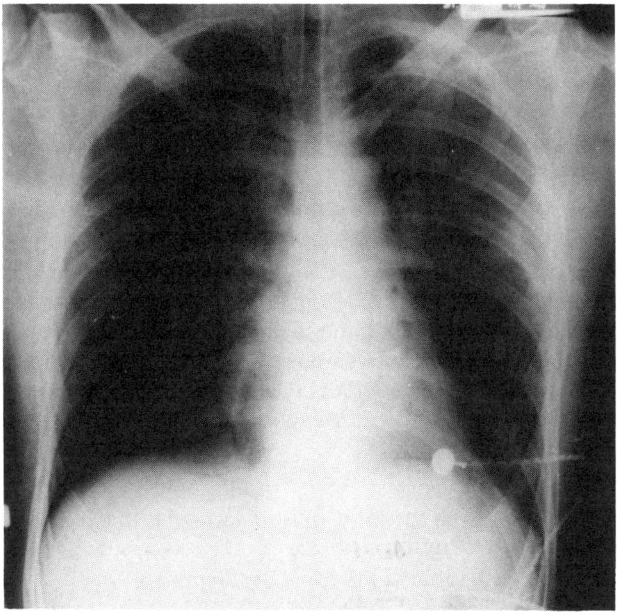

Fig 3–2.—Chest x-ray study showing bilateral chest tubes in the second intercostal spaces and fully expanded lungs. (Courtesy of Hay E, Sternfeld M, Rashid A, et al: *Am J Emerg Med* 10:50-52, 1992.)

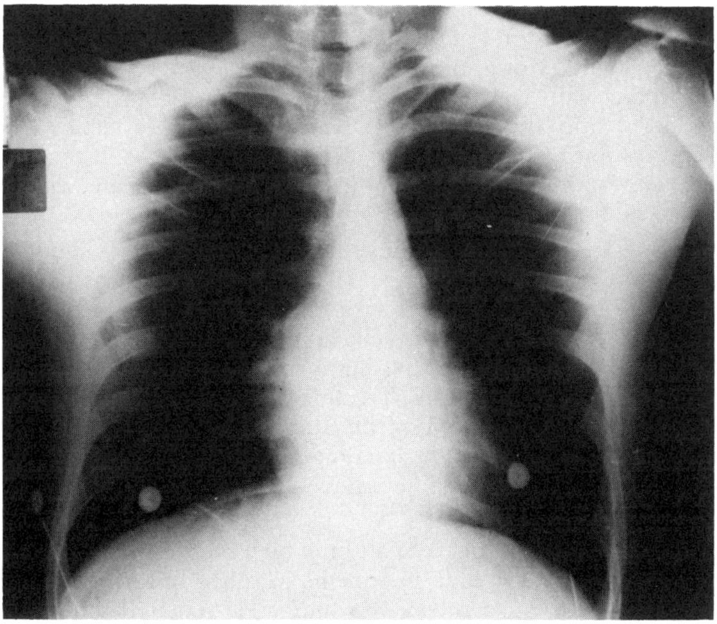

Fig 3–3.—Normal chest x-ray study on discharge. (Courtesy of Hay E, Sternfeld M, Rashid A, et al: *Am J Emerg Med* 10:50–52, 1992.)

asthmatic attack, but chest x-ray studies confirmed the diagnosis of SBSP.

Conclusion.—Simultaneous bilateral spontaneous pneumothorax may mimic bronchial asthma or other lung diseases. The use of CT is recommended in patients with spontaneous pneumothorax in order to assess the etiology of the condition.

▶ One point of curiosity in this article is that the authors in Rehovot, Israel, chose to place chest tubes bilaterally at the second intercostal space. More likely in North America, all forms of decompression and chest tubes would have been placed laterally through the fourth intercostal space at the anterior axillary line. Although the authors emphasize the importance of CT to determine the etiology of these conditions, this extends beyond the interest and needs of the emergency physician (see Abstract 3–63).—E.J. Reisdorff, M.D.

Value of Computed Tomography of the Lung in the Management of Primary Spontaneous Pneumothorax

Warner BW, Bailey WW, Shipley RT (Univ of Cincinnati, Ohio)

Am J Surg 162:39–42, 1991 3–17

Background.—Primary spontaneous pneumothorax is usually caused by the rupture of an apical subpleural bleb. Commonly, the patient receives tube thoracostomy until the air leak stops. Thoracostomy is reserved for patients with prolonged or recurrent leaks; however, it is difficult to predict who will ultimately require thoracostomy. A procedure that would identify this subset of patients would be desirable. Whether CT identification of the number and size of apical blebs in the lungs of patients with spontaneous pneumothorax would correlate with recurrence or need for thoracostomy was analyzed.

Methods.—Twenty-six consecutive patients with primary spontaneous pneumothorax underwent a single CT scan without the use of contrast media within 48 hours of the insertion of a thoracostomy tube. Physicians calculated the number of blebs and determined a bleb score that was calculated by multiplying the number of blebs by a numeric value assigned to a range of bleb sizes. Treating physicians were blinded to the results of the scan. At the end of the study, results of the CT scan were correlated with the patient's hospital course. Patients were followed by telephone or written survey to determine recurrence or the need for further treatment.

Results.—The number of blebs and the bleb score in the affected lung were both significantly greater in patients who had histories of recurrent pneumothorax and/or in those who ultimately required thoracostomy.

There were no significant differences between the "complicated" group, (e.g., those who had either prior pneumothorax, recurrent pneumothorax at follow-up, or a need for thoracostomy) and the "uncomplicated" group in terms of age, gender, duration of hospitalization, or time of follow-up.

Conclusions.—Computed tomography of the lung may help to identify those patients who will ultimately require thoracostomy. A prospective study of many patients might determine the critical number and size of blebs that would predict the absolute risk of recurrence with a high degree of accuracy.

▶ The idea that CT may be used to predict the prognosis of patients with spontaneous pneumothorax is intriguing. The beneficiary of improved predictability is the patient. Emergency treatment will be unchanged. Patients with high ipsilateral bleb scores might undergo thoracostomy earlier if these findings are reproduced.

The statistical correlation of increased bleb score and complicated pneumothorax is an interesting finding of the study.

Spontaneous pneumothorax is commonly seen and managed by emergency physicians. Computed tomography of the apices should be considered in these patients.—J.E. Clinton, M.D.

Disposition of Spontaneous Pneumomediastinum

Smith BA, Ferguson DB (Darnall Army Community Hosp, Fort Hood, Tex)

Am J Emerg Med 9:256–259, 1991 3–18

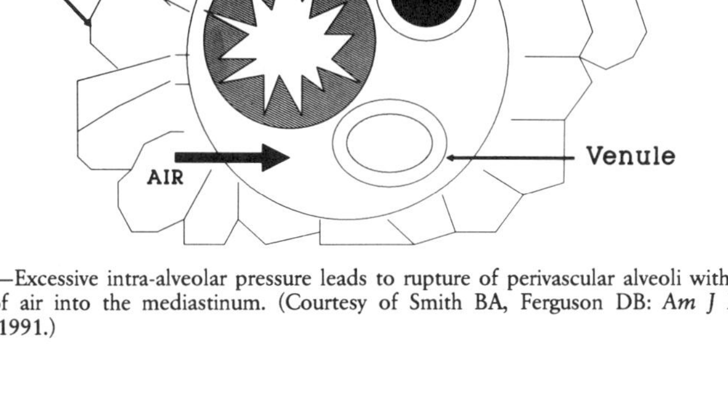

Fig 3–4.—Excessive intra-alveolar pressure leads to rupture of perivascular alveoli with subsequent dissection of air into the mediastinum. (Courtesy of Smith BA, Ferguson DB: *Am J Emerg Med* 9:256–259, 1991.)

Background.—Excluding pathologic causes of pneumomediastinum is important when assessing spontaneous pneumomediastinum. One such cause is Boerhaave's syndrome, which is associated with a high mortality rate. Reports in the literature vary greatly in their recommendations on how to care for patients with presumed spontaneous pneumomediastinum. A patient with spontaneous pneumomediastinum was treated with intravenously administered antibiotics and intensive care unit (ICU) admission despite a normal esophagogram.

Case Report.—A 27-year-old man came to the emergency department with complaints of a 3-day history of pleuritic chest pain, neck pain, dysphagia, and hoarseness. The patient was an active-duty soldier. On physical examination, his neck was remarkably tender on both sides, with a reduced range of motion because of his pain. Chest radiography showed mediastinal air without pulmonary infiltrates, effusion, or pneumothorax. The soft tissues of the neck on cervical plain radiographs contained air. The patient was admitted to the ICU. Intravenous administration of gentamicin and clindamycin was begun. Two days later, a CT scan of the neck showed generalized emphysema of the muscular, prevertebral, and subcutaneous compartments of the neck. There were no masses or abscesses. His cough went away in several days, with no more blood-tinged mucus production. On day 5, a follow-up chest radiograph showed near resolution of the pneumomediastinum. The patient's chest and neck pain diminished gradually. On day 7, he was discharged home.

Conclusions.—The pathophysiology of spontaneous pneumomediastinum is related to excessive pressures resulting in rupture of perivascular alveoli. Air escapes into the perivascular connective tissue, subsequently dissecting into the mediastinum (Fig 3–4). Because there is no evidence that patients with spontaneous pneumomediastinum have poor outcomes, the literature does not support ICU admission for them. Such patients are routinely admitted for observation, but they may do just as well with close outpatient follow-up

▶ The literature varies greatly in the care of patients with presumed spontaneous pneumomediastinum. The fact that this is a relatively uncommon problem with only a slim possibility of a fatal outcome makes it a relatively safe bet to treat patients with less than ICU admission or perhaps even with outpatient follow-up as these authors support.

As long as serious entities such as Boerhaave's syndrome, pneumothorax, and airway foreign bodies are considered with each case and ruled out, the prognosis is indeed good, and I agree that close outpatient follow-up is (for most of these patients) very appropriate.—J.J. Kelly, D.O., F.A.C.E.P.

Etiology and Diagnosis of Pneumonia Requiring ICU Admission
Potgieter PD, Hammond JMJ (Univ of Cape Town, South Africa)
Chest 101:199–203, 1992 3–19

Background.—Clinical setting—including the duration of hospitalization, immune status, the presence of underlying disease, and the accuracy of routine microbiologic evaluation—is important in planning antibiotic therapy for pneumonia. It is unknown whether these factors apply in the intensive care unit (ICU), however. The spectrum of infectious agents and the effectiveness of routine bacteriologic methods in diagnosing severe pneumonia requiring ICU admission were assessed.

Methods.—The study included 178 patients with severe pneumonia who were admitted to a 10-bed respiratory ICU over a 3-year period. The diagnosis was made on clinical grounds and the etiologic diagnosis on microscopy and culture of sputum or tracheal aspirate. The patients were 117 males and 61 females with a mean age 45 years. There were 95 cases of primary pneumonia, 31 of nosocomial pneumonia, and 28 of aspiration pneumonia; 24 patients were immunocompromised.

Findings.—In general, the agents isolated conformed to the typical patterns for the different types of pneumonia; *Streptococcus pneumoniae* was most common in all types except aspiration pneumonia, where *Staphylococcus aureus* predominated. However, there was a 15% incidence of gram-negative infections, mainly *Klebsiella pneumonia, S. aureus,* and *Legionella pneumophila.* These were much more common than in studies in the community or general hospital environment. There was only 1 case of *Mycoplasma pneumoniae* pneumonia. In gram-positive and gram-negative primary pneumonias, staining of sputum or tracheal aspirate taken on intubation reliably predicted the causative organism when compared with infections proved by blood culture. If there was no positive microbiologic diagnosis, serologic studies were useful, but fiber-optic bronchoscopy was not particularly useful.

Conclusions.—Severe pneumonia necessitating ICU admission may differ in cause from less severe disease, and this should be remembered when empirical antibiotic therapy is chosen. These patients have a high mortality rate and a high incidence of gram-negative and *S. aureus* infections. Fiber-optic bronchoscopy is useful mainly in immunocompromised patients.

▶ Usually, if a patient with pneumonia is sufficiently critical to warrant ICU admission, broad-spectrum antibiotics are administered. This study is a reminder that *S. aureus,* cloxacillin-resistant *S. aureus* in nosocomial infections, the gram-negatives, and *Legionella* need to be covered when selecting antibiotic therapy.—J.M. Mitchell-Savinsky, M.D.

Cardiac

ISCHEMIA/DYSRHYTHMIAS

Intravenous Adenosine in the Emergency Department Management of Paroxysmal Supraventricular Tachycardia

Cairns CB, Niemann JT (Univ of California, Los Angeles)

Ann Emerg Med 20:717–721, 1991 3–20

Background.—Management of paroxysmal supraventricular tachycardia (PSVT) has greatly changed since verapamil treatment for this condition was approved. However, the endogenous adenine nucleotide adenosine offers several important advantages in the emergency department (ED) management of this common rhythm disturbance. This prospective study assessed the effectiveness of adenosine in ED treatment of PSVT.

Methods.—The subjects were 23 adults with a total of 27 episodes of PSVT suggested on the basis of surface ECG criteria. Those with clinical or hemodynamic evidence of hypoperfusion were excluded. Patients received 6 mg of adenosine intravenously as a rapid bolus, followed by 1 to 4 additional 12-mg doses at intervals of 3 to 5 minutes. The patients' age, sex, PSVT rate, pretreatment blood pressure, history of cardiac disease, chronic drug therapy, and response to adenosine were assessed.

Results.—Three patients were excluded after receiving intravenously administered adenosine—2 had atrial flutter and 1 had ventricular tachycardia. The remaining 21 patients had 24 episodes of PSVT. These were 13 women and 8 men with a mean age 51 years, 16 of whom had a history of cardiovascular disease. During PSVT, their mean QRS rate was 181. In all but 1 episode, conversion to sinus rhythm was achieved within 20 to 45 seconds of adenosine administration. In 13 of these cases, however, PSVT recurred within 5 minutes. In each of the recurrences, some other antiarrhythmic drug was needed for conversion to and maintenance of sinus rhythm. Four patients had complications of adenosine treatment, but these were transient and clinically unimportant.

Conclusions.—Although intravenously administered adenosine can convert PSVT in patients in the ED with spontaneous PSVT, recurrence is common. Thus, these patients should be treated with other anti-arrhythmic agents rather than repeated doses of adenosine. Adenosine may be useful in distinguishing among the tachyarrhythmias. Conversion of PSVT might be more likely if the initial dose of adenosine was doubled to 12 mg.

▶ Adenosine is basically a pharmacologic vagal maneuver. The high recurrence rate noted in this study is typical of my clinical experience with adenosine, and for cost purposes, this drug is probably best reserved as a diagnostic tool or for patients with a marginal blood pressure and PSVT. For wide QRS complex tachycardia in "stable" patients, adenosine may be useful. In 1 study, 24 patients with ventricular tachycardia (VT) did not respond to sequential doses of adenosine (.05 mg/kg, .15 mg/kg, and .25 mg/kg given at 2-minute intervals) (1). In another report, a 20-mg intravenous bolus of adenosine terminated the arrhythmia in 1 of 14 patients with VT and 1 of 10 patients with acessory conduction and a wide QRS complex (2). Most importantly, adenosine did not cause major adverse side effects in the above patients, unlike previous reports of verapamil use in these situations. If the wide QRS complex tachycardia does respond to adenosine, it is highly likely that the atrioventricular node was involved.—R.M. McNamara, M.D.

References

1. Griffith MJ, et al: *Lancet* 336:670, 1990.
2. Sharma AD, et al: *Am J Med* 88:337, 1990.

Sudden Arrhythmic Death Without Overt Heart Disease

Wellens HJJ, Lemery R, Smeets JL, Brugada P, Gorgels AP, et al (Academic Hosp Maastricht, The Netherlands)

Circulation 85:I-92S–I-97S, 1992 3–21

Background.—Sudden arrhythmic deaths in the absence of overt heart disease are rare and, because young persons are usually affected, shocking.

Patients.—Nine patients were referred after at least 1 episode of circulatory collapse in the absence of overt heart disease and other known causes of arrhythmia. Ventricular fibrillation was documented in 7 patients.

Findings.—The mean age at the first collapse was 28 years. All patients but 1 were men. No patient had a relevant history, and with 1 exception, the patients had normal ECG findings. Four patients had frequent, closely coupled ventricular premature beats after collapsing. Only 2 patients exhibited ventricular arrhythmia on exercise testing. Fibrillation was initiated during programmed electric stimulation in 3 instances; at least 3 premature stimuli were necessary.

Management and Follow-Up.—One patient died suddenly 21 months after his first collapse. The other 8 patients are living, 2 after receiving an automatic implantable defibrillator because of continuing episodes of ventricular fibrillation despite medical measures. Four patients are receiving amiodarone, 1 in combination with aprindine and 1 with sotalol. Three patients are receiving β-blockers.

Discussion.—Long-term ECG monitoring and exercise testing are of limited value in these patients. In only 1 of the present cases did sympathetic stimulation appear to be important in the genesis of arrhythmia. The world literature suggests an 11% rate of sudden death within a year of diagnosis. Implantation of a defibrillator if the arrhythmia recurs during drug treatment is recommended.

▶ This report of sudden death is particularly disturbing since patients admitted to the study were those without cardiac structural abnormalities, pre-excitation syndromes, electrolyte disturbances, and exposure to arrhythmogenic medications, drugs, or alcohol. Only 1 person was noted to have a family history of sudden death. Given the paucity of risk factors, it seems unlikely that one could predict which patients will suffer from this event. These patients *were* documented to be in ventricular arrhythmia, however, and thus they should not be confused with the young, healthy syncopal victim with whom we are often confronted.—H.D. Unger, M.D.

Clonidine for Patients With Rapid Atrial Fibrillation

Roth A, Kaluski E, Felner S, Heller K, Laniado S (Sackler School of Med, Tel Aviv, Israel)

Ann Intern Med 116:388–390, 1992 3–22

Objective.—Atrial fibrillation is usually treated with digoxin, β-blocking agents, or calcium channel blocking agents. However, many patients may develop adverse reactions to these drugs. Clonidine, a centrally acting selective α-agonist was studied to determine whether it can slow the ventricular rate in hemodynamically stable patients who come to the emergency department with rapid atrial fibrillation.

Patients.—Of 18 hemodynamically stable patients who were evaluated for rapid atrial fibrillation, 9 were randomly assigned to receive clonidine .075 mg orally at baseline and again 2 hours later if the heart rate had

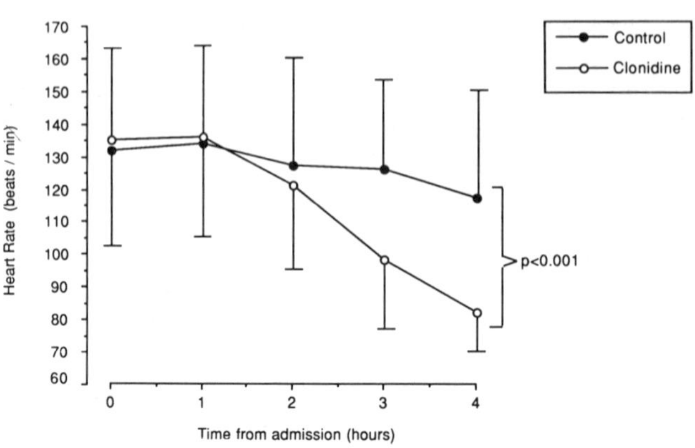

Fig 3–5.—Heart rate. Change in heart rate of 18 patients with rapid anti-fibrillation who were assigned to either oral clonidine (n=9) or no treatment (n=9). (Courtesy of Roth A. Kaluski E, Felner S, et al: *Ann Intern Med* 116:388–390, 1992.)

not decreased by at least 20%, and 9 received no treatment. Patients were monitored for 4 hours.

Results.—During follow-up, the heart rate decreased to below 100 beats per minute in 8 of the 9 clonidine-treated patients and in 2 of the 9 untreated controls (Fig 3–5). The difference in the mean decreases in heart rate between the 2 groups was 38 beats per minute. Six clonidine-treated patients and 1 control patient reverted to normal sinus rhythm. The systolic blood pressure was not significantly affected during follow-up in either group; the mean difference in the decrease between the groups was 1 mm Hg.

Conclusion.—Low-dose clonidine is effective in the treatment of rapid atrial fibrillation in hemodynamically stable patients.

▶ Does clonidine outperform or perpetuate vagal maneuvers (still very effective in the emergency department)? Were patients discharged home on a regimen of clonidine for maintenance of rate or rhythm? The effect demonstrated here, although real, was not proved superior to adenosine for rapid effect or to digoxin for maintenance of the ventricular rate and so remains a curiosity rather than a new standard of care. We have for years been using large doses for hypertensive "urgencies" that probably require no treatment at all.—T. Stair, M.D.

Verapamil Administration to Patients With Contraindications: Is it Associated With Adverse Outcomes?

Kuhn M, Schriger DL (Flinder Med Ctr, Bedford Park, South Australia; Univ of California, Los Angeles)

Ann Emerg Med 20:1094–1099, 1991 3–23

Introduction.—Verapamil was being administered at the study institution to many patients with contraindications. Emergency department (ED) physicians could have been acting out of ignorance or oversight or in a belief that the department's established process criteria were not valid. In reviewing the charts of patients who received verapamil during the study period, the physicians sought to determine whether adverse outcomes were associated with inappropriate use of the drug.

Methods.—All patients older than 12 years of age who had received verapamil between June 1986 and November 1989 were included in the study. To analyze the effects of the drug, the rhythm and rate documented after the final dose that the patient received were recorded. Blood pressure measurements were obtained from nursing records.

Results.—Verapamil was administered to 187 ED patients during the study period. From the group of 166 evaluable patients, 32 had contraindications to use of the drug. Adverse outcomes occurred in 12 of 166 patients, but no deaths were attributed to the use of verapamil. The most significant adverse outcome related to verapamil administration occurred in a man, aged 36 years, in paroxysmal supraventricular tachycardia with a pretreatment blood pressure of 70 palpated. He went into cardiac arrest after receiving 3 verapamil doses. This patient was resuscitated and ultimately recovered. Altogether, 9 patients became hypotensive after verapamil administration. Adverse outcomes occurred in 25% of the patients with contraindications but in only 3% of patients without contraindications to the drug.

Conclusion.—Verapamil should not be given to patients with contraindicated rhythms, low pretreatment blood pressure, or signs of congestive heart failure. Contraindications to the drug should be used as process measures of quality in ED quality assurance programs.

▶ The discussion (but not the data) of this retrospective review perpetuates the belief that verapamil should not be used for regular wide tachycardias. In older patients with known coronary ischemia or younger patients with known cardiomyopathy, this is sage advice since the rhythm is commonly ventricular tachycardia. Further, a patient who is initially hypotensive or who has poor ventricular filling (e.g., a pretreatment ventricular rate of greater than 180 beats per minute) may also deteriorate as a result of verapamil-induced vasodilation should rapid pharmacologic cardioversion occur. However, an otherwise healthy, young patient with a blood pressure of greater than 90 mm Hg during a wide regular tachycardia (ventricular rate less than 280 beats per minute) is unlikely to be harmed by an appropriate dose of verapamil. This agent should be considered for such patients when adenosine and procainamide are unsuccessful or otherwise contraindicated.

The role of calcium chloride administration for averting symptomatic hypotension, when given prior to verapamil use in the setting of mild hypotension and supraventricular tachycardia, remains to be determined. The authors suggest that some of their hypotensive patients were treated with calcium after verapamil administration, but they do not report calcium administration prior to verapamil use. Hence, the authors' rate of hypotensive complications may have been ameliorated had the common practice of calcium pretreatment been used at their institution.—J.R. Heges, M.D.

Reconsiderations of the Routine and Preferential Use of Lidocaine in the Emergent Treatment of Ventricular Arrhythmias

Wesley RC Jr, Resh W, Zimmerman D (VA Med Ctr, Long Beach, Calif; Univ of California, Irvine Med Ctr, Orange)

Crit Care Med 19:1439–1444, 1991 3–24

Background.—Although it is widely used, lidocaine has questionable value as an anti-arrhythmic and antifibrillatory agent. The recent literature is studied on lidocaine's effects on ischemic and nonischemic ventricular arrhythmias, energy and current requirements for defibrillation, and the propensity for asystole during cardiac arrest.

Effect on Arrhythmias.—Theoretically, lidocaine does appear to have a basis for use in the treatment of acute ischemic arrhythmias. This conclusion is based primarily on its voltage- and pH-dependent binding and inactivation of sodium channels in ischemia. However, experimental and clinical studies show that lidocaine does not prevent lethal ventricular arrhythmias during acute myocardial ischemia. It may be somewhat more effective when given by intracoronary infusion. There is no theoretical basis and no scientific evidence for the use of lidocaine for sustained, life-threatening arrhythmias in patients without acute ischemia.

Effect on Defibrillation.—Lidocaine does increase the ventricular fibrillation threshold, but its efficacy is not uniformly supported. It does appear to have significant detrimental effects on countershock efficacy in that it increases current and energy requirements for defibrillation. Further, especially in acidosis and low membrane potential, lidocaine may promote a conduction block.

Lidocaine-Induced Asystole.—Meta-analysis of controlled studies of prophylactic lidocaine suggests that the drug may increase the propensity for asystole during cardiac arrest. This may result from diminutions in conduction and automaticity that are less apparent in the normally functioning sinoatrial node. Another possible mechanism is attenuation of sympathetic nervous system outflow.

Conclusions.—The clinical relevance of lidocaine's demonstrated antifibrillatory effect is questioned. Its usefulness for patients in cardiac arrest is limited, and it may reduce the efficacy of countershock therapy or induce asystole. Guidelines for the management of cardiac arrest should reconsider the use of lidocaine.

▶ This is a provocative article because it challenges one of our standard practices of cardiac therapeutics. Not many of us were surprised when calcium was recognized as, at best, worthless for cardiac arrest. We perhaps needed to be convinced to largely eliminate sodium bicarbonate from advanced cardiac life support protocols. But lidocaine?

Maybe, this review summarizes the case against using lidocaine for converting ventricular fibrillation and for treating sustained ventricular arrhythmias in the absence of acute ischemia. In fact, the authors argue that lidocaine may render ventricular fibrillation more difficult to convert and may actually cause asystole. They believe that although there is at least a theoretical basis for the effectiveness of lidocaine in treating ischemic ventricular dysrhythmias, both clinical and experimental data fail to establish enhanced survival. They urge a reconsideration of the use of lidocaine in the management of cardiac arrest.

While it is certainly frustrating to read that our standard therapy may be worthless, there is no question that our current modalities are not very effective. It is hoped that they will bear little resemblance to our future practices. The only way to achieve better resuscitation results is to literally question everything—from the mechanics of compression to every one of the drugs.

So what should the clinician do? It is my opinion that at this point in time the case against lidocaine is not yet proved. I believe that we should continue to use lidocaine until its lack of effectiveness is clearly demonstrated (see Abstract 1–7).—M.J. Bresler, M.D.

Clinical and Electrophysiologic Characteristics of Exercise-Related Idiopathic Ventricular Tachycardia

Mont L, Seixas T, Brugada P, Brugada J, Simonis F, et al (Academic Hosp Maastricht, The Netherlands)

Am J Cardiol 68:897–900, 1991 3–25

Background.—It has been suggested that the idiopathic ventricular tachycardia (VT) that appears during or in relation to exercise is a catecholamine-sensitive arrhythmia that cannot be easily reproduced during programmed stimulation unless isoproterenol infusion is given. The clinical and electrophysiologic characteristics of patients having exercise-related idiopathic VT were compared with patients having VT not related to exercise.

Methods.—In a group of 53 patients with VT and no recognizable heart disease, 37 patients in group 1 had episodes of VT mainly related to exercise and 16 patients in group 2 had VT with no relation to exercise. Programmed electric stimulation was performed in all patients, and 49 patients underwent a symptom-limited exercise test on a treadmill with the Bruce protocol.

Findings.—The 37 patients in group 1 with idiopathic VT related to exercise were younger and more often had dizziness during VT as compared with the 16 patients in group 2 with non–exercise-related VT. Four patients in group 1 needed cardioversion to terminate the arrhythmia as compared with 6 patients in group 2. Exercise-related VT induced by programmed ventricular stimulation alone occurred in about 50% in both groups. In group 1, VT was induced more easily by isoproterenol infusion, and electrically induced VT was faster. Anti-arrhythmic therapy was most effective with class III drugs and least effective with β-blocking agents. One patient with non–exercise-related VT died suddenly of unknown causes.

Conclusions.—In this study, most patients with idiopathic VT had episodes related to exercise. Several distinctive clinical and ECG characteristics were observed in these patients, but no differences were observed in their response to anti-arrhythmic drugs. The relation of arrhythmia to exercise had no effect on long-term prognosis.

▶ The most important message in this article for emergency physicians is that our current, commonly used drugs, β-blockers, may have little or no significant effect as prevention of idiopathic VT in younger patients. The article states that "it is possible that β-blockers are partially effective, but fail to prevent VT when a high adrenergic tone is present." Clearly, further studies need to be done.—E.J. Lucid, M.D.

The Use of External, Noninvasive Pacing for the Termination of Ventricular Tachycardia in the Emergency Department Setting

Grubb BP, Temesy-Armos P, Hahn H, Elliott L (Med College of Ohio, Toledo)

Ann Emerg Med 21:174–176, 1992 3–26

Objective.—Recent studies conducted in the electrophysiology laboratory and in-hospital settings have suggested that external noninvasive cardiac pacing may be effective in terminating both ventricular and supraventricular tachycardias. The potential usefulness of external noninvasive pacing in the termination of wide-complex tachycardia was evaluated in the emergency department (ED) setting.

Patients.—Six patients seen in the ED with wide-complex, hemodynamically stable tachycardia (mean rate, 158 beats per minute) presumed to be of ventricular origin were treated. Each patient underwent asynchronous overdrive pacing by using a modified external pacemaker at a pulse amplitude of 120 mA and a rate of 200 pulses per minute. Each patient received 1 to 3 mg. of midazolam intravenously before pacing.

Outcome.—External cardiac pacing successfully terminated tachycardia in all 6 patients; 2 required 2 attempts, and 1 required 3 attempts with external pacing for termination. The procedure was well tolerated and required only a modest amount of sedation (mean midazolam dose, 1.6 mg). There were no complications. Subsequent electrophysiologic studies confirmed the ventricular origin of each tachycardia.

Conclusion.—External overdrive cardiac pacing appears to be a promising method for the termination of sustained, hemodynamically stable ventricular tachycardia in the ED setting. External overdrive pacing should not be attempted unless backup defibrillation capacity is present.

► This article reviews the use of an external pacemaker for termination of ventricular tachycardias by overdrive pacing. At the reporting institution, the investigators modified the external pacemaker to achieve a pulse rate of 200 beats per minute. Most external pacers cannot pulse at that rate. For example, the Physio-Control Life Pack 9P can achieve a rate of only 170 pulses per minute, which is inadequate to overdrive some rhythms. The reported technique does require sedation of the patient. The advantage of the technique over cardioversion is undetermined. However, the authors state that "the relatively low sedative requirements for external pacing make it an attractive option for patients (for those with severe lung diseases who may not tolerate the larger sedative doses usually required in cardioversions)".—E.J. Reisdorff, M.D.

Successful Resuscitation and Neurologic Recovery From Refractory Ventricular Fibrillation After Magnesium Sulfate Administration

Tobey RC, Birnbaum GA, Allegra JR, Horowitz MS, Plosay JJ III (Morristown Mem Hosp, NJ; Mountainside Hosp, Montclair, NJ; Santa Monica Hosp, Calif)

Ann Emerg Med 21:92–96, 1992 3–27

Background.—Magnesium has been useful in treating a wide range of arrhythmias either with or without hypomagnesemia, and studies have shown that an infusion of magnesium can reduce the incidence of arrhythmias occurring after acute myocardial infarction. No literature was found on the efficacy of magnesium sulfate in the treatment of sustained ventricular fibrillation. A patient with refractory ventricular fibrillation responded to a single parenteral dose of magnesium sulfate.

Case Report.—A 46-year-old man collapsed after a brief period of light-headedness and shortness of breath associated with diaphoresis and left arm pain. His medical history included an inferior wall myocardial infarction 8 years earlier. Cardiopulmonary resuscitation was begun immediately, and basic and advanced cardiac life support measures were continued for 62 minutes. He remained in ventricular fibrillation despite treatment with a prehospital defibrillator, lidocaine, bretyllium, and other measures. After intravenous administration of 4 g of magnesium sulfate in the emergency department, successful defibrillation was accomplished. The patient had multiple complications but was alert and neurologically intact at discharge on the 96th hospital day. After 3 years, the only lasting sequela was a mild left-sided limp.

Discussion.—Magnesium's effect on cardiac rhythm may result from its interactions with the sodium-potassium pump or with cell membrane channels, but it is not known whether magnesium is effective only because it repletes an intracellular or extracellular magnesium deficiency or because of some intrinsic anti-arrhythmic property irrespective of magnesium levels. Similarly, the optimal anti-arrhythmic dose of magnesium is not known. Magnesium sulfate has been effective in cases of serious refractory ventricular arrhythmias, and it has been suggested that it may alleviate "reperfusion injury."

► Obviously, we need to study the effects of magnesium sulfate in the cardiac arrest situation in a controlled fashion. But in the meantime, I am going to try using a bolus of magnesium sulfate when treating patients with refractory ventricular fibrillation (see also Abstract 3–11).—E. Ruiz, M.D.

Life-Threatening Ventricular Arrhythmias in Patients With Silent Myocardial Ischemia Due to Coronary Artery Spasm

Myerburg RJ, Kessler KM, Mallon SM, Cox MM, deMarchena E, et al (Univ of Miami, Fla)
N Engl J Med 326:1451–1455, 1992 3–28

Objective.—In patients with coronary atherosclerosis, the occurrence of silent myocardial ischemia may be associated with increased risk of adverse cardiac events, including possible death. Research has yet to define the association between silent ischemia and ventricular arrhythmias, however. The associations among coronary artery spasm, degrees of silent myocardial ischemia, and the onset and mechanisms of potentially fatal ventricular arrhythmias in survivors of cardiac arrest were studied.

Methods.—The patients were drawn from a long-term study of 356 patients who survived out-of-hospital cardiac arrest during an 11-year period. Data on arrhythmias, coronary anatomy, and responses to ergonovine testing to provoke coronary artery spasm were collected in prospective fashion. The patients had no flow-limiting coronary artery lesions, previous myocardial infarctions, or other structural causes of cardiac arrest. Both invasive and noninvasive techniques were used to analyze associations between silent myocardial ischemia caused by coronary artery spasm and the occurrence and characteristics of life-threatening ventricular arrhythmias.

Findings.—In 5 patients with induced and/or spontaneous focal coronary artery spasm, silent myocardial ischemic events were associated with the initiation of potentially fatal ventricular arrhythmias. There were 4 men and 1 woman ranging in age from 43 to 68 years. In 2 of these, the onset of the arrhythmia was correlated with reperfusion, not with ischemia itself. The arrhythmia was inducible during electrophysiologic testing in only 1 patient. The dosage of calcium-entry-blocking agents—verapamil, diltiazem, or nifedipine—was titrated against the ability of ergonovine to provoke arterial spasm in 4 patients. This successfully prevented provocation of the spasm and arrhythmias in all 4 patients.

Conclusions.—In patients without flow-limiting structural lesions of the coronary arteries, silent myocardial infarction resulting from coronary artery spasm can lead to life-threatening arrhythmias. Further studies of more patients with more advanced coronary artery lesions are called for. If these findings are confirmed, it would provide an additional justification for intensive anti-ischemic therapy in patients with silent ischemia.

▶ Silent ischemia is generally detected by continuous mapping of the ECG for ST-segment shifts, a tool that will probably soon find its way to the emergency department (ED). This report identifies 5 patients in a high-risk group with major dysrhythmias due to silent ischemia despite relatively normal coronary arteries. In the ED, the discovery of "silent ischemia" in the future will be predominantly useful in patients with normal ECG findings after an episode of chest pain. These patients will almost all have significant coronary lesions upon further study.—R.M. McNamara, M.D.

Five-Year Follow-Up of Young Adults Visiting an Emergency Unit Because of Atypical Chest Pain

Roll M, Kollind M, Theorell T (Danderyd Hosp; Karolinska Inst, Stockholm, Sweden)

J Intern Med 231:59–65, 1992 3–29

Objective.—In young patients arriving at the emergency department (ED) with chest pain, no obvious organic cause is found in most cases. These patients are generally reassured that they have no serious disease and sent home without follow-up. A 5-year follow-up of young patients with unexplained chest pain was conducted.

Methods.—Over an 8-week period, 64 patients were admitted to the ED for acute chest pain of no obvious organic cause. There were 35 men and 29 women with a mean age of 37.6 years. These patients all underwent thorough medical and psychosocial evaluation. Another group of 51 patients—30 men and 21 women, with a mean age of 34.6 years—who did not undergo the thorough investigation were also studied. A mean of 67 to 68 months later, both groups of patients returned to the hospital for a personal interview. A comparison group of 32 normal subjects was also interviewed.

Findings.—Chest pain was reported by 50% of the investigated patients and 45% of the noninvestigated patients as compared with 13% of the controls. The investigative patients were also more likely to report depressive states—thus the thorough examination performed in the research protocol had no sustained therapeutic effect when compared

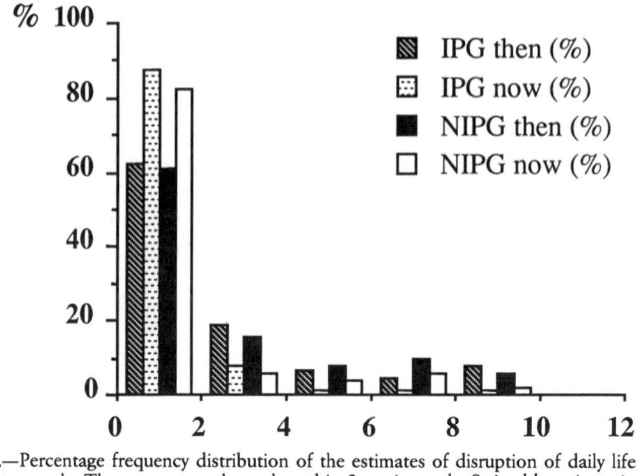

Fig 3–6.—Percentage frequency distribution of the estimates of disruption of daily life on a 12-cm visual analogue scale. The answers are here clusted in 2-cm intervals. *Striped box,* investigation patient (IP) group at emergency visit; *dotted box,* IP group at follow-up; *solid box,* nonvestigation patient (NIP) group at emergency visit; and *white box,* NIP group at follow-up. (Courtesy of Roll M, Kollind M,Theorell T: *J Intern Med* 231:59–65, 1991.)

with routine emergency care. The number of intervening attacks varied greatly, with a median of 5. There was a negative correlation between outcome and tension, anxiety, and the number of physician consultations. Both groups of patients had significantly lower scores for disruption of daily life at follow-up than after the initial examination (Fig 3–6).

Conclusions.—Chest pain of no obvious organic cause in a young patient seems to have an excellent physical prognosis. On the other hand, many of these patients continue to have pain and depression and continue to use medical resources. Some treatment strategy should be devised for these patients, particularly those with psychological symptoms and a history of many physician consultations.

▶ Their definition of "young adults" was less than 40 years old. We know that anxiety attacks and conversion reactions with chest wall muscles as the stress organ are common causes of chest pain in the ED, but is it cost-effective to begin a discussion of these psychological subjects on the initial ED visit? The rare young adult who does have cardiac ischemia missed in the ED in this country is liable to sue, and our experience suggests that he is more likely to sue if psychiatric follow-up is suggested. I concentrate on physical dangers on the first visit and defer discussing patient insight until he makes repeat visits with chest pain.—T. Stair, M.D.

A Tool for Judging Coronary Care Unit Admission Appropriateness, Valid for Both Real-Time and Retrospective Use: A Time-Insensitive Predictive Instrument (TIPI) for Acute Cardiac Ischemia: A Multicenter Study

Selker HP, Griffith JL, D'Agostino RB (New England Med Ctr and Tufts Univ, Boston, Mass)

Med Care 29:610–627, 1991 3–30

Introduction.—Potentially unnecessary coronary care unit (CCU) admissions in the United States may waste up to $3 billion each year in direct costs alone. An acute ischemia—predictive instrument was previously developed, but it was not specifically designed for retrospective use. A time-insensitive predictive instrument (TIPI) that is valid for both real-time clinical use and retrospective review has been developed and assessed.

Methods.—Prospective data at 6 hospitals were collected on 5,773 emergency patients with symptoms of acute cardiac ischemia. The TIPI instrument, based on logistic regression, was developed with use of data from 3,453 patients seen during the first year. The TIPI used 7 easily obtained clinical factors to express a patient's likelihood of having acute cardiac ischemia over a range of 0% to 100%. Four risk categories of similar size were created with cutoff points of 10%, 25%, and 55%, and the instrument was prospectively tested on 2,320 patients seen during the second year.

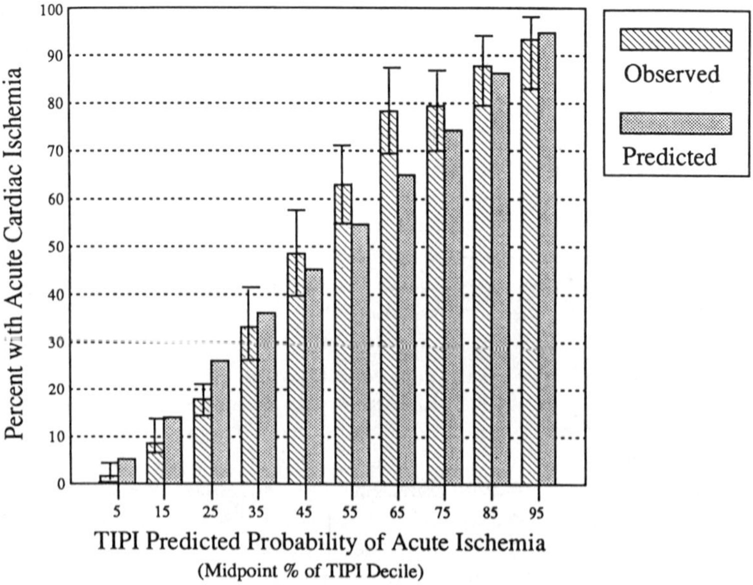

Fig 3–7.—Prospective test of the TIPI's calibration: comparison of the observed percentages of patients with acute cardiac ischemia and the percentage predicted by the TIPI. Bars represent 95% confidence intervals for the observed ACI rate. (Courtesy of Selker HP, Griffith JL, D'Agostino RB: *Med Care* 29:610–627, 1991.)

Results.—Diagnostic performance of the TIPI was excellent, with a receiver-operating characteristic curve area of .88. Average values were 59% for patients who proved to have acute ischemia vs. 21% for those who did not. The difference held even for patients with various dispositions, including inappropriate ones. Ischemia was present in only 1.6% of the low-risk group as compared with 81.6% of the high-risk group (Fig 3–7). Across hospitals, the overall mean value for emergency department patients was 33%, while that for CCU patients was 50%, which reflects a 52% increased likelihood of ischemia in the latter group. For emergency patients who were sent home, the mean TIPI value was 18%. One of the study hospitals had significantly different values for patients seen in the emergency department, admitted to the CCU, or sent home than the others did.

Conclusions.—The TIPI instrument for predicting acute cardiac ischemia has proved accurate and reliable. It can be applied to real-time CCU triage as well as to quality assurance and cost containment; as such, it may enhance cooperation among clinicians, institutions, payers, and review agencies.

▶ When using the authors' earlier version of this tool, I found limitations at both the high and low ends: a chief complaint of chest pain was already positive in 2 categories, and any 1 of the several ECG criteria was good for a night in a monitored bed. Although much evolved, these criteria still leave out many of the risk factors and circumstantial probabilities that emergency physicians actually use to make admission decisions. I was surprised there was not more dispersion of the incidence of cardiac ischemia among hospitals. Their new logistic regression is more accurate than their old linear regression equation, but this methodology has already been eclipsed by the more accurate, artificial neural network published by Baxt (1).—T. Stair, M.D.

Reference

1. Baxt WG: *Ann Intern Med* 115:843–848, 1991.

Effect of Epinephrine on the Ability of End-Tidal Carbon Dioxide Readings to Predict Initial Resuscitation From Cardiac Arrest

Callaham M, Barton C, Matthay M (Univ of California, San Francisco)

Crit Care Med 20:337–343, 1992 3–31

Purpose.—Previous studies have found a decrease in expired end-tidal carbon dioxide (CO_2) tension in patients given epinephrine, particularly large doses. This could decrease the ability of end-tidal CO_2 measurement to predict resuscitation from cardiac arrest. The physicians sought to confirm this effect of epinephrine in patients in cardiac arrest.

Methods.—The subjects were 64 patients in cardiac arrest with a mean age of 70 years. Thirty-five patients were men. Epinephrine doses ranged from 1 to 15 mg intravenously. End-tidal CO_2 was measured on arrival, before the first dose of epinephrine was given, and 4 minutes afterward.

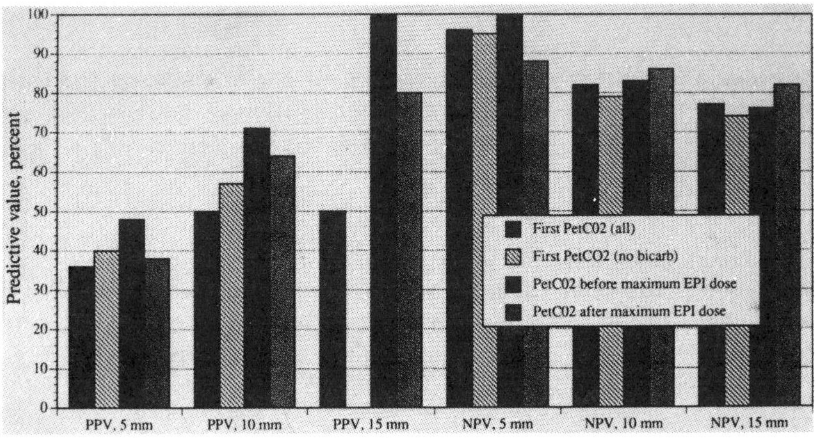

Fig 3–8.—Positive predictive value (*PPV*) and negative predictive value (*NPV*) of end-tidal carbon dioxide (CO_2) for return of spontaneous circulation at various end-tidal CO_2 thresholds (*Pet*CO_2). *Abbreviations: bicarb,* bicarbonate; *EPI,* epinephrine. (Courtesy of Callaham M, Barton C, Matthay M: *Crit Care Med* 20:337–343, 1992.)

Results.—None of the patients lived to be discharged from the hospital. After the administration of epinephrine, end-tidal CO_2 decreased an average of .3 torr. Of patients with a return of pulse, the decrease was 2 torr as compared with an increase of .3 torr for those with no return of pulse. Thirty-three percent of the patients had no change, 28% had an increase, and 39% had a decrease. Alteration in end-tidal CO_2 after epinephrine was not correlated with regaining a pulse, although most patients with a decrease did regain a pulse. A first end-tidal CO_2 of 10 torr had a positive predictive value for a return of pulse of 50% and a negative predictive value of 82%. These values were 71% and 83% just before the administration of epinephrine and 64% and 86% 4 minutes afterward (Fig 3–8). The occurrence of a decrease in end-tidal CO_2 after epinephrine carried a positive predictive value of 53% and a negative predictive value of 92%. The most accurate predictors of resuscitation were readings taken after initial stabilization and before epinephrine administration.

Conclusions.—In patients with cardiac arrest, epinephrine may decrease end-tidal CO_2 tension. However, it does so in an unpredictable way and does not abolish the predictive value of the measurement. The most accurate measurement appears to be that taken after several minutes of initial resuscitation.

▶ The use of end-tidal CO_2 monitoring in cardiac arrest has been somewhat of a disappointment. In the laboratory where it can be carefully controlled, it does seem to have a predictive effect on resuscitation. However, in clinical studies, the results have been mixed at best. This probably has to do with the fact that patients have longer downtimes than do most of the animal studies and have an etiology of cardiac arrest that is different from the laboratory animal.—W.H. Spivey, M.D.

Transesophageal Echocardiography in Emergency Medicine and Critical Care

Shenoy MM, Dhala A, Khanna A (Coney Island Hosp; State Univ of New York, Brooklyn)

Am J Emerg Med 9:580–587, 1991 3–32

Introduction.—A diagnostically adequate echocardiographic examination requires an optimal acoustic window over which the transducer can be applied and the ultrasonic beam can be directed at the heart. In patients with narrow intercostal spaces, emphysema, obesity, or abdominal distension and in post-cardiac surgery patients the images and data obtained with conventional echocardiography may be suboptimal. Because there are virtually no interposing structures between the esophagus and the heart, images obtained with transesophageal echocardiography (TEE) can provide strikingly detailed and clear images. Furthermore, anatomic details that are rarely seen by conventional echocardiography

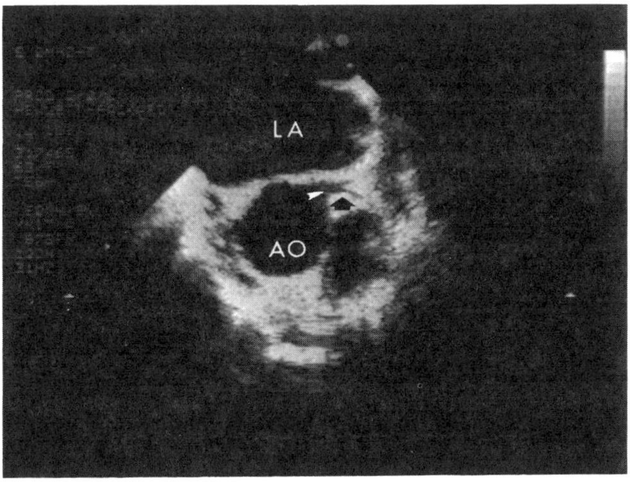

Fig 3–9.—Transesophageal echocardiographic image showing the normal aortic root (AO), the ostium of the left coronary artery (*white arrow*), and its bifurcation (*black arrow*). LA = left atrium. (Courtesy of Shenoy MM, Dhala A, Khanna A: *Ann Emerg Med* 9:580–587, 1991.)

such as the proximal coronary arteries, the atrial appendages, and the pulmonary veins are easily visualized (Fig 3–9).

Indications.—Transesophageal echocardiography can be used in any clinical situation where conventional echocardiography is not feasible but where obtaining information is imperative. There are also many evolving indications for the usefulness of TEE in emergency medicine, such as in suspected aortic dissection. A multicenter study that compared the diagnostic accuracy of TEE, CT, and aortography in diagnosing acute aortic dissection revealed that echocardiography had high sensitivity and high negative predictive value and was not inferior to either CT or angiography. When echocardiography was negative, no dissection was detected by CT or angiography. Moreover, TEE was superior in providing rapid diagnosis since the examination usually took only 15 minutes. TEE is a safe procedure, and major complications such as esophageal perforation are extremely rare.

Outlook.—Because instruments with smaller tips and calibers incorporating multiplane transducers have already been developed and 360-degree imaging transducers are currently being developed, it is expected that the imaging capability and diagnostic accuracy of TEE will be greatly enhanced in the near future.

▶ Transesophageal echocardiography in emergency medicine provides another acronym (TEE) for hospital vernacular. It is hoped that it will prove to be a superior, rapid technique for diagnosing suspected aortic dissection and be user friendly as well—G.V. Anderson, M.D.

Aortic Pressure During Human Cardiac Arrest: Identification of Pseudo-Electromechanical Dissociation

Paradis NA, Martin GB, Goetting MG, Rivers EP, Feingold M, et al (New York Univ, NY; Henry Ford Hosp, Detroit, Mich)

Chest 101:123–128, 1992 3–33

Background.—Electromechanical dissociation (EMD) is defined as electrical activity of the heart without cardiac output and has a grim prognosis. Often considered a single clinical entity, EMD is actually a *heterogeneous* pathophysiologic state. In this prospective study of adult patients who underwent cardiac arrest and died suddenly, patients were classified on the basis of whether or not they had aortic pulse pressures. The ECG findings and rates of return of spontaneous circulation were compared in the 2 groups.

Patients.—Two hundred consecutive patients with a mean age of 67 years were designated as having pseudo-EMD if they had regular aortic pulse pressures < 60 mm Hg synchronous with ECG depolarizations or as having true EMD if they were without aortic pulse pressures. Fifty-four patients were seen in EMD, and EMD later developed in 40 during their resuscitation. Of these 94 patients with EMD, 39 were found to have pseudo-EMD.

Results.—Patients with pseudo-EMD had significantly more witnessed arrests, higher oxygen pressure (arterial) values, and lower carbon dioxide pressure (arterial) values than did those in true EMD. Patients with pseudo-EMD had shorter QR and QRS durations than did those in true EMD. The resting aortic pressure was 28 mm Hg for patients with pseudo-EMD, significantly higher than that of 18 mm Hg for patients in true EMD. Patients with pseudo-EMD had resting aortic pressures ranging from 8 to 58 mm Hg, with a mean aortic pulse pressure of 6.3 mm Hg. Their pulse rates ranged from 15 to 180 beats per minute, with a mean of 65 beats per minute. Fourteen of 39 patients in pseudo-EMD experienced a return of spontaneous circulation after standard therapy including epinephrine doses of 1 mg, significantly more than the 8 of 55 patients in true EMD who responded to low-dose epinephrine. Similarly, 14 of 18 patients with pseudo-EMD had a return of spontaneous circulation after high-dose epinephrine, significantly more than the 6 of 26 patients in true EMD who responded to high-dose epinephrine. All patients who experienced a return of spontaneous circulation died after intensive therapy was terminated.

Conclusions.—Patients with EMD can range from those with normotension to those with complete absence of perfusion. Patients with detectable aortic pulse pressures appear to respond better to epinephrine than do those with true EMD, and high-dose epinephrine may be considered in the treatment of these patients.

▶ This article required careful reading to accurately interpret. The choice of the term "pseudo-EMD" is unfortunate because it implies that these patients are not in EMD when, in fact, the conclusion of the article is that they are in EMD. The most important thing to gain from reading this article is that the definition of EMD should be expanded to include patients who have some cardiac output and that these patients have a better prognosis than those with no cardiac output. The article is well worth reading carefully.—E.J. Lucid, M.D.

Systolic and Diastolic Time Intervals in the Critically Ill Patient
Máttar Z, Shoemaker WC, Diament D, Lomar A, Lopes AC, et al (Hosp São Luiz, São Paulo, Brazil; King/Drew Med Ctr, Los Angeles)
Crit Care Med 19:1382–1386, 1991 3–34

Background.—Early investigations of cardiac failure focused solely on the inotropic or systolic behavior of the heart, but it is clear that both systolic and diastolic dysfunction can produce hemodynamic abnormalities. The first derivative of impedance waveform provided by the thoracic electric bioimpedance technique permits evaluation of the diastolic period. The application of impedance waveform tracing and its use in evaluating both systolic and diastolic time intervals were reviewed.

Patients.—Nine hundred thirteen thoracic electric bioimpedance tracings were obtained from 15 normal controls and 85 critically ill adult patients. The monitor was coupled to a 2-channel strip-chart recorder in 86% of the tracings. The waveform of the first derivative of thoracic electric bioimpedance was used to calculate systolic time intervals of the cardiac cycle, or the pre-ejection period–left ventricular ejection time ratio, and diastolic time intervals, or the isovolumic relaxation period–filling time ratio.

Findings.—The normative values in the control subjects were a mean pre-ejection period–left ventricular ejection time ratio of .4 and a mean ratio of the isovolumic relaxation period–filling time of .35. In a subgroup of 17 critically ill patients, systolic functions compared by the ejection fraction displayed on the thoracic electric bioimpedance monitor and by the radionuclide technique were 57 and 58, respectively. In 9 of the 17 patients with a low systolic index, increased diastolic time ratios with normal or near-normal systolic time intervals were documented.

Conclusions.—Both systolic and diastolic time intervals can be investigated noninvasively by the thoracic electric bioimpedance technique. A study of both time intervals can provide a better understanding of left ventricular heart function and may have therapeutic implications.

▶ As more emergency physicians become involved with highly monitored patients, in formal critical care units as well as observation centers adjacent to emergency departments, familiarity with available technology becomes imperative. The authors identify a means to provide noninvasive cardiac output monitoring utilizing thoracic electric bioimpedance measurements. Of importance to this technique was their finding that suggests that a low-stroke volume index was due to a reduction in left ventricular diastolic function rather than a compromising contractility. The effect of currently employed drugs could similarly be noninvasively investigated to better understand their overall impact on the cardiac-compromised patients.—D.K. Wagner, M.D.

Postpericardiotomy and Postmyocardial Infarction Syndrome Presenting as Noncardiac Pulmonary Edema

Kassanoff AH, Martirossian MG (Presbyterian Hosp, Dallas, Tex)

Chest 99:1410–1414, 1991 3–35

Background.—Symptoms of postpericardiotomy and post–myocardial infarction syndromes classically occur 1 to 4 weeks after heart injury. In the 3 patients described, acute pulmonary edema developed with no apparent cause within 2 to 3 days of cardiac injury.

Case 1.—A 75-year-old man had an acute myocardial infarction requiring a temporary pacemaker. During hospitalization he became progressively hypoxemic despite the administration of oxygen, intravenous nitroglycerine, diuretics, and captopril, and pulmonary edema developed. There was no mitral regurgitation, ventricular septal defect, or pericardial effusion. The patient improved dramatically after receiving methylprednisolone.

Case 2.—A 57-year-old woman had undergone coronary artery bypass surgery. She had no apparent problems in the immediate postoperative period, but pulmonary edema developed 48 hours after surgery. There was no evidence of congestive heart failure. Corticosteroid administration led to prompt improvement.

Case 3.—A 56-year-old man had also undergone coronary artery bypass surgery. Progressive hypoxemia developed on the second postoperative day. Pulmonary edema was found without evidence of volume overload. Dramatic improvement followed prednisone therapy.

Conclusion.—Because all 3 patients had a history of myocardial or pericardial damage, pulmonary edema may have resulted from an acute autoimmune mechanism precipitated by acute heart injury in the presence of already existing antiheart antibodies. Without recognition of the autoimmune possibility and prompt high-dose corticosteroid therapy, the patients might not have survived. This syndrome may not be uncommon and should not be confused with congestive heart failure, adult respiratory distress syndrome, or other causes of pulmonary edema.

▶ Autoimmune postpericardiotomy and post–myocardial infarction pulmonary edema may represent an additional cause of pulmonary edema in the absence of heart failure. Emergency physicians should suspect this condition when patients with a prior history of pericardial or myocardial injury develop pulmonary edema in the setting of a new cardiac event and they do not respond to standard measures for heart failure. The diagnosis is supported by the finding of good ventricular function on the echocardiogram or cardiac output catheter and by an elevated sedimentation rate. Intravenous steroids appear to be effective therapy.—J.R. Hedges, M.D.

Incidence and Characteristics of Preventable Iatrogenic Cardiac Arrests

Bedell SE, Deitz DC, Leeman D, Delbanco TL (Harvard Med School, Boston; Beth Israel Hosp, Boston, Mass)

JAMA 265:2815–2820, 1991 3–36

Introduction.—Iatrogenic disorders often result in major morbidity and mortality for hospitalized patients. Cardiac arrest which is a major complication of iatrogenic illness, was studied in 1 hospital to determine whether the cardiac arrest in resuscitated patients could have been avoided if early signs and symptoms had been recognized and treated appropriately.

Methods.—All patients undergoing CPR in a university teaching hospital in 1981 were assessed within 24 hours of cardiac arrest. Data were retrospectively obtained from the medical record of each patient to determine the possible relationships between iatrogenic complications and cardiac arrest: Reasons for an iatrogenic illness included complications from procedures, medication errors, and insufficient response to physiologic parameters. One investigator reviewed all 201 in-hospital arrests, and 3 reviewers examined a random group of 58 patients whose cardiac arrests were not thought to be iatrogenic at the initial screening.

Results.—Twenty-eight (14%) of the 203 patients with cardiopulmonary arrest in whom resuscitation was attempted had an iatrogenic cardiac arrest. Resuscitation successfully restored the pulse and blood pressure in 20 (71%), whereas 8 (29%) of the patients died. Nine of the 20 survived, and 11 were discharged from the hospital, a 39% (11 of 28 patients) survival rate among patients with iatrogenic cardiac arrest. This is statistically better than the overall survival rate of 11% (20 of 175 patients). Survival rates were the same for both groups after 3 years of follow-up, however. Demographic factors and previous cardiac illness did not influence the outcome. Patients with iatrogenic arrest had less of a chance of cardiogenic shock before the arrest but were more likely to be using digoxin or other anti-arryhthmic medications than those not having an iatrogenic arrest. The most frequent mechanism of arrest was ventricular tachycardia or fibrillation. Fifteen (54%) of the iatrogenic cardiac arrests were caused by drugs, usually in the form of avoidable medication errors. Four procedures and 7 cases of omission errors led to iatrogenic cardiac arrest.

Implications.—Fourteen percent of cardiac arrests in a group of resuscitated hospitalized patients during 1981 were iatrogenic. The most common causes of the arrests included medications, procedures, and a lack of attention to clinical signs and symptoms of patient difficulty. These findings suggest that many cases of iatrogenic cardiac arrest can be prevented by heightened awareness of drug toxicity and increased attention to patient monitoring.

▶ I would have suspected that the risk of iatrogenic disease stemming from medication errors and toxic drug effects would have been greater in patients with renal failure. This was not the case in this study. I presume that since physicians *expect* complications in this subset of patients, we are particularly mindful of the type and dose of medication we prescribe to this group. Unfortunately, we do not pay the same close attention to the interactions of age and weight on the pharmacodynamics of drugs we prescribe to patients with normal renal function. This type of neglect was responsible for 44% of the potentially unavoidable arrests.

It was disturbing that twice as many patients on the surgical service (on a percentage basis) suffered an iatrogenic arrest as those on the medical service. The commonly held misconception that surgical housestaff are less attentive to "details" of patient management is not helped by these data.

Despite the fact that the frequencies of iatrogenic and potentially avoidable deaths remained the same in this hospital when the initial study was repeated 5 years later, there is hope that ongoing quality assurance in this area will improve a hospital's performance. At my institution, the "code 99" committee is responsible for reviewing all resuscitations. To date, we have concerned ourselves with monitoring compliance with family notification, code sheet completion, etc. After reading this article, I think that the chairman of the committee (HDU) will suggest that we begin evaluating the medical care prior to the code and look for these potentially avoidable errors in practice.—H.D. Unger, M.D.

Emergency Department Interpretation of Electrocardiograms
Westdorp EJ, Gratton MC, Watson WA (Univ of Missouri, Kansas City)
Ann Emerg Med 21:541–544, 1992 3–37

Background.—Little is known about how emergency physicians compare with cardiologists in the interpretation of ECG results. The concordance of these 2 groups' interpretations of ECG results was investigated.

Methods.—Seven hundred sixteen ECG recordings were reviewed in a retrospective cohort study. One hundred forty-three patients with an abnormal emergency department ECG result had been discharged from the emergency department. The results were interpreted by both an emergency physician and a cardiologist. The cardiologist's final interpretation was defined as the correct one. Discordance was defined as any abnormality that the emergency physician did not identify.

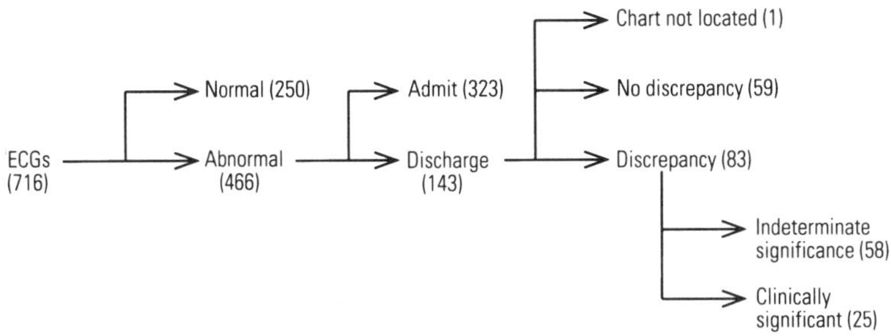

Fig 3–10.—Results of emergency department ECG recordings. (Courtesy of Westdorp EJ, Gratton MC, Watson WA: *Ann Emerg Med* 21:541–544, 1992.)

Findings.—The overall discordance between the 2 physician groups was 58%. Twenty-five discordant interpretations were probably significant clinically (Fig 3–10) and represented missed ischemia, infarct, and abnormal rhythm. Emergency physicians most often missed evidence of ischemia or infarct of the anterior wall and atrial fibrillation. Of the 83 patients with discordant interpretations, 21 were lost to follow-up. Two had a discrepancy that would have changed patient care.

Conclusions.—The overall discordance between emergency physician interpretation and cardiologist interpretation of ECGs was 58%. Most emergency department misinterpretations were judged unlikely to be clinically signifiant. More research is needed to identify variables contributing to emergency department ECG misinterpretation and to develop ways to resolve these difficulties.

▶ This study seems to say that emergency department (ED) physicians are astonishingly poor at reading ECGs. The authors state that of patients discharged from the emergency department, 18% had a clinically significant misreading of their ECG in the ED. More than 10% had ischemia or an infarct that was missed!

This study is very disturbing. However, there are some serious problems with the methodology of this study, and we need to see better-designed studies of the same subject before we worry too much about it.—J. Schoffstall, M.D.

The Ability of Physicians to Predict Hyperkalemia From the ECG
Wrenn KD, Slovis CM, Slovis BS (Univ of Rochester, NY)
Ann Emerg Med 20:1229–1232, 1991 3–38

Background.—Hyperkalemia can be difficult to diagnose since its symptoms and findings on physical examination are nonspecific. It has been suggested that the ECG is a sensitive indicator of hyperkalemia and is a better predictor as the severity of hyperkalemia increases.

Methods.—Two experienced emergency department physicians independently read the ECGs of 220 consecutive by admitted adult patients with retrospective diagnoses of hyperkalemia or renal insufficiency. The physicians, blinded to all laboratory values, the particular diagnosis, and previous ECG tracings, predicted the presence or absence of hyperkalemia and, if present, whether hyperkalemia was mild, moderate, or severe. Their interpretations were compared with laboratory values for serum potassium concentrations.

Results.—Forty percent of the 220 patients had hyperkalemia, including 58 with mild hyperkalemia, 20 with moderate hyperkalemia, and 9 with severe potassium level elevations. Although the readers had 90% agreement with each other on the presence of hyperkalemia, the sensitivity was .43 for 1 reader and .34 for the other, and the specifities were .85 and .86. The better positive predictive value was .65, and the better negative preditive value was .69. When only patients with potassium levels of more than 6.5 mmol/L were analyzed, the sensitivities of the readers increased to .62 and .55. Readers' judgments of the severity of hyperkalemia were generally inaccurate.

Conclusions.—On the basis of a large study using 2 multiply blinded readers and high-risk patients, ECG analysis does not seem to be a sensitive predictor of the presence of hyperkalemia, and its negative predictive value is only .69. When treatment can safely be delayed, serum values should be obtained before treatment for hyperkalemia is initiated.

▶ The authors have shown that there is a variable ECG response to hyperkalemia, thus making clinical management of hyperkalemia difficult on the basis of the ECG alone. Other investigators have shown that peaked T-waves can occur in the presence of metabolic acidosis without hyperkalemia. Hence, while it may be best to await laboratory results before treating stable patients with peaked T-waves, a patient with the same ECG findings and hypotension or rhythm abnormalities in a setting suggesting hyperkalemia (e.g., diabetic ketoacidosis or renal failure) may warrant empirical treatment with sodium bicarbonate. Whether the ECG changes are due to metabolic acidosis or hyperkalemia, the alkali should be beneficial.—J.R. Hedges, M.D.

Usefulness of ST-Segment Changes in ≥ 2 Leads on the Emergency Room Electrocardiogram in Either Unstable Angina Pectoris or Non-Q-Wave Myocardial Infarction in Predicting Outcome

Cohen M, Hawkins L, Greenberg S, Fuster V (City Univ of New York, NY)

Am J Cardiol 67:1368–1373, 1991 3–39

Background.—Like patients with angina at rest, patients with non–Q-wave myocardial infarction are susceptible to recurrent ischemia, infarction, or both. This raises the question of whether all patients with ischemic chest pain at rest should have early catheterization and coronary arteriography. A study was conducted to determine whether an admission ECG obtained in the emergency department was a reliable predictor of an adverse clinical outcome.

Methods.—The study sample comprised patients with angina pectoris at rest or non–Q-wave myocardial infarction who were participating in a prospective trial of antithrombotic therapy. There were 55 men and 35 women with a mean age of 62 years and a mean interval from the onset of angina or first infarction of 47 months. Subjects were randomized to receive aspirin, heparin, or both in addition to their anti-anginal medication. They were followed prospectively for 3 months. Each patient had an admission ECG in the emergency department that was analyzed for ST-segment deviations of 1 mm or more per lead and for T-wave changes. Each patient who had coronary arteriography was assigned a myocardium-in-jeopardy score based on the number and location of stenoses.

Results.—In the series as a whole, ST-segment deviation in 2 or more leads had a positive predictive value for adverse clinical events of 79% and a negative predictive value of 64%. In 62 patients without left ventricular hypertrophy, the ECG was recorded during an episode of chest pain; for this group, the positive predictive value of ST deviation was 89%, and the negative predictive value was 72%. In the 53 patients who had coronary arteriography, a positive linear correlation was seen between the number of leads with ST-segment deviation and the myocardium-in-jeopardy score.

Conclusions.—An admission ECG recorded during pain in patients with unstable angina or non–Q-wave infarction can provide valuable information predicting outcome. ST-segment changes in 2 or more leads reliably predict major clinical events. The extent of myocardium in jeopardy can be reliably predicted by the total number of leads with ST changes.

▶ This article is interesting, the results not particularly surprising, and its applicability to emergency medicine uncertain. What the authors found is that in patients arriving at the emergency department with chest pain, ST-segment elevation or transient depression of at least 1 mm in at least 2 leads is predictive of future cardiac sequelae. This finding is particularly predictive if recorded during an episode of chest pain.

The overall positive predictive value of this criterion for adverse clinical events was 79%. For patients without left ventricular hypertrophy (which can cause ST-segment changes by itself) and whose ECGs were recorded during an episode of chest pain, the positive predictive value increased to 89%.

The major difficulty in applying these findings to clinical reality is that the overall negative predictive value was only 64%. For the subset of patients without left ventricular hypertrophy and with concurrent chest pain, the negative predictive value rose to only 72%. These values, in my opinion, are simply not sufficient to rely on a "negative" test, i.e., the absence of ST changes in no way rules out a significant danger of impending ischemic complications.

The authors point out several other limitations of the study. All of their patients received antithrombotic therapy consisting of aspirin, heparin, or both, a fact that might significantly alter the results. They acknowledge that the presence of left ventricular hypertrophy reduces the reliability of ST changes. They also admit that the absence of chest pain significantly reduces the sensitivity of criteria.

So what do we do with this information? Certainly, ST elevation or depression of at least 1 mm in 2 leads in a patient complaining of chest pain must be taken seriously, particularly if the tracing is obtained during an episoide of pain. However, the absence of these ST changes does *not* reliably rule out an impending ischemic event, especially if the patient is no longer experiencing chest pain at the time the ECG is obtained.

The lesson? Once again, we must rely on history and "gestalt" in evaluating patients with chest pain—hardly a satisfying situation.—M.J. Bresler, M.D.

Myocardial Infarction

Do CK-MB Results Affect Chest Pain Decision Making in the Emergency Department?

Young GP, Hedges JR, Gibler WB, Green TR, Swanson R (Portland VA Med Ctr; Oregon Health Sciences Univ, Portland; Univ of Cincinnati, Ohio)
Ann Emerg Med 20:1220–1228, 1991 3–40

Background.—Emergency physicians examining patients complaining of chest pain must consider the possibility of an acute myocardial infarction (AMI). In assessing the probability of AMI, physicians must rely on relatively subjective information (e.g., the patient's description of the pain) and on fairly insensitive data such as obtained through ECG. The availability of creatine kinase isoenzyme (CK-MB) levels, when used to supplement clinical examination, may enhance emergency physicians' recognition of AMI. The effects of CK-MB results on decision making in emergency department patients with chest pain were studied.

Methods.—Patients included in the prospective, controlled observational study were older than 30 years of age and complained of chest discomfort that warranted an ECG. Three hundred seventy-six patients met these criteria. Initial assessment consisted of ECG but not CK-MB data. After initial assessment, physicians answered questions about the estimated probability of AMI and disposition plans. Creatinine kinase isoenzyme levels were then determined every hour for up to 3 hours. Physicians could admit their patients at any time. After a second ECG and with all available CK-MB data, the physicians were asked the same questions about AMI probability and disposition plans. Physicians then rank-ordered the contribution of initial and serial clinical examinations and initial and serial CK-MB enzymes concentrations to their decision making.

Findings.—Twenty-nine patients, or 7.7%, had AMI. Physicians said that CK-MB levels were useful for decision making in more than one third of the cases. When considered useful, CK-MB findings strengthened the impression of AMI in patients with AMI and lessened the impression of AMI in patients without it. Creatinine kinase isoenzyme findings also correlated with the perceived need for cardiac care unit admission in patients with AMI and with a decreased need to admit non-AMI patients. The use of CK-MB did not significantly raise emergency department release rates.

Conclusions.—The rapid availability of serial CK-MB results in the emergency department appears to affect decision making in one third of the patients with chest pain and nondiagnostic ECGs. Creatinine kinase isoenzyme levels seem to complement clinical assessment of patients in the emergency department with chest pain in a fashion analogous to the ECG.

▶ One of the most exhausting aspects in the practice of emergency medicine is the toll of repetitive decision making. This is especially true when the presenting dilemma is common, the cost of overtriage is great, and the risk of undertriage is deadly and disastrous.

Even though chest pain accounts for approximately 5% of all initial chief complaints, the decision-making energy required for those patients with chest pain and nondiagnostic ECGs seems to account for at least 30% of the struggle in any 1 shift. If CK-MB results can reduce the load a third of the time, let's get the test in every emergency center as soon as possible (see also Abstracts 3–41 and 3–50).—E.H. Taliaferro, M.D.

Use of Rapid Serial Sampling of Creatine Kinase MB for Very Early Detection of Myocardial Infarction in Patients With Acute Chest Pain

Marin MM, Teichman SL (Cornell Univ, New York, NY; Genentech, Inc, South San Francisco, Calif)

Am Heart J 123:354–361, 1992 3–41

Background.—Preliminary diagnostic evaluations using serum creatine kinase MB patterns to determine the presence of myocardial infarction have been encouraging. Characteristic serum creatine kinase-MB patterns have been observed as early as 2 to 6 hours after the onset of chest pain and abnormal patterns of the subforms of creatine kinase-MM and -MB as early as early as 1 to 6 hours after symptom onset.

Methods.—Serial creatine kinase-MB concentrations were sampled in 313 patients during triage of acute chest pain of less than 12 hours. The "rule out myocardial infarction" protocol included daily ECG recordings for 3 days, baseline serial determinations of total creatine kinase at admission and determinations 8 hours for the first 24 hours of the hospital stay, determinations of the MB fractional precentage of total creatine phosphokinase when the total creatine kinase content was elevated, and real-time ECG monitoring for arrhythmias. Creatine kinase-MB concentrations were analyzed for their ability to detect infarction.

Results.—Infarction was present in 22% of patients and was diagnosable from the index ECGs in 39% of those patients. Sensitivity for the detection of infarction was 76%, and specificity was 72% as determined from baseline MB values only. The sensitivity increased to 92% and the specificity to 96% in all 4 samples. Analysis of serum samples taken 2 hours apart showed a sensitivity of 94% and a specificity of 91%.

Conclusions.—The temporal creatine kinase-MB pattern can be used to differentiate patients with acute chest pain caused by myocardial infarction from patients with chest pain resulting from other causes within 2 to 4 hours of hospital arrival. Improving initial diagnostic accuracy in patients with acute chest pain may conserve resources through more appropriate triage when the initial or index clinical suspicion of myocardial infarction is low, identify patients with infarction appropriate for early intervention, and avoid premature hospital discharge of patients with infarction.

▶ The authors were careful to note that clinical judgment will continue to be very important in evaluating patients with chest pain. However, the test described looks promising, and I look forward to being able to apply it. This is an area in which I need all of the help I can get.—E. Ruiz, M.D.

Use of an Artificial Neural Network for the Diagnosis of Myocardial Infarction

Baxt WG (Univ of California, San Diego)
Ann Intern Med 115:843–848, 1991 3–42

Background.—Physicians have been slow to accept electronic data-processing technologies that aid in clinical diagnosis. Most of these technologies have not been able to perform consistently better than physicians, but artificial neural network-based pattern recognition has potential in the clinical setting. A retrospective study showed better sensitivity and specificity for the artificial neural network in diagnosing acute myocardial infarction than for either physicians or other computer-based methods. The first prospective testing of the network on 331 adult patients seen with anterior chest pain was studied.

Methods.—The artificial neural network is a group of interconnected mathematical equations that calculate an output on the basis of input data. The network is trained by creating patterns based on data from numerous patients with anterior chest pain who are proved to have had or not to have had acute myocardial infarction. In this study, 10,000 iterations were run. Both the network and physicians used the same data as the basis for diagnosis.

Results.—Network testing of 331 patients yielded .03773 error per patient. Myocardial infarction was correctly diagnosed in 28 patients for a sensitivity of 77.7%. No myocardial infarction was correctly diagnosed in 250 patients for a specificity of 84.7%. The network incorrectly diagnosed myocardial infarction in 1 patient for a sensitivity of 97.2%. It incorrectly diagnosed no myocardial infarction in all 11 patients for a specificity of 96.2%.

Conclusions.—An artificial neural network trained to identify myocardial infarction in adult patients may be an important aid to clinical diagnosis in patients seen in the emergency department with chest pain. However, prospective testing should be done on larger patient samples before this conclusion can be confirmed.

▶ Unfortunately, the 11 patients who were incorrectly diagnosed as not having had a myocardial infarction would have been discharged home by the computer. This is another reason an emergency physician is required, that is, to prevent this from happening.—G.J. Ordog, M.D.

Importance of Two-Dimensional Echocardiographic Assessment of Left Ventricular Systolic Function in Patients Presenting to the Emergency Room With Cardiac-Related Symptoms

Sabia P, Abbott RD, Afrookteh A, Keller MW, Touchstone DA, et al (Univ of Virginia, Charlottesville)

Circulation 84:1615–1624, 1991 3–43

Background.—Although many clinical and ECG variables are diagnostically and prognostically valuable in evaluating emergency department patients with cardiac symptoms, the usefulness of evaluating left ventricular systolic function in this setting is unknown. Two-dimensional ECG (2DE) was used to study the relationship between left ventricular systolic function and cardiac events occurring during or soon after emergency department visitation, as opposed to those occurring later.

Methods.—The subjects were 171 consecutive patients seen in the emergency department with cardiac-related symptoms over a 2-year period. Eighty-eight were men with a mean age of 59 years, and 83 were women with a mean age of 62 years. For each patient, 1 of the investigators obtained a complete history and physical examination, 12-lead ECG and serum enzyme measurements, and 2DE study. Emergency department physicians treated the patient without knowledge of the results of 2DE. All patients were contacted at 2 years for follow-up. Cardiac events occurring within 48 hours of the emergency room visit were considered early and those occurring thereafter as late.

Results.—Some major cardiac event occurred during follow-up in 32% of the patients; of these 55 events, 32 were early and 23 late. The age-adjusted rate of early events was 26.9% for patients with left ventricular systolic dysfunction (LVSD) as compared with 3.3% for patients without LVSD. The rate of late cardiac events was 23.9% for those with LVSD and 6.4% for those without. An ECG that was diagnostic of myocardial infarction was the most important confounder in predicting early events, other than advanced age. For late events, advanced age and a history of hypertension were important confounders. However, after controlling for other risk factors, the only parameter associated with both types of events was LVSD. The presence or absence of LVSD based on a combination of historical, clinical, ECG, and 2DE findings greatly improved the prediction of cardiac events.

Conclusions.—In the emergency department, LVSD as shown by 2DE is a valuable diagnostic and prognostic finding in patients who are seen with cardiac-related symptoms. The physician may wish to admit patients with LVSD in whom an acute event is suspected. The absence of LVSD can ease the decision to discharge, especially in those with a normal ECG. Those with the finding of LVSD should be followed aggressively.

▶ A number of studies indicate that 5% to 7% of patients arriving at the emergency center with chest pain will be sent home and later be diagnosed as having had an acute myocardial infarction (AMI). Although "missed" AMI represents the sixth most common cause for litigation against emergency physicians, it ranks first in dollars awarded. In recent years, many investigations have attempted to improve the sensitivity and specificity of diagnosing AMI in patients presenting with chest pain. Such studies include the measurement of serum myoglobin, rapid measurement of creatine kinase MB isoenzymes, the use of computer-based ECG scoring systems, "early" cardiac radionuclide scanning, and echocardiography. It remains uncertain whether any of these studies have improved the diagnostic acumen of the emergency physician or whether such tests are cost-effective in the broadest sense of the term. This study by Sabia et al. is rather unique in that AMI is not the major concern. Rather, LVSD was the major study variable. LVSD, due to whatever cause, is an indicator of early and late cardiac mortality. This observation is not unexpected, and the value of emergency center cardiac echocardiography remains uncertain in the typical patient with acute chest pain.—J.T. Niemann, M.D.

Estimating the Size of Myocardial Infarction by Magnetic Resonance Imaging

Turnbull LW, Ridgway JP, Nicoll JJ, Bell D, Best JJK, et al (Royal Infirmary, Edinburgh, England)

Br Heart J 66:359–363, 1991 3–44

Background.—The outcome for patients with acute myocardial infarction depends on the extent of myocardial damage and residual left ventricular function. A method of examining infarct size with MRI was developed and compared with pyrophosphate positron-emission tomography.

Methods.—The patients were 14 men and 5 women who had their first myocardial infarction. None had been treated with thrombolytic drugs. Five to 7 days after the onset of symptoms, the patients underwent both MRI and pyrophosphate scanning to measure the size of the infarct. The patients also underwent measurement of creatine kinase MB release and assessment of ventricular performance by radionuclide ventriculography.

Results.—Both techniques showed the infarct clearly and identically. Volume measurements of the infarct agreed well, with a mean difference of 2.7 cm^3. Correlations with creatine kinase MB release were best when total rather than peak release was used. There was also a close correlation between the imaging studies and the patients' subsequent ventricular performance.

Conclusions.—In patients with acute myocardial infarction, MRI is an accurate technique of measuring infarct size. It agrees well with pyrophosphate scanning, ventricular function assessments, and total creatine kinase MB release. Use of a 128 × 128 pixel matrix and reduced slice thickness should improve precision, although they will lengthen examination time.

▶ Magnetic resonance imaging to determine infarct size might be useful for primary care physicians or cardiologists in care of post–myocardial infarction patients. It may also be a tool for research on the impact of interventions on infarct size. For emergency department management and evaluation, I find this of limited clinical usefulness at the present time.—J.M. Mitchell-Savinsky, M.D.

Effects of Intravenous Magnesium in Suspected Acute Myocardial Infarction: Overview of Randomised Trials

Teo KK, Yusuf S, Collins R, Held PH, Peto R (Natl Heart, Lung, & Blood Inst, Bethesda, Md; Univ of Oxford, England)

BMJ 303:1499–1503, 1991 3–45

Introduction.—A number of studies have demonstrated a relationship between low magnesium concentrations and ischemic heart disease. Several actions of the magnesium ion could afford cardiac protection. Because certain anti-arrhythmic drugs may have adverse effects, magnesium offers an attractive alternative. Treatment regimens are simple and apparently safe; furthermore, there are few known contraindications to magnesium. Seven randomized trials were reviewed to determine the effects of intravenous magnesium administration on mortality in suspected acute myocardial infarction.

Methods.—The randomized, placebo-controlled trials involved 1,301 patients. Treatment was generally started within 12 hours of the onset of chest pain. Short-term follow-up, at least on mortality, was obtained for 99.4% of the patients. Five studies used an infusion of magnesium sulfate; 2 used magnesium chloride. The duration of the infusions ranged from 24 to 48 hours.

Results.—There were 25 deaths (3.8%) among 657 patients who received magnesium and 53 deaths (8.2%) among the 644 control patients. Magnesium use was thus associated with a 55% reduction in the odds of death. Serious ventricular arrhythmias were more common among the control patients. This difference was significant in 2 of the 7 studies. Flushing and hypotension were reported in some patients treated with magnesium, but these effects did not require discontinuation of the infusion.

Conclusion.—Intravenous magnesium therapy appears valuable in reducing mortality in patients with acute myocardial infarction. Larger trials now under way should provide more information regarding magnesium regimens.

▶ There have been several overviews of randomized trials of therapeutics in acute myocardial infarction. The individual investigations of intravenous magnesium have similar problems as those that studied nitroglycerin, β-blockers, lidocaine, and calcium channel blockers: the study populations are small, timing of therapy is not uniform and is often delayed beyond a window of maximal benefit, and the end points vary (early mortality, late mortality, infarct size). They point out that prophylactic lidocaine in suspected myocardial infarction was widely used in small studies, but 2 separate overviews indicated that this practice may actually be associated with increased total mortality.

The present overview of magnesium therapy shows promise for reduced mortality from acute myocardial infarction. The concept is not particularly new, with one of the individual reports as early as 1981, but was probably overshadowed by the development of thrombolytic techniques. It is unclear how mortality is reduced, and as pointed out by the authors, larger studies need to be done (see Abstracts 3–11 and 3–46).—J.M. Mitchell-Savinsky, M.D.

Resuscitation From Prolonged Cardiac Arrest With High-Dose Intravenous Magnesium Sulfate

Craddock L, Miller B, Clifton G, Krumbach B, Pluss W (Rose Med Ctr, Denver, Colo)

J Emerg Med 9:469–476, 1991 3–46

Background.—Patients in prolonged cardiac arrest have a dismal prognosis with standard therapy. Intravenous administration of magnesium sulfate may help convert fibrillation (VT/VF) to normal rhythm and contraction. Successful resuscitation from prolonged cardiac arrest associated temporally with the intravenous administration of 8 g of magnesium sulfate, was acheived.

Case Report.—A 41-year-old woman was generally healthy. At the completion of liposuction surgery, however, she had bradycardia and a drop in oxygen tension after reversal of general anesthesia with physostigmine. Her ECG rhythms degenerated to ventricular asystole. Standard treatment consisting of multiple boluses of epinephrine, atropine, wide-open dopamine, and attempts at right heart pacing was ineffective. External CPR was maintained continuously while the patient was intubated on 100% oxygen. When VT/VF occurred, multiple electric countershocks and lidocaine were administered, but that treatment too was unsuccessful. About 1 hour into the resuscitation, 8 g of magnesium sulfate was given and countershock repeated. Although the 7 preceding countershocks had been unsuccessful, the eighth countershock resulted in a stable pulse and normal sinus rhythm within 4 minutes. The patient recovered without neurologic deficit and was discharged in stable condition.

Conclusions.—A patient was in cardiac arrest for 70 minutes with no evidence of spontaneous perfusion. In such cases, the probability of surviving to hospital discharge is estimated to be less than 4%. This patient's dramatic recovery after intravenous magnesium administration indicates the need for a controlled clinical trial of this treatment in patients with cardiac arrest.

▶ The literature is replete with articles describing the use of magnesium in the treatment of ventricular arrhythmias. A case report from Morristown Memorial Hospital (1) sounds frighteningly similar to this article. In it, the authors describe the successful resuscitation, without neurologic sequelae, of a cardiac arrest victim who received 62 minutes of basic and advanced life support. Following 4 g of magnesium, he was successfully defibrillated. Other studies have described a marked decrease in complex ventricular arrhythmias in patients with myocardial ischemia who have received magnesium therapy (2).

Perhaps the most remarkable aspect of this paper and the case report by Tobey et al. is not the successful conversion of ventricular fibrillation to sinus rhythm, but rather the complete neurologic recovery seen in both patients. Successful CNS recovery following prolonged euthermic cardiac arrest is virtually nonexistent. Does magnesium have a neuroprotective effect in addition to its cardiac activity?—H.D. Unger, M.D.

References

1. Tobey RC, et al: *Ann Emerg Med* 21:92, 1992.
2. Keren A, et al: *PACE* 13:937, 1990.

Diagnostic Testing in Acute Myocardial Infarction: Does Patient Age Influence Utilization Patterns? The Worcester Heart Attack Study

Gurwitz JH, Osganian V, Goldberg RJ, Chen Z, Gore JM, et al (Beth Israel Hosp, Boston; Univ of Massachusetts, Worcester)

Am J Epidemiol 134:948–957, 1991 3–47

Introduction.—Although ischemic heart disease is the leading cause of death among the elderly in the United States, few studies have considered the impact of patient age on the use of diagnostic tests and procedures among patients with acute myocardial infarction. This question was addressed in a review of the charts of 4,109 patients hospitalized with acute myocardial infarction.

Methods.—Data were obtained from the 16 hospitals in the Worcester, Massachusetts, metropolitan area between 1975 and 1986. The records were abstracted for demographic and clinical data and for information about the use of selected cardiac tests. Patients were stratified according to 5 age groups: younger than 55, 55 to 64, 65 to 74, 75 to 84, and 85 years or older. The study population was 62% male.

Results.—There were significant differences in demographic and clinical characteristics among patients of different ages with acute myocardial infarction. In-hospital mortality was directly related to patient age. Older patients were more likely to be female and to have a history of angina, hypertension, and diabetes mellitus. The older patients were more likely to have congestive heart failure, cardiogenic shock, and atrial fibrillation. Acute myocardial infarction in the older age groups tended to be recurrent, anterior, and non-Q wave. Younger patients were significantly more likely to undergo exercise testing, radionuclide ventriculography, pulmonary artery catheterization, and coronary arteriography.

Conclusion.—Patient age appears to determine the use of diagnostic testing in patients with acute myocardial infarction. This finding raises an issue requiring further study—whether there is an underuse of medical resources in the older patient.

▶ In this study, the authors present data that strongly suggest that physicians manage patients with acute myocardial infarction differently with advancing age: less diagnostic testing is used in older patients. They also showed that this trend did not change between 1975, when such procedures as pulmonary artery cannulation and peri-infarct coronary angiography were considered "big deals," and 1986. However, when one reflects on how differently we approach out-of-hospital cardiac arrest in elderly vs. younger patients, it would appear that old age is considered a terminal disease.

For me, the study raises two questions: what was the functional status of the older patients, and what was the purpose of the diagnostic tests? The authors addressed the first question and felt that a true answer was unavailable in their retrospective study. Good functional status in independent elderly patients without other physical or mental disabilities might warrant more aggressive approaches. Functional status might also limit the ability to perform exercise testing. My 82-year-old grandmother underwent monthly chemotherapy, and it wasn't the Adriamycin she dreaded, but pedaling the bicycle for the multiple gated acquisition scan!

The purpose of doing specific testing is an important consideration. For example, if coronary angiography is performed to determine the presence of surgically correctable lesions, patients in the older age groups might be excluded. However, since age is a relatively limiting factor for the use of systemic thrombolysis, selected elderly patients might be candidates for angiography with balloon reperfusion techniques. Why were the other studies done? Since more elderly patients had complications such as cardiogenic shock, why were fewer pulmonary artery cannulations done to guide management? Are we afraid of "torturing" old people?

I would like to see a similar study done prospectively with a description of the functional status of the patients and what data were sought from the diagnostic tests.—J.M. Mitchell-Savinsky, M.D.

Accuracy of 22-Lead ECG Analysis for Diagnosis of Acute Myocardial Infarction and Coronary Artery Disease in the Emergency Department: A Comparison With 12-Lead ECG

Justis DL, Hession WT (Fairview Southdale Hosp, Edina, Minn)

Ann Emerg Med 21:1–9, 1992 3–48

Background.—The differentiation of chest pain in the emergency department is based in part on a resting 12-lead ECG, although this test may have only a 50% sensitivity for the diagnosis of acute myocardial infarction (AMI) and coronary artery disease. This often results in needless, expensive admissions for ruling out myocardial infarction as well as exclusions for patients who might benefit from early thrombolytic therapy. The diagnostic accuracy for AMI of a new 22-lead ECG procedure was compared with the standard 12-lead ECG in patients with chest pain who were seen in the emergency department.

Methods.—One hundred sixty-three admitted patients with chest pains underwent 12-lead ECGs as well as 22-lead ECGs using digital cardiac electrogram technology. The accuracy of the results was assessed by comparisons with serum creatine kinase MB analyses and subsequent angiography.

Results.—On the basis of serum enzyme analyses, 41 of 163 patients had an AMI. The sensitivity of the 22-lead ECG was 83%, significantly greater than that of 51% with the 12-lead. The specificity of the 22-lead ECG was 76%, whereas that of the 12-lead ECG was 99%. The 22-lead ECG had a significantly higher positive predictive value than the 12-lead ECG, but the differences in their negative predictive values were not significant. For the diagnosis of coronary artery disease, the 22-lead ECG had significantly higher sensitivity and comparable specificity to the 12-lead ECG.

Conclusions.—Together with clinical judgment, the use of the 22-lead ECG adds significant diagnostic accuracy in the evaluation of AMI to the 12-lead ECG with or without clinical judgment. With retrospectively modified output rules to optimize the 22-lead ECG for diagnosis of AMI, the emergency department physician could have achieved a 97% sensitivity. At the same time, unnecessary admissions would have been cut by more than two thirds. Prospective trials should be done to validate the accuracy of the 22-lead ECG in the diagnosis of AMI.

▶ The investigators describe a new approach to ECG signal analysis. Several cautionary notes must be sounded. First, a select group of patients, largely hospital admissions, was examined. The applicability of this device to all emergency department (ED) patients with chest pain is unknown, but it is likely that additional false-positive cases will be found were this test to be used on all patients with chest pain. Second, the cutoff thresholds for AMI are empirical and have been revised by the investigators who used their own data to improve sensitivity. It is imperative that the recommended cutoff values be validated on a larger, more diverse, independent patient population. Third, many of the positive 22-lead ECGs were obtained on patients with diagnostic ST-segment elevation on the 12-lead ECG. The real issue is how well the device works for those patients who are missed by the 12-lead ECG. The authors' data suggest that the device had an 80% sensitivity for AMI patients without a diagnostic 12-lead ECG, but this estimate is based on a sample of only 20 patients. Fourth, the 22-lead ECGs were always obtained after the 12-lead ECG, an average of 2.5 hours following ED arrival. Therefore, it is possible that some of the 12-lead ECGs may have become diagnostic for AMI in the interim. Fifth, the speculation that physicians would use the device as supportive evidence to release patients is unfounded. In summary, 22-lead ECG conduction velocity analysis is promising but requires further clinical study.—J.R. Hedges, M.D.

Early Prediction of Acute Myocardial Infarction From Clinical History, Examination and Electrocardiogram in the Emergency Room

Karlson BW, Herlitz J, Wiklund O, Richter A, Hjalmarson Å (Sahlgrenska Hosp, Göteborg, Sweden)

Am J Cardiol 68:171–175, 1991 3–49

Purpose.—Of all the patients who are admitted to an emergency room (ER) with chest pain or other symptoms suggestive of acute myocardial infarction (AMI), only a minority will have a confirmed AMI. The possibility of early prediction of which patients admitted to the ER with chest pain and symptoms of an AMI would actually have one was examined in 7,157 patients during a 21-month study.

Patients.—On the basis of history, clinical examination, and a standard 12-lead ECG recorded soon after admission to the ER, all patients were classified prospectively into 4 categories depending on the degree of initial suspicion of AMI.

Results.—Of the 7,157 patients, 4,690 (66%) were admitted to the hospital, and 921 of them had an AMI during the first 3 days in the hospital. Of the 4,690 patients admitted, 1,576 (34%) had a normal admission ECG, and 90 of them (6%) had an AMI. Of the 1,964 patients with an abnormal ECG who had no signs of acute ischemia, 268 (14%) had an AMI. Of the 1,109 patients with acute ischemia on the ECG, 563 (51%) had an AMI. Of the 466 patients with no suspicion of AMI, only 6 (1%) had one. Thus, only very few patients with a normal initial ECG or a vague initial suspicion of AMI will actually have a confirmed AMI.

Discussion.—Overall, only 20% of the patients admitted to the hospital actually had an AMI. Only 1% of patients with a normal ECG had an AMI. Other methods of early diagnosis of AMI are cardiac enzyme determinations and thallium scintigraphy. However, enzyme analysis has not proved useful in the ER and scintigraphy is time-consuming. The physician's estimate of the probability of infarction remains a good predictor of infarction.

▶ While this prospective study offers no new insights into the early diagnosis of AMI, it does support a previously reported study that I do think is particularly useful. In 1985, Brush et al. prospectively followed patients admitted for suspected myocardial infarction (1). They noted that although patients with normal ECGs did rule in for infarction, they had virtually no complications while in the hospital. My inference from that study is that while physicians must admit even the "class 3" patients about whom there is only a "vague suspicion" of infarction, they may be observed in a lower-acuity telemetry setting and do not need to be admitted to the intensive care unit.—W.P. Burdick, M.D.

Reference

1. Brush JE, et al: N *Engl J Med* 312:1137, 1985.

The Potential Utility of a Rapid CK-MB Assay in Evaluating Emergency Department Patients With Possible Myocardial Infarction

Green GB, Hansen KN, Chan DW, Guerci AD, Fleetwood DH, et al (Johns Hopkins Univ; Johns Hopkins Hosp, Baltimore, Md)

Ann Emerg Med 20:954–960, 1991 3–50

Background.—Because myocardial infarction (MI) may be difficult to distinguish from benign conditions, some cases of MI are misdiagnosed. A new rapid creatine kinase MB assay may be of use in the emergency department (ED) setting when the diagnosis of MI is unclear. The sensitivity, specificity, and predictive values of the rapid creatine kinase MB assay vs. the current standard creatine kinase MB assay were evaluated.

Methods.—The Johns Hopkins Hospital, which serves a socioeconomically disadvantaged population, sees approximately 1,800 patients with possible MI per year in the ED. Of this group, 10% to 12% are subsequently diagnosed as having had an MI. The study subjects were drawn from all adult patients with excess sera and 1 of several defined conditions seen during a 4-month period.

Results.—The final study population included 271 patients, 54.2% women and 45.8% men, with a mean age of 62 years. Most (67.5%) were black persons. Chest pain was the most common (63.1%) presenting symptom. Most of these patients (71.2%) were admitted to the hospital, 28.4% were discharged from the ED, and 1 patient left against physician advice. The rapid creatine kinase MB assay was performed in 10 minutes, whereas the standard creatine kinase MB assay required 2 hours. The rapid creatine kinase MB assay had a sensitivity of 100%, a specificity of 96.8%, a positive predictive value of 75%, and a negative predictive value of 100%.

Conclusion.—The rapid creatine kinase MB assay is recommended for evaluating ED patients with possible MI, but for whom a coronary care unit or intensive care unit admission is not considered. The assay is fast and simple to use and may identify unsuspected MI and prevent the discharge of such patients or admission to unmonitored beds.

▶ This paper presents very useful information for emergency physicians. The accurate diagnosis of MI is a major risk management area for emergency physicians (see also Abstract 3–51).

The authors are careful not to overstate their conclusions. The recommendation to use the test in patients who would otherwise be discharged or placed in unmonitored beds is a prudent recommendation. As experience with this approach is gained, more aggressive use of the test may be warranted.

Every emergency physician who practices for some time has witnessed or been involved in the misdiagnosis of myocardial infarction. The rapid creatine kinase MB test is a welcome tool to help us in this high-risk area of emergency medicine.—J.E. Clinton, M.D.

Ruling Out Acute Myocardial Infarction: A Prospective Multicenter Validation of a 12-Hour Strategy for Patients at Low Risk

Lee TH, Juarez G, Cook EF, Weisberg MC, Rouan GW, et al (Brigham and Women's Hosp, Boston, Mass; Harvard Med School, Boston; Yale-New Haven Hosp, Conn; Univ of Cincinnati Hosp, Ohio)

N Engl J Med 324:1239–1246, 1991 3–51

Background.—Studies have suggested that 24 hours is needed to rule out acute myocardial infarction in patients admitted to the coronary care unit for evaluation of acute chest pain. It was hypothesized, however, that 12 hours might be sufficient for patients whose probability of infarction was low at admission. Patients from the Multicenter Chest Pain Study were evaluated to test this hypothesis.

Methods.—A bayesian model involving a derivation set of 976 patients with acute chest pain who were admitted to 7 hospitals was used to identify candidates for a shorter period of observation. In those patients, those whose clinical characteristics in the emergency department predicted a 7% or lower probability of infarction had only a .4% risk of infection if they had neither abnormal cardiac enzyme levels nor recurrent ischemic pain in the first 12 hours. An independent set of 2,684 patients was tested, 957 of whom were classified as candidates for this period of observation.

Results.—Seven hundred seventy-one of the patients did not have either enzyme abnormalities or recurrent pain during the first 12 hours. Of that group, .5% subsequently had acute myocardial infarction. Only .4% died after primary cardiac arrests, and all of those occurred 3 to 5 days after admission. Low rates of other major cardiovascular complications were noted in patients who might have been transferred from the coronary care unit after 12 hours. The standard strategy of 24-hour observation identified all but 11 of the 739 myocardial infarctions in patients with a higher initial risk of infarction.

Conclusions.—Clinical data from the emergency department can identify a large subgroup of patients in whom acute myocardial infarction can be excluded in a 12-hour observation period. This allows progression of specific evaluation and treatment measures without restrictions imposed by protocols to rule out myocardial infarction. Patients at low risk should not be discharged at 12 hours because they do not necessarily have a low risk of unstable angina.

▶ This study does *not* suggest that patients who meet the criteria to rule out a myocardial infarct after 12 hours of observation should be discharged home. Rather, it recommends that select patients be transferred out of a monitored setting at that point and begin the remainder of their inpatient workup i.e., exercise testing. The impact on the emergency department would optimally be a decrease in the length of time other admitted patients would have to wait for a monitored bed to become available.—H.D. Unger, M.D.

THROMBOLYTIC THERAPY

ISIS-3: A Randomised Comparison of Streptokinase *vs* Tissue Plasminogen Activator *vs* Anistreplase and of Aspirin Plus Heparin *vs* Aspirin Alone Among 41 299 Cases of Suspected Acute Myocardial Infarction

Third International Study of Infarct Survival Collaborative Group (Radcliffe Infirmary, Oxford, England)

Lancet 339:753–770, 1992 3–52

Background.—The overall clinical efficacy of fibrinolytic and antithrombotic regimens in the treatment of acute myocardial infarction is defined not only by the speed of coronary recanalization and its persistence but also by the rate of hemorrhagic complications. The multicenter ISIS-3 trial was designed to compare the benefits and risks of 3 different fibrinolytic and 2 different antithrombotic regimens.

Study Design.—A total of 41,299 patients entering 914 hospitals within 24 hours after the onset of suspected acute myocardial infarction were randomly allocated to streptokinase (SK), tissue plasminogen activator (tPA), or anisoylated plasminogen-streptokinase activator complex (APSAC) in a 3×2 factorial study design (Fig 3–11). Half of all patients were randomized to take aspirin daily for 1 month, and the other half were randomized to take aspirin plus subcutaneous calcium heparin for 7 days. Because SK is the most widely tested of the 3 fibrinolytic agents, tPA and APSAC were each compared with SK.

Results.—The addition of heparin to aspirin was associated with an excess of transfused or other major noncerebral bleeds and an excess of definite or probable cerebral hemorrhage. However, there were no substantial differences in mortality rates between these regimens either in days 0 to 35 or during the 6 months of follow-up. When compared with SK, there was a slight excess of strokes with APSAC and a significant excess of strokes with tPA. There were significiantly fewer reinfarctions

SK	tPA	APSAC	
SK + ASPIRIN PLUS HEPARIN (6893 patients)	tPA + ASPIRIN PLUS HEPARIN (6870 patients)	APSAC + ASPIRIN PLUS HEPARIN (6893 patients)	Subtotal 1: 20 656 patients allocated ASPIRIN PLUS HEPARIN
SK + ASPIRIN ALONE (6887 patients)	tPA + ASPIRIN ALONE (6876 patients)	APSAC + ASPIRIN ALONE (6880 patients)	Subtotal 2: 20 643 patients allocated ASPIRIN ALONE
Subtotal A: 13 780 patients allocated SK	Subtotal B: 13 746 patients allocated tPA	Subtotal C: 13 773 patients allocated APSAC	Total: 41 299 patients

Fig 1—Factorial design of ISIS-3.

Fig 3–11.—Factorial design of ISIS-3. There were 41,299 patients: 36,381 in whom the responsible clinician considered there to be a "clear indication" for fibrinolytic therapy, plus half of the 9,475 in whom the indication was considered "uncertain." (Courtesy of The Third International Study of Infarct Survival Collaborative Group: *Lancet* 339:753–770, 1992.)

with tPA than with SK or APSAC. There was no significant difference in 35-day mortality or in 6-month survival rates between the 2 antithrombotic regimens or between the 3 fibrinolytic regimens.

Conclusions.—Any differences in mortality between different antithrombotic regimens or between different fibrinolytic regimens are unlikely to be large.

▶ The magnitude of difference between the regimens studied in terms of the incidence of cerebral hemorrhage was a matter of a few cases per thousand, far outweighed by the potential benefit of thrombolytic treatment. Nevertheless, continued surveillance and testing is necessary to produce a regimen with the best possible benefit-to-risk ratio. I am sure that further refinements will be made.—E. Ruiz, M.D.

One-Year Results of the Thrombolysis in Myocardial Infarction Investigation (TIMI) Phase II Trial

Williams DO, for the TIMI Phase II Trial (Rhode Island Hosp, Brown Univ, Providence)

Circulation 85:533–542, 1992 3–53

Background.—The Thrombolysis in Myocardial Infarction (TIMI) Phase II Trial was designed to compare 2 management strategies for patients with acute myocardial infarction (AMI) treated with thrombolytic therapy. The results of this trial were assessed after 1 year.

Methods.—The TIMI Phase II Trial included 3,339 patients randomly assigned in roughly equal numbers to invasive or conservative treatment after intravenous recombinant tissue-type plasminogen activator for AMI. The invasive strategy involved routine cardiac catheterization and, when appropriate, percutaneous transluminal coronary angioplasty (PTCA) or coronary artery bypass grafting 18 to 48 hours after infarction. Patients assigned to the conservative strategy underwent those procedures only in response to spontaneous or provoked ischemia. One-year follow-up data were available for 99.3% of the patients enrolled.

Findings.—The primary trial end points were death and nonfatal reinfarction. Those occurred in 14.7% of patients in the invasive strategy group and in 15.2% of those in the conservative strategy group. Analyzed individually, there were no significant differences in death or recurrent infarction between the 2 groups. Seven percent of those in the invasive group and 7.4% in the conservative group died, and 9.4% in the invasive group and 9.8% in the conservative group suffered nonfatal reinfarctions. The groups also had similar anginal status at 1 year. Cardiac catheterization and PTCA were done more often in patients assigned to the invasive strategy than in those assigned to the conservative arm. The cumulative number of patients who had coronary bypass surgery at 1 year was also similar in the 2 groups.

Conclusions.—The 2 strategies compared in this trial resulted in similar favorable outcomes at 1 year. Mortality and reinfarction rates did not differ and were impressively low in both groups. The data suggest that in patients with a history of AMI, 1-year mortality was lower in the invasive strategy group than in the conservative strategy group.

▶ Thrombolytic therapy is a major breakthrough in the management of AMI. Morbidity and mortality have been reduced. In this study, patients who had aggressive, invasive strategies fared better. However, many emergency medicine physicians in community hospitals have no access or limited access to aggressive invasive therapies (e.g., catheterization, PTCA) for their patients.—S.B. Repasky, D.O.

Safety of Thrombolysis in Association With Cardiopulmonary Resuscitation

Cross SJ, Lee HS, Rawles JM, Jennings K (Aberdeen Royal Infirmary; Univ of Aberdeen, Scotland)

BMJ 303:1242, 1991 3–54

Introduction.—Thrombolysis is not recommended after prolonged or traumatic CPR because it can induce a temporary systemic fibrinolytic state. Bleeding complications were sought in patients with acute myocardial infarction before or after receiving thrombolysis.

Patients.—Thirty-nine patients with acute myocardial infarction who were treated by thrombolysis and had a cardiac arrest within 24 hours were divided into 3 groups. Patients in group I (10) had a cardiac arrest before receiving thrombolysis. Four patients in group I had chest compression with cardioversion, and the rest had cardioversion only. One patient died a week later. Patients in group II (18) had a cardiac arrest within 24 hours after receiving thrombolysis and could not be resuscitated despite chest compression in all cases and cardioversion when appropriate. There were no bleeding complications in this group. Group III patients (11) had a cardiac arrest within 24 hours after receiving thrombolysis and were successfully resuscitated by chest compression in 2 patients and cardioversion alone in the others. One patient sustained a chest wall hematoma after a precordial blow.

Results.—There was no clinically significant bleeding complication in patients receiving thrombolysis before or after cardio-pulmonary resuscitation. All but 1 patient who received thrombolysis after resuscitation survived. Group II patients had signficantly more arrests secondary to electromechanical dissociation and asystole and significantly fewer from ventricular fibrillation and tachycardia as compared with group III patients.

Conclusion.—Although the study group was small, the results suggest that CPR is not a clear contraindication to thrombolysis.

▶ This is an important topic, although because of the small number of subjects in each study group, the results are insignificant. A larger series of this type needs to be studied.—G.J. Ordog, M.D.

Safety and Efficacy of a New Regimen of Intravenous Recombinant Tissue-Type Plasminogen Activator Potentially Suitable for Either Prehospital or In-Hospital Administration

McKendall GR, Attubato MJ, Drew TM, Feit F, Sharaf BL, et al (Brown Univ, Providence, RI; New York Univ, NY; Genentech, Inc, South San Francisco, Calif)

J Am Coll Cardiol 18:1774–1778, 1991 3–55

Introduction.—The intravenous administration of recombinant tissue-type plasminogen activator (rt-PA) appears to be safe and effective in lowering death from myocardial infarction. An inverse relationship exists between the effectiveness of rt-PA in preventing further cardiac tissue damage and death and the time between the infarction and the administration of this drug. The results of the development of an initial bolus rt-PA dose followed by a later infused dose of the thrombolytic agent that can be used before hospitalization in patients having a heart attack were evaluated.

Methods.—Patients arriving at the emergency department of a hospital who had an onset of myocardial infarction symptoms within 6 hours were selected for study participation. They first received a 20-mg rt-PA bolus injection, followed 30 minutes later by a 2-hour infusion of 54 mg of rt-PA during the first hour and 20 mg of rt-PA during the second hour. The patients also received 5,000 units of heparin intravenously after the initial bolus of rt-PA. Each patient underwent serial coronary angiography soon after the first rt-PA dose.

Results.—Sixty-three patients with suspected myocardial infarction entered the study, but 3 were eventually excluded. Of the 60 remaining patients, 80% were male, and all had an average age of 55 years. The mean time between the first administration of rt-PA and the initial symptom onset was 166.7 minutes. The infarct-affected artery was identified in each individual. Of the 60 patients, 20 underwent coronary angiography 30 minutes after receiving the 20-mg bolus of rt-PA, whereas 53 of the patients underwent the procedure 60 minutes after receiving the drug. The patency rate 30, 60, 90, and 120 minutes after rt-PA administration was 50%, 75.5%, 91.7%, and 84.9%, respectively. Twenty-six patients underwent follow-up angiography an average of 9 days after the first angiography procedure that showed a Thrombolysis in Myocardial Infarction (TIMI) grade 3 flow in 22 individuals and a TIMI grade 2 flow in 4 other patients. Fourteen patients experienced possible recurrent ischemia.

Conclusions.—Recombinant tissue-type plasminogen activator can effectively reduce the outcome of a myocardial infarction if given before arriving at the hospital emergency department. The regimen should not be used until verified by a large clinical trial.

▶ Emergency medical service systems should carefully evaluate two major components of prehospital administration of thrombolytics: (1) the reduction in time from field transmission of 12-lead ECGs to the receiving hospital and (2) the additional incremental reduction in time by administration of the agent in the field. The implementation of (1) may provide the largest time reduction, while the addition of the drug to the regimen provides a smaller incremental reduction. All this is, of course, based on the underlying assumption that "time is muscle" and that, in short, transport systems that shave minutes off the time to administration reduce eventual morbidity or mortality. Once a system has decided to proceed and decides to introduce the agents in the field, this article addresses the bolus administration of rt-PA to eliminate the need for prehospital infusion. This is an interesting study but one that, as mentioned above, needs further collaborative study.—W.J. Koenig, M.D.

Clot-Selective Coronary Thrombolysis With Low-Dose Synergistic Combinations of Single-Chain Urokinase-Type Plasminogen Activator and Recombinant Tissue-Type Plasminogen Activator

Kirshenbaum JM, for the Pro-Urokinase for Myocardial Infarction Study Group (Brigham and Women's Hosp, Boston, Mass)

Am J Cardiol 68:1564–1569, 1991 3–56

Background.—Results of animal studies suggest that tissue-type plasminogen activator (t-PA) and single-chain urokinase-type plasminogen activator (scu-PA) work together to produce synergistic lytic effects. Both agents were simultaneously infused in patients with acute myocardial infarction to determine whether a synergistic effect of t-PA and scu-PA would reduce the total dose needed for thrombolysis.

Methods.—The study was designed as an open-label prospective trial. Twenty-three patients with a mean age of 61 years satisfied eligibility criteria. All had myocardial infarction documented by elevated plasma levels of myocardial-specific enzymes. The average time from the onset of chest pain to the administration of thrombolytic therapy was 2.6 hours. Upon enrollment, patients immediately received a 5,000-IU heparin bolus. Thrombolysis was started with a low (20-mg) dose of t-PA administered intravenously as a 10-mg bolus followed by a 10-mg infusion over a period of 60 minutes. A separate line was used for the simultanous infusion of scu-PA, which was administered as a 4-mg bolus followed by a 60-minute infusion of 12.3 mg.

Results.—After the 1-hour infusion of t-PA and scu-PA, infarct artery patency was achieved in 16 patients (70%). The fibrinogen concentration had decreased, although not significantly, at 90 minutes. Plasminogen had decreased to 69% and α-antiplasmin to 77% of pretreatment values.

There were no bleeding episodes requiring termination of drug infusion or transfusion. The only hospital death occurred in a 66-year-old man who had an intraventricular and cerebral hemorrhage.

Conclusion.—Concerns regarding increased bleeding risks and high costs may inhibit the use of thrombolytic agents. Combination therapy with t-PA and scu-PA may achieve effective thrombolysis with substantially lower doses than those required in monotherapy.

▶ The final story on thrombolytic therapy will probably not be written for some time, but this paper is certainly an interesting chapter. Bleeding complications are certainly our greatest fear in using these agents, and this paper highlights an intriguing combination of drugs that by acting synergistically, allow for lower doses of each drug. Certainly, much larger studies must be performed to verify this study.—E.J. Lucid, M.D.

Accuracy of Computer-Interpreted Electrocardiography in Selecting Patients for Thrombolytic Therapy

Kudenchuk PJ, for MITI Project Investigators (Univ of Washington, Seattle)

J Am Coll Cardiol 17:1486–1491, 1991 3–57

Background.—Early treatment with thrombolytic therapy is desirable in selected patients with acute myocardial infarction. Patients with ST-segment elevation are known to benefit from thrombolytic therapy, whereas the benefit in patients with other ECG abnormalities has not been clearly demonstrated. Reliable computer-interpreted ECG could minimize the time to treatment in appropriate patients.

Methods.—Paramedics used a checklist of history and physical examination criteria to evaluate patients with chest pain to select patients who might be suitable candidates for a prehospital ECG and consideration for treatment with thrombolytic therapy. Patients aged 74 years or younger with symptoms of less than 6 hours duration who had a low risk of serious bleeding received an ECG. Paramedics used a battery-powered ECG with both computer-interpretive and cellular-telephone transmission capabilities. In the emergency room, the receiving unit printed a record for review by a physician. The acquisition-to-reading process took no longer than 30 seconds. Paramedics obtained ECGs a mean of 1.5 hours after the onset of symptoms.

Results.—Paramedics performed prehospital ECGs on 1,189 consecutive patients with chest pain. Of 391 patients with evidence of acute myocardial infarction, a computer-interpreted ECG identified 202 as having ST-segment elevation. An electrocardiographer identified 259 patients. Of 798 patients with chest pain but no infarction, 785 (98%) were correctly excluded by computer, whereas the electrocardiographer excluded only 757. The positive predictive value of computer-interpreted

ECGs was 94% vs. 86% for physician-interpreted ECGs. The negative predictive values were 81% for the computer and 85% for the physician.

Conclusions.—Prehospital computer-interpreted ECG to screen potential candidates for thrombolytic therapy is feasible and highly specific. Further improvement in the currently available algorithm should promote speedy and appropriate treatment of patients with acute myocardial infarction.

▶ This study dramatically demonstrates the positive predictive value of computer interpretation of myocardial infarction patterns on ECGs.

In the overall algorithm of time delays between the onset of symptoms and the initiation of thrombolytic therapy, prehospital transport time is a contributor, but the time from emergency department arrival to drug administration frequently results in at least twice as much wasted time (1). If medics can communicate the computer-generated diagnosis in advance of a patient's arrival, thrombolytic therapy could be ready and waiting for immediate administration. Medic administration of the drug is also possible but will probably be useful only when the logistics of administration are minimized.—W.P. Burdick, M.D.

Reference

1. Kereikes DJ, et al: *Am Heart J* 120:773, 1990.

Hemorrhagic Events During Therapy With Recombinant Tissue-Type Plasminogen Activator, Heparin, and Aspirin for Acute Myocardial Infarction: Results of the Thrombolysis in Myocardial Infarction (TIMI), Phase II Trial

Bovill EG, Terrin ML, Stump DC, Berke AD, Frederick M, et al (Univ of Vermont, Burlington; Maryland Med Res Inst, Baltimore; Columbia Univ, New York, NY; Univ of Massachusetts, Worcester; Univ of Texas, Dallas)

Ann Intern Med 115:256–265, 1991 3–58

Introduction.—Thrombolytic therapy is often effective in early acute myocardial infarction, but hemorrhagic complications continue to occur. Rates as high as 30% are reported when invasive procedures are part of the protocol.

Study Design.—A multicenter trial included 3,339 patients with ischemic chest pain who received recombinant tissue plasminogen activator (rt-PA) in a dose of 150 or 100 mg. Patients were randomly assigned either to an invasive approach entailing coronary angiography with percutaneous angioplasty, if feasible, 18 to 48 hours after the start of thrombolysis, or to conservative management. The latter patients had angiography if ischemia recurred. Patients also were randomized to immediate intravenous β-blocker therapy or deferred treatment.

Results.—Among patients given 100 mg of rt-PA, hemorrhage was more frequent in those assigned to invasive management than in those managed conservatively (18.5% vs. 12.8%). Hemorrhage correlated with the degree of fibrinogen breakdown, the peak rt-PA level, thrombocytopenia, an activated partial thromboplastin time exceeding 90 seconds, and signs of cardiac decompensation. Women and patients weighing 70 kg or less had hemorrhagic events more frequently. Intracranial bleeding was more common in patients given the higher dose of rt-PA, and a greater hemostatic defect developed in these patients.

Implications.—Many factors contribute to the occurrence of hemorrhage in patients given thrombolytic treatment for myocardial infarction. Invasive management was associated with more frequent hemorrhage in this study.

▶ The investigators found that coronary angiography 18 to 48 hours after study entry was associated with increased hemorrhage both at puncture sites and in the gastrointestinal system. No explanation is offered for the latter. Perhaps stress ulcers associated with the additional emotional and physical insult of the percutaneous coronary angiography may play a role.

This study, coupled with the investigators' earlier TIMI-II clinical outcome report, suggests that for most patients with myocardial infarction, diagnostic angiography should be postponed beyond 48 hours postthrombolysis. However, if patients do not demonstrate evidence of reperfusion and a large portion of previously viable myocardium remains in jeopardy, invasive procedures (i.e., therapeutic angiography or coronary bypass graft surgery) may be needed, even before the 18-hour period described in this report. Emergency physicians should prepare for emergency blood replacement in all patients receiving thrombolytic therapy, minimize puncture wounds, and reduce associated psychological and physical patient stress (see also Abstracts 3–59 and 3–60).—J.R. Hedges, M.D.

Massive Upper Airway Bleeding After Thrombolytic Therapy: Successful Airway Management With the Combitube®

Klauser R, Röggla G, Pidlich J, Leithner C, Frass M (Wahringer Gurtel, Vienna, Austria)

Ann Emerg Med 21:431–433, 1992 3–59

Introduction.—In patients who are not breathing, endotracheal tube insertion may sometimes be difficult. The use of the Combitube airway in a patient in whom endotracheal intubation failed was studied.

Case Report.—A 63-year-old man with severe chronic obstructive pulmonary disease was admitted to the intensive care unit with acute dyspnea and chest pain. Physical examination and chest radiography suggested the diagnosis of acute pulmonary embolus, and thrombolytic therapy with anisoylated plasminogen streptokinase activator was begun. However, as a result of confusion over

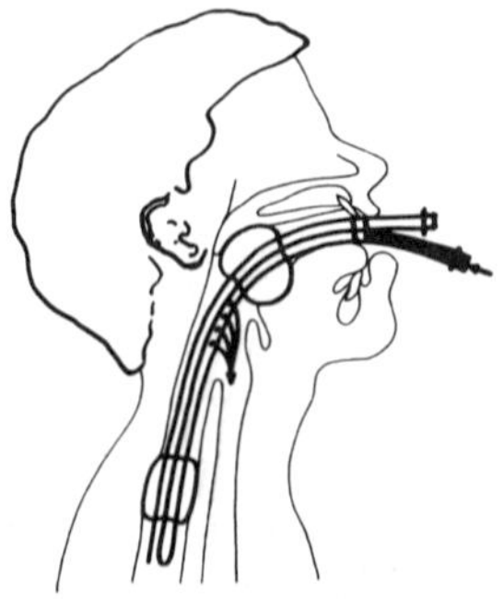

Fig 3–12.—Combitube after esophageal placement. (Courtesy of Klauser R, Röggla G, Pidlich J, et al: *Ann Emerg Med* 21:431–433, 1992.)

the protocol, 2 doses of 230 mg were accidentally infused during 1 hour. Massive bleeding from the pharynx followed 4 hours after the start of therapy. The patient was aspirating large amounts of blood, and endotracheal intubation failed because the glottis could not be visualized. Blind and fiber-optic intubation also failed, and cricothyroidotomy was deemed inadvisable. The Combitube was then inserted, and the patient was mechanically ventilated; his blood gas analysis reflected adequate ventilation. Prothrombin complex concentrate and antithrombin were also given. A conventional endotracheal tube was inserted in place of the Combitube 30 minutes later. At this time, direct laryngoscopy showed sublingual hematomas in the soft palatal and right pharyngeal regions. The patient was weaned and extubated after 2 days, and he was discharged with no signs of neurologic deficit in 1 week.

Discussion.—The Combitube may provide for adequate ventilation in nonbreathing patients for whom endotracheal intubation fails. This twin-lumen tube can be inserted esophageally or endotracheally (Figs 3–12 and 3–13) and allows adequate ventilation without having to worry about the face-mask seal, as with the esophageal obturator airway. The

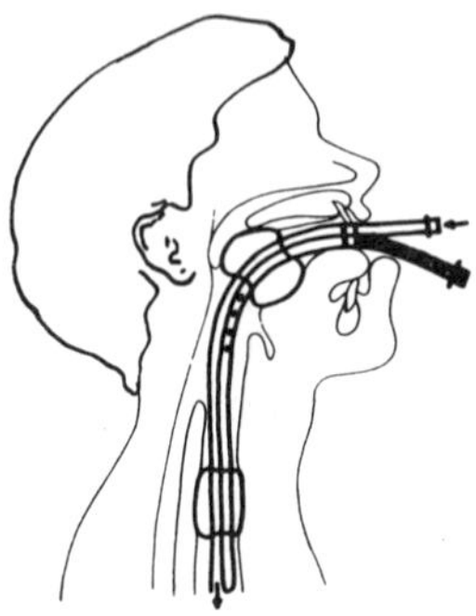

Fig 3–13.—Combitube after endotracheal placement. (Courtesy of Klauser R, Röggla G, Pidlich J, et al: *Ann Emerg Med* 21:431–433, 1992.)

device is quickly and easily inserted, although the physician must be familiar with airway management and know how to determine the correct position by auscultation or other means.

► At my institution, a patient underwent nasotracheal intubation in the coronary care unit shortly after receiving thrombolytic therapy resulting in severe bleeding from the nasopharynx. This made tracheal intubation difficult. Such complications will occur, and we should be prepared for it. The Combitube should lend itself to this situation. Our colleagues in Vienna should be complimented for their quick thinking.—E. Ruiz, M.D.

Bleeding Complications Following Initiation of Thrombolytic Therapy for Acute Myocardial Infarction: A Comparison of Helicopter-Transported and Nontransported Patients

Fromm RE Jr, Hoskins E, Cronin L, Pratt CM, Spencer WH III, et al (Baylor College of Medicine; Methodist Hosp, Houston, Tex)

Ann Emerg Med 20:892–895, 1991 3–60

Introduction.—Thrombolytic therapy is widely used in patients with acute myocardial infarction (AMI) and ST-segment elevation. Prehospital treatment may save time and improve left ventricular salvage, but there are concerns about the risk of bleeding in patients being transported. The effect of helicopter transport on bleeding complications in AMI patients who have been started on thrombolytic therapy was evaluated.

Methods.—During the 2-year study period, 95 patients were transported by helicopter within 12 hours of the initiation of thrombolytic therapy with recombinant tissue-type plasminogen activator. These patients were compared with 119 nontransported AMI patients treated in a similar manner.

Results.—The mean time from the initiation of thrombolytic therapy to transport was 44.4 minutes. Seventy-eight of the transported patients were also moved by ground ambulance during a period when the hospital's rooftop heliport was unavailable. Fifteen patients had hypotension requiring intravenous fluid challenge during transport, but on the whole, the helicopter trip was well tolerated. Through the time of hospital discharge, bleeding complications were observed in 43.2% of the transported patients and 49.6% of the nontransported patients. Bleeding at catheterization, intravenous line, or other vascular puncture sites was common in both groups.

Conclusion.—When accomplished by a highly skilled team, the helicopter transport of AMI patients after initiation of thrombolysis does not appear to increase the risk of bleeding or other complications. The nurse-physician teams at the study institution have received extensive education in the use of thrombolytic drugs and their potential adverse effects.

▶ As the title suggests, this article specifically addresses bleeding complications as a result of interfacility transport. While bleeding complications were statistically not significantly different between the groups, the transferring physicians should be familiar with both the indications for transport and the capabilities of the flight crew. In addition to the complications stated above, 9 patients received atropine for bradycardia, and 1 required external pacing. Patients sustaining an AMI can be very unstable en route. The authors describe using a "highly trained" physician and nurse crew.—W.J. Koenig, M.D.

Medical, Ethical and Legal Issues Regarding Thrombolytic Therapy in the Jehovah's Witness

Sugarman J, Churchill LR, Moore JK, Waugh RA (Duke Univ Med Ctr, Durham, NC; Johns Hopkins Med School, Baltimore, Md; Univ of North Carolina, Chapel Hill)

Am J Cardiol 68:1525–1529, 1991 3–61

Background.—Care was provided recently for a patient receiving thrombolytic treatment for an acute myocardial infarction. The patient was a Jehovah's Witness who refused blood transfusion and subsequently bled to death. Medical, ethical, and legal questions about the use of thrombolytic treatment in persons refusing blood transfusions a priori were raised.

Case Report.—A 57-year-old woman came to an emergency department with complaints of chest discomfort. An acute inferior myocardial infarction was diagnosed, and the patient was asked to participate in a study on thrombolysis and angioplasty in myocardial infarction. On her consent, she was randomly assigned to receive thrombolysis with tissue plasminogen activator and urokinase followed by acute cardiac catheterization. She had clearly stated her religious objection to the use of any blood products in her care. Over a period of several days, she became hypotensive. Her stool was melenic, and her hematocrit, 20%. She was told that her condition was life-threatening, but she again refused transfusion. Despite treatment with sucralfate and an H_2 blocker, her gastrointestinal bleeding continued. Her hematocrit dropped to 14%. She deteriorated mentally and became incapable of making decisions. Her family confirmed her prior refusal of blood transfusion and knew that she could die without the treatment. She subsequently died.

Implications.—A review of medical, ethical, and legal in the use of thrombolytic therapy in Jehovah's Witnesses stresses the need for informed consent that highlights the possible need for blood transfusion. Physicians in similar situations may wish to consider various factors, such as the likely hemodynamic consequences of the infarction and the use of treatment modalities that may minimize the need for blood transfusions. Researchers may consider excluding such patients from studies on the efficacy of thrombolytic therapy.

▶ The inclusion criteria for thrombolysis appear to be ever-broadening. This article underlines several important points. One is that not all myocardial infarctions (MIs) are alike. A relatively uncomplicated inferior wall MI benefits little by thrombolysis; neither left ventricular function nor morbidity is greatly improved. Given this, one should carefully balance the risk-to-benefit issues in treating an inferior wall MI with thrombolytic agents. However, withholding thrombolytic therapy implies a selection bias and potentially prohibiting access to valuable, potentially lifesaving treatment. In all cases, a careful discussion of the benefits and risks must occur, and the patient and family must be integral partners in the decision making.—E.J. Reisdorff, M.D.

Outcome of Patients With Acute Myocardial Infarction Who Are Ineligible for Thrombolytic Therapy

Cragg DR, Friedman HZ, Bonema JD, Jaiyesimi IA, Ramos RG, et al (William Beaumont Hosp, Royal Oak, Mich)

Ann Intern Med 115:173–177, 1991 3–62

Introduction.—Intravenous thrombolytic therapy may reduce mortality from acute myocardial infarction (AMI) by as much as 50%. However, when traditional eligibility criteria are applied, thrombolytic therapy is used in only a minority of patients with AMI. The proportion of patients admitted with AMI who were not eligible for thrombolytic therapy was calculated and the outcome in those excluded patients determined.

Patients.—During a 27-month period, 1,471 patients were admitted with AMI, 230 (16%) of whom received thrombolytic therapy according to the protocol and an additional 97 (7%) of whom received non-protocol thrombolytic therapy, coronary balloon angioplasty, or both. The remaining 1,144 patients (78%) did not receive reperfusion therapy because of one or more exclusion criteria. Excluded patients were older, were less likely to be men, and had a higher rate of non-Q-wave infarction. An average of 1.9 reasons for exclusion were identified per excluded patient.

Outcome.—The overall mortality rate in excluded patients with AMI was 19% vs. 4% in those who received thrombolytic therapy on the study protocol. The in-hospital mortality rates for patients excluded from thrombolytic therapy were 28% in elderly patients, 29% in those with stroke or bleeding risk, 17% in those with delayed presentation, 14% in those ineligible on the basis of an ECG, and 26% in those with a miscellaneous reason for exclusion. Age greater than 76 years, stroke or other bleeding risk, ineligible ECG, or the presence of 2 or more exclusion criteria were independent predictors of increased mortality.

Conclusion.—Only patients with AMI who have low-risk prognostic characteristics are currently eligible for thrombolytic therapy. Investigations to broaden the application of thrombolytic agents are warranted.

▶ The largest groups excluded from thrombolytic use were patients with nondiagnostic ECGs those arriving more than 4 hours after the onset of symptoms, and patients over 76 years of age. Almost half of the 1,400 patients with AMI in this retrospective study had nondiagnostic ECGs—a humbling reminder about the importance of the history. Optimally, this group will be made smaller in the future by the use of earlier chemical markers of infarction such as troponin and myoglobin and the development of quicker assays for creatine kinase. The use of thrombolytic therapy beyond 4 hours of the onset of symptoms is now more widely accepted than during the period covered by this chart review, although the outer limit of intervention is still very much open to further study.

About 20% of the patients were excluded from thrombolytic therapy in this study because they were elderly. This supports data from another study by Weaver et al. in which patients with AMI under the age of 75 years were 6 times as likely to receive thrombolytic therapy as patients over 75 (1). While the risk of intracerebral bleeding is reported to be higher in older patients, the potential benefits are also higher since the mortality rate in patients over 75 is 18% vs. only 2% among those less than 55 years of age. Therefore, once those with specific disease-based contraindications have been excluded, elderly patients should be considered eligible for thrombolytic therapy.—W.P. Burdick, M.D.

Reference

1. Weaver DW, et al: *J Am Coll Cardiol* 18:657, 1991.

Gastrogenital and Urogenital

Spontaneous Haemopneumothorax: A Rare Clinical Entity

Baas P, Stam J (Free Univ Hosp, Amsterdam, The Netherlands)
Eur Respir J 4:1027–1028, 1991 3–63

Background.—Early recognition and surgical intervention resulted in successful treatment of a patient with spontaneous hemopneumothorax.

Case Report.—A 39-year-old man had acute right-sided chest pain and shortness of breath of sudden onset with no history of trauma. Findings on physical examination of dyspnea, a hyperresonant percussion note, and reduced breath sounds on the right side suggested a right-sided pneumothorax. A spontaneous pneumothorax was confirmed by chest radiography, and findings suggested a tension pneumothorax. On initial pleural drainage, 120 mL of hemorrhagic fluid was collected. Within 24 hours, after re-expansion of the lung, shock developed, and 1,200 mL of hemorrhagic fluid was spontaneously collected. A right-sided thoracotomy was performed, and the remnants of a ruptured, continuously bleeding vessel in the lung apex were found and coagulated.

Discussion.—An air fluid line in a sitting or standing chest radiograph and the development of hemorrhagic pleural effusion and shock signal hemopneumothorax. Treatment of spontaneous hemopneumothorax can be conservative or operative, but in cases of high initial blood loss or recurrence of bleeding or shock, thoracotomy is mandatory. Death occurs mainly in the first 48 hours. Close monitoring of a patient with pneumothorax and early surgical intervention for hemopneumothorax are recommended.

▶ This article is a timely reminder that serious complications can result from spontaneous pneumothorax even after full expansion of the lung has been achieved. The availability of small chest tubes inserted with the Seldinger technique and the pressure to keep patients out of the hospital must not cause us to discharge such patients prematurely without a careful study of potential problems (see also Abstract 3–16).—E. Ruiz, M.D.

Prevention of Stress Gastritis With Tissue Preservation Solution

Fenton AH, Clark TW, Meyer MS, Moorman DW (Northeastern Ohio Univ, Akron; Akron Gen Med Ctr, Ohio)

Am Surg 58:250–254, 1992 3–64

Background.—Decreased gastric mucosal blood flow appears to be central to the production of stress gastritis in critically ill patients. Prevention of ischemia might prevent the gastritis. A study was conducted in rats to determine whether topically applied synthetic organ preservation solution can inhibit the development of stress gastritis.

Methods.—The study included 18 similar male Sprague-Dawley rats divided into 2 groups. One group of animals received only 5% dextrose and water (D_5W) for 72 hours, and the other received D_5W and a 50% solution of University of Wisconsin cold preservation solution (UWS), an isoosmolar, non-glucose-based solution that minimizes hypothermia-induced cell swelling while preventing intracellular acidosis and oxygen free radical injury harvested organs. After 72 hours, the animals were anesthetized and stressed according to the cold-restraint model for 4 hours at 4°C. They were then killed and examined for signs of gastric ulcers.

Findings.—Animals that received UWS solution had nearly half as many ulcers as those in the D_5W-only group. They also had a significantly lower mean total ulcer length and ulcer index. Grade 0 to 1 gastritis was present in most of the UWS group, whereas grade 3 gastritis was found in more than half the D_5W-only group. The groups had similar gastric mucosal pH.

Conclusions.—Topically applied UWS organ preservation solution can decrease the severity and incidence of stress gastritis. The consistent mucosal pH suggests that this might occur by alteration of the effects of gastric mucosal ischemia at a cellular level.

▶ Stress ulceration of the gastric mucosa is a common complication of many sorts of critical illness, including severe burns, trauma, mechanical ventilation, and cardiac resuscitation. It is at least partially mediated by gastric acid, and it is commonly recommended to administer H_2 blockers prophylactically to critically ill patients. These authors tried a different approach: orally feeding their rats a cocktail originally designed for the vascular perfusion of organs in cold storage awaiting transplantation (1). It is unclear to me whether the reduction in stress ulcers they saw resulted from local action of the UWS on the gastric mucosa or systemic absorption of its components.

The composition of the UWS solution includes an inhibitor of xanthine oxidase, a scavenger of free radicals and peroxides, ATP substrate, buffers, and magnesium. This reflects current thinking about the mechanisms of cellular injury during ischemia (2). Similar "resuscitation cocktails" have been proposed for use in patients resuscitated from cardiac arrest to blunt the effect of ischemic injury to the brain and other organs. Their use in the manner described in this paper is a new twist, one that bears further investigation.—J. Schoffstall, M.D.

References

1. Belzer FO, Southard JH: *Transplantation* 45:673, 1988.
2. Krause GS, et al: *Crit Care Med* 16:714, 1988.

Omeprazole Versus Placebo for Acute Upper Gastrointestinal Bleeding: Randomised Double Blind Controlled Trial

Daneshmend TK, Hawkey CJ, Langman MJS, Logan RFA, Long RG, et al (Univ and City Hosps, Nottingham, England)

BMJ 304:143–147, 1992 3–65

Background.—Profound suppression of gastric acid secretion with the proton pump inhibitor omeprazole may reduce morbidity and mortality associated with acute upper gastrointestinal bleeding. The possible therapeutic role of omeprazole in unselected patients with upper gastrointestinal bleeding was assessed in a double-blind placebo-controlled study.

Methods.—Subjects included 1,147 patients aged 18 years or older and consecutively hospitalized for acute upper gastrointestinal bleeding during a 40-month period. Omeprazole, 80 mg, was given intravenously immediately, then in 3 doses of 40 mg intravenously every 8 hours, followed by 40-mg doses orally every 12 hours. Treatment was begun within 12 hours of admission and continued for 4 days or until surgery, discharge, or death.

Findings.—No significant differences were found between the group given omeprazole and the group given placebo in transfusion rates, rebleeding rates, the need for surgery, or death rates. However, patients treated with omeprazole had a significant, unexpected reduction in endoscopic signs of upper gastrointestinal bleeding when compared with those given placebo. The percentages of patients with those signs were 45% in the placebo group and 33% in the omeprazole-treated group.

Conclusions.—Omeprazole does not reduce mortality, rebleeding, or transfusion requirements in patients hospitalized with acute upper gastrointestinal bleeding. However, a decrease in endoscopic signs of bleeding suggests that acid inhibition may influence intragastric bleeding. The routine use of acid-inhibiting drugs in patients with hematemesis and melena is not justified.

▶ This is an interesting study, but no new treatment modality for gastrointestinal bleeding comes of it. Upper gastrointestinal bleeding will be managed in the traditional way in the emergency center for the time being, including gastrointestinal decompression and volume replacement followed by endoscopic evaluation and direct control of identified bleeding points.—S.B. Repasky, D.O.

Sonographic Detection of the Normal and Abnormal Appendix

Rioux M (Hôpital Saint-François d'Assise, Québec, Canada)

AJR 158:773–778, 1992 3–66

Background.—The use of sonography in diagnosing appendicitis has been the subject of much research. In the current study, the author tried to optimize visualization of the appendix in patients with suspected acute appendicitis and assess whether visualization improved the overall accuracy of sonography in the diagnosis of a normal or abnormal appendix.

Methods.—One hundred seventy patients were prospectively studied. All had suspected appendicitis. Wall thickness, appendix compressibility, and echogenicity of surrounding fat were the main criteria used to determine the status of the appendix. Of the 60 patients who had surgery, 45 were proved to have appendicitis. The remaining 110 patients who did not have surgery were contacted by telephone. These patients had no clinical follow-up evidence of acute appendicitis.

Findings.—A normal appendix was clearly identified on sonography in 82% of 125 patients without acute appendicitis. Sonography had a sensitivity of 93% in detecting appendicitis. Its specificity was 94%, and its accuracy was 94%. The predictive value of a positive test was 86%, and the predictive value of a negative test was 98%. In all 11 cases, ruptured appendicitis was predicted sonographically.

Conclusions.—A normal appendix can be visualized on sonography much more often than has been previously thought. Wall thickness was a useful index of appendix status, with 3 mm or less being normal. The search for sonographic visualization of normal as well as abnormal appendix seems to significantly decrease the percentage of false-negative results.

▶ This is an article worth sending to the radiology department of every hospital. It never ceases to amaze me how the diagnosis of appendicitis is a purely clinical diagnosis after 5:00 P.M., but between 8:00 A.M. and 5:00 P.M., it can be made with ultrasound. This is just another paper that demonstrates that diagnosis can be assisted with ultrasound. An ultrasound should be available either in the emergency department 24 hours a day or by a radiologist 24 hours a day.

Since missed appendicitis is one of the most common reasons why emergency physicians are sued, it certainly makes sense to be aggressive in using every tool at one's disposal to make the correct diagnosis.—W.H. Spivey, M.D.

Arterial-Venous pH Differences and Tissue Hypoxia in Patients With Fulminant Hepatic Failure

Wendon JA, Harrison PM, Keays R, Gimson AE, Alexander G, et al (King's College Hosp, London, England)

Crit Care Med 19:1362–1364, 1991 3–67

Introduction.—A recent study suggests that acid-base status in hypotensive patients is best assessed by simultaneous estimates of arterial pH, mixed venous pH, and bicarbonate. This method would be useful in detecting covert tissue hypoxia, a condition characteristic of patients with fulminant hepatic failure. The arterial-venous pH difference as an indicator of tissue hypoxia was evaluated in 22 patients with fulminant hepatic failure, and findings were compared with the results of an infusion of prostacyclin to uncover tissue hypoxia.

Methods.—Hepatic failure was caused by acetaminophen toxicity in 19 patients and by non-A, non-B hepatitis in 3. All but 2 patients were undergoing artificial ventilation. Blood samples taken from the pulmonary artery and radial artery were analyzed to determine oxygen delivery and consumption. An oxygen flux test was used to compare arterial pH, mixed venous pH, and bicarbonate.

Results.—The pH and bicarbonate differences in arterial and mixed venous blood samples were not indicative of tissue hypoxia. After an infusion of prostacyclin, however, the measurement of oxygen consumption, which demonstrated an increase in oxygen uptake, was more accurate in detecting cover tissue hypoxia.

Conclusion.—The oxygen flux test, as performed with prostacyclin, can demonstrate tissue hypoxia and hypoperfusion in patients with fulminant hepatic failure better than evaluation of an arterial-venous pH difference.

▶ This article is interesting but not very relevant to the setting of the emergency department since it concludes that an oxygen flux test is necessary to truly measure the "correct" tissue hypoxemia in patients with fulminant hepatic failure.—E.J. Lucid, M.D.

Massive Rectal Bleeding From a Dieulafoy's Type Ulcer of the Rectum: A Review of This Unusual Disease

Franko E, Chardavoyne R, Wise L (Long Island Jewish Med Ctr, New Hyde Park, NY)

Am J Gastroenterol 86:1545–1547, 1991 3–68

Background.—Dieulafoy's ulcer is an uncommon lesion whose cause remains unknown. Most reported ulcers have occurred in the stomach. In 1 patient, apparently the first, Dieulafoy's ulcer occurred in the rectum.

Case Report.—A 20-year-old man entered the emergency room with a 6-hour history of bleeding from the rectum. The patient remained normotensive, and an abdominal examination was unremarkable. Rigid sigmoidoscopy revealed a small mucosal ulceration with a spurting artery at its base. Endoscopic coagulation and rectal packing were ineffective in controlling the hemorrhage. The patient underwent wide suture ligation of the vessel under general anesthesia. No recurrence of bleeding had occurred at 9 months of follow-up.

Discussion.—A review of the literature showed the average age of patients with Dieulafoy's ulcer to be about 50 years. There is a male preponderance and an association, according to some studies, with alcohol abuse. The lesion has had a high mortality rate until recent years. One study suggested that the ulcer results from a congenital vessel malformation. Surgery is the treatment of choice, although endoscopic therapy has been recommended for gastric Dieulafoy's ulcers.

Conclusion.—Hemorrhage associated with Dieulafoy's ulcer of the rectum probably results from mechanical damage of the mucosa combined with erosion of the vessel by fecal flow. Rigid sigmoidoscopy should diagnose the ulcer, although angiography may be necessary with high rectal ulcers. Widely oversewing the rectal lesion was recommended as the primary treatment.

▶ Dieulafoy's ulcer is characterized by massive hemorrhage from an abnormally large submucosal artery with an overlying small mucosal defect. Although most commonly described within the gastric mucosa, it has been reported infrequently throughout the gastrointestinal tract. This report indicates that it may also occur in the rectum and should be considered in the differential diagnosis of massive hematochezia (see Abstract 9–25).—J.T. Niemann, M.D.

Comparative Study of the Efficacy of Dipyrone, Diclofenac Sodium and Pethidine in Acute Renal Colic

Garcia-Alonso F, for the Collaborative Group of the Spanish Society of Clinical Pharmacology (Ministerio de Sanidad y Consumo, Madrid, Spain)
Eur J Clin Pharmacol 40:543–546, 1991 3–69

Background.—Opiate analgesics are usually used to treat patients with acute renal colic. However, opiates have side effects, and their use would be best restricted to patients not responding to conventional analgesics. Several nonopiate analgesics have been proposed. The effects of dipyrone, diclofenac sodium, and pethidine in acute renal colic were investigated.

Methods.—Four hundred fifty-one patients in 13 Spanish hospitals were enrolled in the randomized, double-blind clinical trial. Patients received dipyrone, 1 or 2 g; (intramuscularly administered) intramuscularly administered diclofenac sodium; or intramuscularly administered pehidine. Pain severity was assessed by physicians and patients using visual analogue scales. Drug efficicy was judged according to the need for rescue treatment—pethidine, 100 mg intramuscularly administered 30 minutes after the experimental treatment was delivered.

Findings.—Ninety-three patients required rescue treatment: 24.1% of the 1-g dipyrone group, 22.3% of the 2-g dipyrone group, 16.4% of the diclofenac sodium group, and 19.5% of the pethidine group. Between-group differences were nonsignificant. In the remaining 358 patients, there were no differences among the treatment conditions.

Conclusions.—In patients with acute renal colic, dipyrone, 1 g, appears to be just as effective as dipyrone, 2 g. Thus, giving 2 g of dipyrone is not justified. Diclofenac has a similar analgesic effect and is a valid alternative in this patient population.

▶ This study revealed various forms of pharmacologic therapy that are unavailable in the United States for the treatment of acute renal colic. As a matter of reference, dipyrone is related to phenylbutazone, pethidine is an opioid, and diclofenac is a nonsteroidal anti-inflammatory drug (NSAID) which, in tablet form, is Voltaren. Some forms of pethidine produced in the Middle East and in Europe are meperidine-containing compounds. These agents were given intramuscularly. This study demonstrated that the parenteral use of nonopioid analgesics can be very effective in the treatment of renal colic. Currently, in North America, the NSAID ketorolac (Toradol), 60 mg, intramuscularly, is effective in the treatment of renal colic. Concurrent use of ketorolac and narcotics may decrease the dose requirements for opioids.—E.J. Reisdorff, M.D.

Renal Colic: Utility of the Plain Abdominal Roentgenogram

Mutgi A, Williams JW, Nettleman M (Med College of Ohio, Toledo; Duke Univ, Durham, NC; Univ of Iowa, Iowa City)

Arch Intern Med 151:1589–1592, 1991 3–70

Background.—Physicians routinely use the plain abdominal roentgenogram (PAR) to evaluate patients with suspected renal stones and renal colic. However, a recent study suggested a relatively low sensitivity for PAR and poor predictive value in diagnosing renal stones. This study assessed the sensitivity and specificity of PAR in detecting renal stones in 85 consecutive patients with acute renal colic during a 2-year period.

Methods.—Physicians retrospectively studied demographic data, clinical history, laboratory results, and results from PAR and intravenous pyelography (IVP). They calculated the sensitivity, specificity, and positive and negative predictive values of PAR. They also evaluated the value of a simple clinical scoring system in predicting the presence of stones as compared with PAR.

Results.—With positive IVP results and/or stone retrieval as the gold standard, 72 patients had documented stones; 68 patients had positive IVP findings, but an additional 4 patients had stones retrieved during follow-up. Nine patients had negative IVP results, and 4 had indeterminate results. Forty-six patients had positive PAR findings. Of these, 4 were false-positive. Of 39 negative PARs, 30 were false-negative. The sensitivity of PAR was 58%, and its specificity was 69%. In a population with a stone prevalence of 85%, the positive predictive value for PAR was 91%, whereas the negative predictive value was only 23%. In comparison, the clinical system using a score of ≥ 3 to indicate presence of a stone and ≤ 2 to indicate the absence of a stone yielded a sensitivity of 73% and a specificity of 46%. The positive predictive value was 88%, and the negative predictive value was 24%.

Conclusions.—A clinical scoring system based on signs and symptoms compared favorably with PAR. Clinical scoring plus selective use of IVP is more cost-effective than PAR. Because PAR has low sensitivity and specificity and little added predictive value, its routine use cannot be justified in terms of cost.

▶ The routine use of PAR for screening patients with possible ureteral colic is commonplace in emergency centers. This paper provides useful information for the emergency physician to limit this test.

Analysis of the sensitivity, specificity, and predictive value of PAR was carried out in a straightforward fashion. A comparison with a clinical scoring system shows no advantage to PAR over clinical evalution with urinalysis.

This paper confirms my clinical experience. Clinical impressions routinely override PAR findings, especially when the film is negative. PAR in this setting seems to be another example of reflex ancillary testing that does little but increase the cost of medical care. I expect to see decreasing use of PAR in the future.—J.E. Clinton, M.D.

Urinary Bladder Distention Presenting as Venous Obstruction and Hypovolemic Shock

Bouachour G, Tirot P, Varache N, Dauphin M, Alquier P (Centre Hospitalier Universitaire, Angers, France)
Am J Emerg Med 9:563–564, 1991 3–71

Background.—Urinary bladder distension is usually an obvious diagnosis. However, in exceptional cases, the clinical presentation can simulate neurologic, digestive, or vascular disorders. A patient with clinical vascular complications secondary to acute urinary retention is described.

Case Study.—A 63-year-old man with previous history of head injury and neurologic sequelae was admitted with hypovolemic shock. His blood pressure was 80/40 mm Hg, and his heart rate was 130 per minute. Physical examination revealed signs of arterial and venous obstruction of the left leg. Arterial pulses were not palpable, and there was cyanosis, major diffuse edema, and petechial purpura of the knee. The patient was confused, but he had no neurologic deficit. The belly was rigid on abdominal palpation. Rectal examination revealed a markedly enlarged and firm prostate gland. Phlegmasia cerulea dolens secondary to venous thrombosis was diagnosed. The emergency physician began vascular expansion. Radiologists performed phlebography, which disclosed extrinsic removal of the right primitive and external iliac venae. There was also complete compression without opacification of the left iliac vessels by a large pelvic mass that proved to be the distended urinary bladder. A radiogram showed bilateral distension of the calyces. Symptoms resolved after insertion of a Foley catheter that evacuated 3,000 mL of urine.

Discussion.—In the absence of the usual clinical manifestations, a distended bladder may be revealed by its complications. In this case, the clinical picture was similar to the typical features of phlegmasia cerulea dolens. The hypovolemic shock experienced by the patient was due to sequestration of fluid in the lower extremities.

► A distended bladder is common in the emergency center setting. However, for the distended bladder to function as a solid mass and compress and displace the iliac veins and arteries without rupture suggests a thickening of the bladder wall such as occurs in chronic interstitial cystitis.—G.V. Anderson, M.D.

Co-Morbidity Associated With Fabricated Illness (Munchausen Syndrome by Proxy)

Bools CN, Neale BA, Meadow SR (St James's Univ Hosp, Leeds, England)

Arch Dis Child 67:77–79, 1992 3–72

Background.—In Munchausen syndrome by proxy, a parent fabricates an illness in a child and seeks medical attention for it. The comorbidity associated with this syndrome was studied.

Patients and Outcomes.—Fifty-six children with fabricated illnesses and 82 of their 103 siblings were assessed. Sixty-four percent of the index children had had other illnesses fabricated by their mothers in addition to the index fabrication. Twenty-nine percent of the index children had a history of failure to thrive. Twenty-nine percent had a history of nonaccidental injury, inappropriate medication, or neglect. At least 1 of these additional problems occurred in 73% of the index children. Eleven percent of the siblings studied had died in early childhood. Causes of death could not be identified. Thiry-nine percent of the siblings had also had illnesses fabricated by their mothers. Seventeen percent had had failure to thrive, had nonaccidental injury, had been given inappropriate medication, or had been neglected.

Conclusions.—When Munchausen syndrome by proxy occurs, all children in the index family should be considered at high risk for abuse and neglect. The relevant professionals must carry out a detailed assessment of the children and the parenting behavior of the mother and father. Professional involvement will usually be needed to ensure the safety and development of the children in such a family.

▶ Munchausen syndrome by proxy was originally described in 1977 (1). It is a difficult condition to define during a brief encounter in the emergency department. Nevertheless, it is an important diagnosis to establish. This importance is emphasized since the authors of this article have demonstrated a risk of injury and neglect to the siblings. Although the study is from the United Kingdom, the dynamics of this syndrome should be similar in North America.—E.J. Reisdorff, M.D.

Reference

1. Meadow R: *Lancet* ii:343, 1977.

Neurologic

Cerebral Dural Sinus Thrombosis

Pannke TS (Univ of Illinois, Peoria)

Ann Emerg Med 20:813–816, 1991 3–73

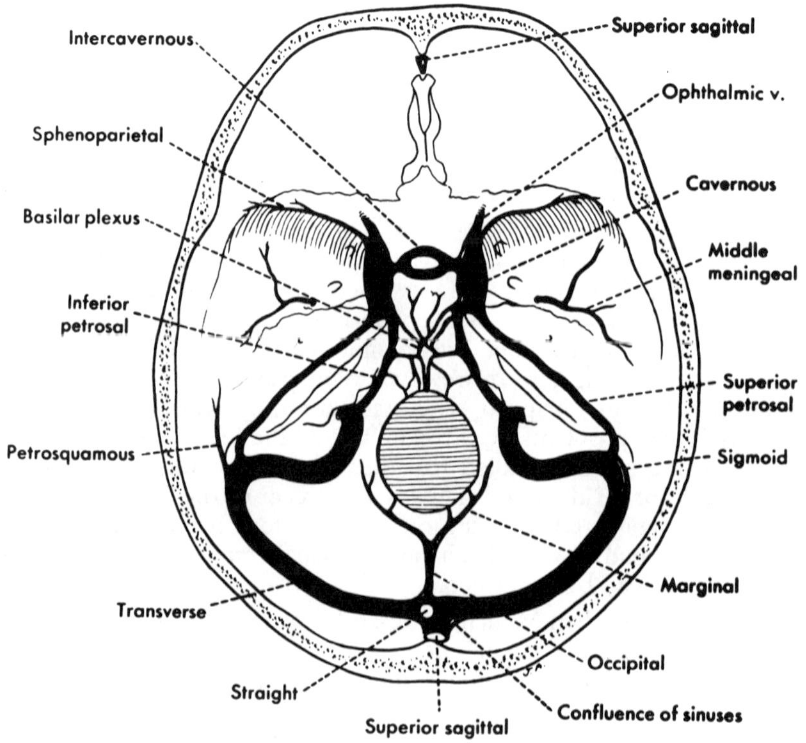

Fig 3–14.—Diagram of cerebral dural sinuses. (From Pannke TS: *Ann Emerg Med* 20:813–816, 1991. Courtesy of Hollinshead WH, Rosse C: *Textbook of Anatomy*, ed 4. Philadelphia, JB Lippincott Co, 1985, p 925.)

Introduction.—Severe headache is a fairly common complaint from emergency department patients. Cerebral dural sinus thrombosis (CDST) is an uncommon syndrome that can cause severe headache. A woman with a previous history of migraines was given a diagnosis of CDST.

Case Report.—A 31-year-old woman with a significant history of recurrent migraines experienced a severe headache and vomiting. There were no other neurologic symptoms. Medications included oral contraceptive pills, prazepam, and piroxicam. Although the appropriate diagnostic workup for suspected CDST was performed, no etiology was found. The headache improved, and the patient was discharged. A day later, the patient was readmitted with generalized tonic-clonic seizures and subsequent dense right hemiplegia. Magnetic resonance imaging studies showed extensive thrombosis in the sagittal, straight, and jugular sinuses (Fig 3–14), which was confirmed on cerebral angiography. Heparin, mannitol, and phenytoin were administered, and the patient improved.

Discussion.—Cerebral dural sinus thrombosis may be evidenced by severe headache alone or generalized seizures followed by focal deficits. A review of 38 previously reported cases of CDST show 2 groups of patients with CDST: the first group typically has headache and papilledema representing a thrombus in the sinus alone, while a second group with headache, papilledema, vomiting, seizures, and focal neurologic deficits represents extension of the thrombus into the cortical veins. The present case demonstrates the natural history of a typical presentation of CDST. There are several known or suspected predisposing factors to CDST, including hypercoagulability. Diagnostic studies include enhanced CT, MRI, and cerebral angiography. Therapy remains controversial, although combination therapy with antiseizure and anticoagulant medication and an osmotic diuretic was successful in the case above. The prognosis for patients with CDST is fairly good.

▶ Although the author concludes that the patient had a CDST that escaped detection despite appropriate diagnostic workup on the first admission, it is possible that the process was in an early phase at that time. Since there is no mention that oral contraceptive use was discontinued and acetazolamide was recommended, it is possible that an oral diuretic by relative dehydration through induced diuresis would contribute to a hyperviscous state.—G.V. Anderson, M.D.

Warning Signs in Subarachnoid Hemorrhage: A Cooperative Study

Bassi P, Bandera R, Loiero M, Tognoni G, Mangoni A (Univ of Milan; Inst of Pharmacological Research M Negri, Milan, Italy)

Acta Neurol Scand 84:277–281, 1991 3–74

Background.—Because patients with ruptured aneurysms have better prognoses if intervention is performed early, it is important to reduce diagnostic and admission delays. Avoidable mortality in patients with subarachnoid hemorrhage (SAH) from intracranial aneurysms was identified in this study. Whether a classification of warning signs represents a proper clinical nosographic identity or a misdiagnosis of SAH was investigated. The best strategy for shortening delays in referral and diagnosis was evaluated.

Methods.—Sixteen neurosurgical units and 8 neurologic departments participated in the study. Warning signs preceding major hemorrhage were analyzed in 364 patients with intracranial aneurysms confirmed by angiography and clinical history. Clinical features were compared in misdiagnosed patients and in patients with correct diagnoses of SAH and clinical grade 1 disease at admission.

Results.—Seventy-four patients had a history of warning signs preceding major rupture of an intracranial aneurysm. Eight patients had 2 or more episodes of warning signs. In both men and women, there was a peak of warning signs in the group aged 51 to 60 years. The percentage of warning signs was higher in young men than in women, but the percentage was higher for women older than 60 years of age. Of 290 patients without a history of warning signs, 78 were in grade 1 at admission. The percentage of nonidentified cases increased from 36.7% in patients younger than 40 years of age to 61.2% in patients aged 51 to 60 years. Symptoms of warning signs were generally clear enough to be considered a misdiagnosis of intracranial aneurysm. Severe, unusual, and a sudden thunderclap headache was the principal symptom in all patients. However, patients with correct diagnoses and early admission more frequently also had other associated symptoms.

Conclusions.—Approximately 50% of warning signs can be considered to be caused by a minor leak. In these cases, a CT scan followed by lumbar puncture (LP) if the CT scan is negative constitutes the best diagnostic strategy if done within 72 hours of the episode. In this study, the CT scan was positive in every case when performed within 3 days; LP was positive even when performed after 1 week.

▶ The patient with a thunderclap headache should be investigated by an immediate CT scan, LP if the CT is negative, and then angiography if the LP is negative. This may include or be followed by MRI and MRI angiography. The latter three were not included in this article. Unfortunately, we have seen many CT scans performed that were negative, only to be positive at a later date. This symptom is so highly indicative of an impending catastrophe that the patient, at a minimum, should be admitted to the hospital so that this workup can be done.—G.J. Ordog, M.D.

A Double-Blind Comparison of Granisetron and Placebo for the Treatment of Acute Migraine in the Emergency Department

Rowat BMT, Merrill CF, Davis A, South V (The Toronto Hosp; SmithKline Beecham Pharma Inc, Oakville, Ont, Canada)

Cephalalgia 11:207–213, 1991 3–75

Background.—A variety of therapies are used for control of migraine headaches in the emergency department, but their efficacy has not been sufficiently assessed in controlled studies. The selective serotonin receptor agonist granisetron has been shown to eliminate nausea and vomiting after cisplatin treatment without significant adverse effects. The effectiveness of granisetron in acute migraine attacks was studied in the emergency department.

Methods.—For this randomized, double-blind, placebo-controlled study, 397 patients arriving at the emergency department with acute migraine headaches over a 10-month period were screened. Of these, 28 met the stringent eligibility requirements and completed the study protocol. Patients were randomized into 3 groups: granisetron, 40 or 80 μg/kg administered intravenously, or placebo. Evaluation continued for 4 hours or until alternative treatment was indicated. Patients completed a

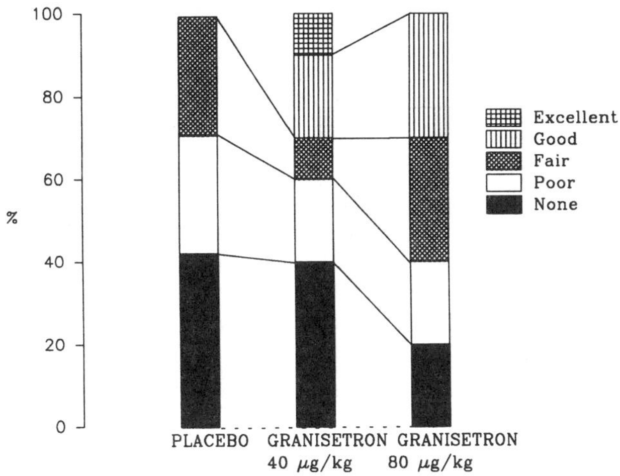

Fig 3–15.—The global evaluation of efficacy as assessed by the patient at the conclusion of the study. The percentage of patients in each category is stacked per treatment group. (Courtesy of Rowat BMT, Merrill CF, Davis A, et al: *Cephalalgia* 11:207–213, 1991.)

global evaluation of treatment before discharge and returned 3 days later for follow-up evaluation.

Results.—Rescue medication was needed at 2 hours by 80% of the 40 μg/kg granisetron group, 50% of the 80 μg/kg granisetron group, and 75% of the placebo group. Patients receiving the higher dose of granisetron showed significant improvement in pain on visual analogue and categorical scales, and both granisetron groups showed improvement on the sensory and affective components of the Hunter headache scale. The placebo group showed significantly worse nausea at 30 minutes than the active treatment groups, but there were no differences in vomiting or photophobia. In both granisetron groups, 30% of patients rated the treatment as good or excellent (Fig 3–15). There were no significant adverse effects and no significant abnormal laboratory findings.

Conclusions.—Granisetron may help relieve symptoms of acute migraine; however, other than nausea, there were few significant differences from placebo. Headache pain relief seems to be more consistent with a dose of 80 than 40 μg/kg, but the optimal dose is unknown. Future studies should employ larger groups and higher doses of granisetron.

▶ Granisetron appears to be a promising new approach to the treatment of migraine headaches. There are patients who do not get satisfactory relief with out current regimens, and it will be good to have an alternative to narcotics for this group.—E. Ruiz, M.D.

Prospective Versus Retrospective Methods of Identifying Patients With Delirium

Johnson JC, Kerse NM, Gottlieb G, Wanich C, Sullivan E, et al (Univ of Pennsylvania, Philadelphia; Philadelphia VA Med Ctr)

J Am Geriatr Soc 40:316–319, 1992 3–76

Purpose.—Delirium is an important problem in elderly patients. Accurate definition of this problem is crucial for research and clinical purposes, but it is difficult. Because of the concern that a retrospective approach does not identify all patients with delirium, cases identified by a prospective method were compared with those identified by 3 retrospective approaches.

Methods.—The study sample comprised 235 elderly patients with medical illness. Patients with potential delirium as well as a group of control patients were identified by a nurse clinician. Both groups were then interviewed by a psychiatrist, who used DSM-III criteria to make the diagnosis of delirium. After discharge, the records of all prospectively identified delirious patients were examined for different types of evidence of delirium.

Findings.—The psychiatrist identified 47 delirious patients. On chart review, only 4 patients were found to have ICD-9 codes suggestive of delirium, for a sensitivity of .09. On evaluation of physicians' diagnoses, only 8 patients were identified as being delirious or acutely confused; the sensitivity of this type of evidence was .17. In 10 cases, the specific criteria for a DSM-III diagnosis of delirium could be determined from the medical record, for a sensitivity of .21.

Conclusions.—Retrospective methods of establishing the diagnosis of delirium by medical chart review are shown to be highly imprecise. It cannot be determined whether physicians simply fail to recognize delirium or whether they recognize it but fail to document it. This condition carries high morbidity and mortality and must be recognized, appropriately monitored, and treated. Prospective designs will be needed as research on delirium moves into the area of pathogenesis and treatment.

▶ This article will have its main impact on delirium research since it is clear that retrospective identification through ICD-9-CM codes will miss most patients. The clinicians most frequently used the terminology altered mental status, confusion, and dementia when delirium was not accurate.—R.M. McNamara, M.D.

Endocrine and Hypertension

Oral Labetalol Versus Oral Clonidine in the Emergency Treatment of Severe Hypertension

Atkin SH, Jaker MA, Beaty P, Quadrel MA, Cuffie C, et al (Univ of Medicine

and Dentistry of New Jersey, Newark)
Am J Med Sci 303:9–15, 1992 3–77

Objective.—The treatment of mildly symptomatic or asymptomatic patients with severe hypertension (diastolic blood pressure greater than 120 mm Hg) without acute end-organ dysfunction is not clear. The clinical efficacy and safety of orally administered clonidine and orally administered labetalol in the treatment of these patients in the emergency department were evaluated.

Treatment.—In a randomized, double-blind prospective study, 36 patients with a mean baseline blood pressure of 199/132 mm Hg without acute end-organ dysfunction were treated with either orally administered labetalol or orally administered clonidine. All but 2 patients were black

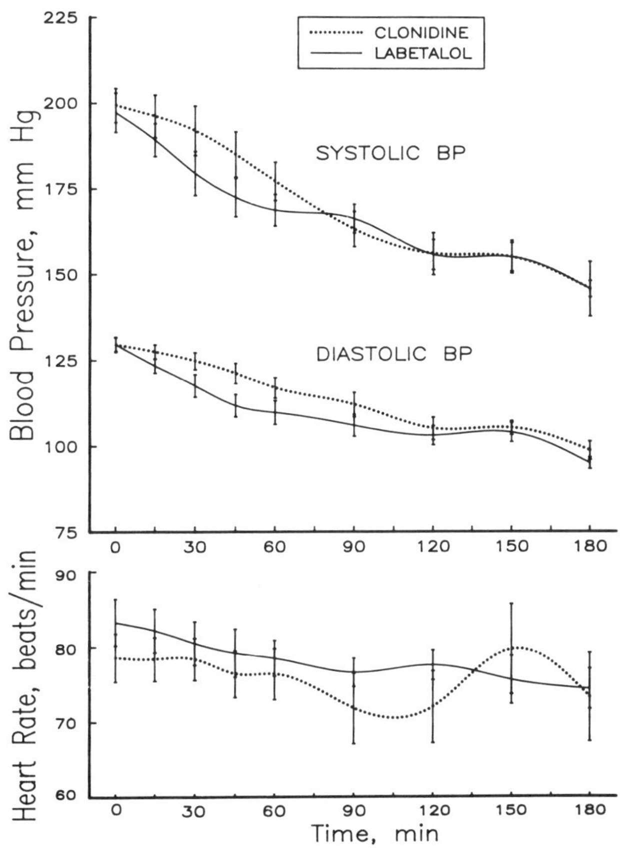

Fig 3–16.—Mean systolic and diastolic blood pressures and heart rates for each group of patients receiving either labetalol (*solid line*) or clonidine (*dotted line*) who achieved goal diastolic blood pressure within 3 hours. Labetalol, n = 12; clonidine, n = 10. (Courtesy of Atkin SH, Jaker MA, Beaty P, et al: *Am J Med Sci* 303:9–15, 1992.)

persons, and 56% had mild symptoms. Labetalol was administered initially at a dose of 200 mg, followed by hourly 200-mg doses up to a maximum of 1,200 mg at 6 hours. Clonidine was given initially at .2 mg followed by hourly .1-mg doses up to .7 mg.

Outcome.—Within 6 hours of treatment, labetalol decreased diastolic blood pressure in 94% of the patients, with a mean reduction in blood pressure of 54/37 mm Hg (Fig 3–16). Of these, 71% achieved the target diastolic blood pressure within 3 hours on a total dose of 600 mg or less of labetalol. Likewise, clonidine reduced diastolic blood pressure in 83% of the patients, and all 15 responders achieved the target blood pressure within 4 hours. The mean reduction in blood pressure was 57/32 mm Hg. Except for 1 patient in the labetalol-treated group who experienced transient hypotension, side effects were mild in both groups.

Conclusion.—Orally administered labetalol is comparatively as effective and safe as orally administered clonidine and provides a useful alternative for the treatment of severe hypertension in an emergency department setting. Further studies are recommended to define the most effective dosing regimen for orally administered labetalol in this setting.

▶ The approach to a *mildly* symptomatic and asymptomatic patient with severe hypertension is controversial. My primary goal is to convince the patient of the need for long-term therapy. The short-term morbidity of mildly or initially asymptomatic severe hypertension is probably greater with aggressive treatment than with no treatment. The authors note new drowsiness, dizziness, and orthostatic hypotension in their treatment groups. If I initiate antihypertensive therapy for these patients in the emergency department, I administer the standard daily dose only (i.e., no loading process as described in this article). I then arrange for a 48-hour re-evaluation and medical adjustment (if needed). This affords the opportunity to establish and reinforce further follow-up through a long-term care provider.—J.R. Hedges, M.D.

Isolated T-Wave Abnormalities and Evaluation of Left Ventricular Wall Motion After Nifedipine for Severe Hypertension

Phillips RA, Goldman ME, Ardeljan M, Eison HB, Shimabukuro S, et al (Mount Sinai Med Ctr, New York, NY)

Am J Hypertens 4:432–437, 1991 3–78

Background.—Vasodilators are commonly used in the emergency department to achieve rapid blood pressure reduction in patients with severe hypertension. The use of these drugs has been associated with T-wave inversion, the significance of which, without chest pain or other signs of ischemia, is unknown. A prospective study was done to ascertain the effects of immediate blood pressure reduction with nifedipine on the ECG and on wall motion.

Methods.—The subjects were 23 patients with severe hypertension, defined as an average sitting diastolic blood pressure of 120 mm Hg or higher on 3 determinations in 3 minutes. There were 13 women and 10 men with a mean age of 52; 13 patients were black. The mean body mass index was 29 kg/m^2, and the mean serum creatinine level was 1.3 mg/dL. Patients were studied by ECG and 2-dimensional echocardiographic left ventricular wall motion studies before and after rapid blood pressure reduction with nifedipine, 10 mg orally.

Results.—The average blood pressure was reduced from 189/117 to 151/91 mm Hg 1 hour after nifedipine treatment. Twenty-six percent of patients showed new T-wave inversions, but their echocardiograms showed no new abnormalities of wall motion. Eleven patients had an abnormal wall motion score before treatment. After treatment, the mean score improved from 1.4 to 1.2.

Conclusions.—Nifedipine used for quick blood pressure reduction causes asymptomatic T-wave inversions in many patients. These changes are not associated with left ventricular wall motion abnormalities and thus probably not with any significant myocardial ischemia. The mechanism of the repolarization abnormalities is unknown.

► This study confirms the previous observations that a rapid reduction in blood pressure to an "acceptable" level in the setting of "severe" hypertension may be associated with ECG repolarization abnormalities. However, after echocardiographic assessment of left ventricular wall motion, this study suggests that these ECG changes are not due to myocardial ischemia resulting from the abrupt decrease in myocardial perfusion pressure. This study does not address an important issue, namely, what is "severe" hypertension or a hypertensive urgency as opposed to hypertensive emergency? Would the results have been different in a study population who had chest pain, ECG evidence of acute myocardial infarction, or pulmonary edema?—J.T. Niemann, M.D.

Emergency Department Presentation of Renal Dialysis Patients: Indications for EMS Transport Directly to Dialysis Centers

Sacchetti A, Harris R, Patel K, Attewell R (Our Lady of Lourdes Med Ctr, Camden, NJ; Thomas Jefferson Univ, Philadelphia, Pa)

J Emerg Med 9:141–144, 1991 3–79

Objective.—There is little information on the patterns of presentation for emergency care of patients who require renal dialysis. Emergency department (ED) visits by patients who undergo renal dialysis at a regional dialysis center were analyzed.

Methods and Findings.—The study took place at a tertiary-care and regional dialysis facility to which all dialysis patients requesting emergency care are transported. Data were collected for all dialysis center patients seen in the ED over a 3-month period. One hundred patients with an average age of 51 years were included in the analysis. Eighty were treated by hemodialysis and 10 by peritoneal dialysis. Shortness of breath was the most common presenting complaint, followed by chest pain, abdominal pain, and vomiting. Twenty-three patients had a diagnosis of congestive heart failure; the next most common diagnoses were chest wall pain and electrolyte abnormalities. Thirty patients required interventional dialysis (ID), defined as dialysis performed as quickly as possible for treatment of the presenting complaint. In this group, the most common complaints were shortness of breath, weakness, and chest pain. Only shortness of breath was a significant predictor of the need for ID: the positive predictive value was .63, and the negative predictive value was .85.

Conclusions.—Many patients with chronic renal failure who are admitted to the ED will require ID. Some presenting complaints, expecially shortness of breath, should alert the physician to consider preparing for ID. Patients complaining of shortness of breath should be taken directly to dialysis centers.

▶ Dr. Michael J. Krentz, referring to protocols in *Principles of EMS Systems* published by the American College of Emergency Physicians (1989), states that "triage protocols probably are the most controversial and the ones that attract the most attention in the course of their development."

In the past, this was based on a lack of evidence of increased efficacy of specialty centers and the monetary issues involved in bypassing potential receiving facilities.

Currently, prehospital transport of patients to "appropriate" facilities (i.e., trauma centers) is an accepted practice in protocol development. This article should be welcomed by the emergency medical service community because it describes a group of patients who may benefit by transport to a speciality center (i.e., one in which dialysis is available).

Care should be taken to avoid making prehospital triage decisions to transport to a facility in which *only* dialysis is available on the basis of this study because patients may also need more extensive resuscitative measures.—D.J. Cionni, M.D.

4 Special Emergencies

AIDS/Infections

An Analysis of Emergency Department Use by Patients With Minor Illness

Shesser R, Kirsch T, Smith J, Hirsch R (George Washington Univ; George Washington-Georgetown Emergency Medicine Residency, Washington, DC)

Ann Emerg Med 20:743–748, 1991 4–1

Purpose.—Several retrospective investigations of the reasons for the current increase in nonemergency patient visits to hospital emergency departments (EDs) reported a high rate of appropriate ED use but also left the impression of inappropriate use for minor complaints by patients of low socioeconomic status who do not have an established health care provider. The reasons why patients with minor illnesses chose to come to the ED were examined.

Methods.—The study sample consisted of 325 adults aged 18 to 65 years who consulted the ED for minor illnesses during 15 randomly selected weekdays. The control sample consisted of 224 patients seen in the ED for any reason during 2 randomly selected 24-hour periods not overlapping with the sampling days. Patients in the study sample were interviewed on socioeconomic background, reasons for using the ED, and how they perceived the urgency of their condition. Demographic and socioeconomic data were collected on the control patients.

Results.—The study group contained more men, more self-pay patients, and fewer Medicare patients than the control group. Study patients also tended to have higher incomes than controls. There was no significant differences in racial, marital, employment, or educational backgrounds between the 2 groups. Eighty-three percent of the study patients had no chronic medical problems, and 42.5% reported that their current problem had originated within the 24 hours before the ED visit. The main reasons listed for choosing the ED rather than alternative health care sources were convenience (23.7%), absence of previous provider relationship (22.1%), and the inability to get a prompt appointment with the regular health care provider (19%).

Conclusions.—Demographic and social class parameters of patients with minor illnesses are similar to those of the general ED population. Disproportionate ED use by patients with minor illness from lower socioeconomic classes was not observed. Rapid access to professional attention and convenience were the most often cited reasons for choosing the ED.

▶ Surprising to many, the authors' data show similar use patterns for minor illnesses in both economically advantaged and disadvantaged patients. Contrary to conventional wisdom, a utilization of the emergency center for minor illness by patients from lower socioeconomic classes did not occur. The unanswered question is whether such care is most efficiently and optimally given by a facility within the hospital or whether such care should be promoted in non–hospital-based ambulatory facilities. Of additional interest was the fact that more men were involved in minor care episodes than women, contrary to other statistics that identify that over two thirds of all physician encounters involve the female gender.—D.K. Wagner, M.D.

The Management of HIV-Related Illness in the Emergency Department

Talan DA, Kennedy CA (Olive View/UCLA Med Ctr, Sylmar, Calif; Naval Hosp, San Diego)

Ann Emerg Med 20:1355–1365, 1991 4–2

Background.—Approximately 1 to 1.5 million Americans are infected with HIV. As the epidemic continues to grow, more patients with AIDS and with unrecognized HIV infection will be treated in the emergency department (ED). Diagnostic and management issues related to the AIDS epidemic that are unique to the ED setting were discussed.

Risk for HIV Infection.—Patients at risk who have tested HIV antibody-negative may still harbor the infection. Many physicians, however, do not routinely screen patients for risk behavior. Risk may be assessed through direct questioning or by an assessment of general demographics and clues from clinical evaluation. Opportunistic infections are the most frequent problems for which HIV-infected patients come to the ED. Common symptoms are fever, chills, night sweats, and rigors. Psychosocial problems are often seen; for example, the relative risk of suicide in the HIV-infected men is 66 times that in the general population.

Specific Infections.—Pulmonary infections, including *Pneumocystis carinii* pneumonia (PCP), are commonly seen. The clinical diagnosis is not difficult in patients with defined HIV risk factors and characteristic radiographic findings. The therapies of choice for PCP are trimethoprim/sulfamethoxazole and pentamidine. Corticosteroids may prevent respiratory deterioration in patients with moderate-to-severe PCP. Any CNS-related complaints should also prompt immediate evaluation in any patient at risk for HIV infection. In addition, AIDS patients are at risk for serious bacterial disease, gastrointestinal problems (such as refractory diarrhea), cytomegalovirus (CMV) retinitis, the acute retroviral syndrome (which appears 1 to 6 weeks after exposure to HIV and mimics mononucleosis), and metabolic and drug complications.

Conclusion.—Although many of the patterns of disease, subtleties of diagnosis, and therapies for the varied manifestations of AIDS have been clarified, numerous questions remain. Much of the existing clinical research in HIV-related illness, however, is applicable to the diagnostic and management problems that arise in the ED.

▶ Every emergency physician should read *The Medical Letter* 33:95, 1991. This issue dealt with "Drugs for AIDS and Associated Infections." It can be quickly read and addresses areas of controversy. Drug regimens for various infections are listed on the last two pages. I photocopied it and carry it in my white coat (see also Abstract 4–30).—J.T. Niemann, M.D.

Prophylaxis With Zidovudine (AZT) After Exposure to Human Immunodeficiency Virus: A Brief Discussion of the Issues for Emergency Physicians

Callaham ML (Univ of California, San Francisco)

Ann Emerg Med 20:1351–1354, 1991 4–3

Introduction.—Emergency medical personnel, especially those in urban areas, are at risk of being infected with HIV. The Centers for Disease Control recommends the use of universal precautions in emergency department (ED) care, but many health care workers do not observe them, and it is probably impossible to follow precautions 100% of the time. The use of zidovudine (AZT) is explored as a preventive agent once exposure of the health care worker has occurred.

Background.—Zidovudine prevents HIV replication but does not kill the virus, eliminate infection, or prevent ultimate progression of the disease. No clinical studies have defined the effectiveness of AZT in prophylaxis against HIV infection. Decisions about the prophylactic use of the drug must therefore be based upon risk-benefit assessments. Some individuals may chose to take AZT or any prophylactic regimen that might delay a positive antibody response, thereby delaying possible job termination. This strategy might result, however, in exposure of sexual partners to infection. Another consideration is the fact that the long-term health consequences of AZT in healthy persons is not known, and it should not be used in pregnancy, regardless of possible HIV exposure. Finally, although a 6-week course of AZT is expensive ($1,150), this sum is small when weighed against the cost of illness and lost earnings.

Conclusion.—Current knowledge on the efficacy of AZT for prophylaxis does not provide an easy answer. Emergency department directors should study prophylaxis programs so that immediate decisions can be made in the event of HIV exposure. It is suggested that the potential benefits of AZT outweigh the risks for potentially infected health care workers.

Management Guidelines for Health Care Workers Exposed to Blood and Body Fluids

Go GW, Baraff LJ, Schriger DL (Univ of California, Los Angeles)

Ann Emerg Med 20:1341–1350, 1991 4–4

Introduction.—For health care workers (HCWs), exposure to possibly contaminated blood and body fluids is an occupational hazard. General guidelines for management of these exposures and considerations for particular infections were reviewed.

Guidelines.—An HCW should seek attention as soon as possible after parenteral exposure to blood and body fluids. Management guidelines should be agreed on by the emergency and occupational health departments. Detailed information must be gathered on the nature of the exposure, preferably on a checklist or complaint-specific medical record. Open, contaminated wounds should be treated as necessary, with copious irrigation. Immunization should be begun for HCWs who are not immunized for tetanus and diphtheria.

Specific Infections.—Susceptible HCWs have an overall incidence of hepatitis B infection of 26% after exposure to hepatitis B surface antigen–contaminated blood. All nonimmunized workers are recommended to receive the hepatitis B vaccine. The risk of infection must be determined by the infectivity of the source and the immune status of the exposed worker. There is controversy as to the best revaccination policy for transient responders. There are no data on the incidence of infection after needlestick exposure to hepatitis C virus. Immune globulin is not specifically recommended for use as postexposure prophylaxis. Antibody testing is unnecessary. It was recommended that the exposed worker be given immune globulin if the source has non-A, non-B hepatitis and the worker is not given hepatitis B immune globulin. The risk of HIV infection per exposure has been estimated as 0.29%. Blood and body fluids from all patients should be considered hazardous. Zidovudine chemotherapy may be given as prophylaxis, but its efficacy has not been determined. Its use was cautiously recommended. The exposed worker may be distraught and needs information and sometimes psychological counseling. The source and exposed worker should be tested for HIV antibody.

Discussion.—Comprehensive guidelines for occupational exposure to blood and body fluids are needed for proper management. Institutions should establish their own guidelines, with treatment plans based on specific patient considerations and preferences.

Prevalence of HIV Antibody in a Noninner-City University Hospital Emergency Department

Baraff LJ, Talan DA, Torres M (Univ of California, Los Angeles)

Ann Emerg Med 20:782–786, 1991 4–5

Background.—Emergency department (ED) health care workers often do not adhere strictly to the universal precautions recommended by the Centers for Disease Control. The prevalence of HIV antibody in a non-inner-city university hospital ED was determined.

Methods.—Patients in the University of California, Los Angeles, Emergency Medicine Center between the ages of 18 and 59 years were studied. These patients had injuries that met trauma center triage criteria or had non–trauma-related illness. They had blood drawn for physician-requested laboratory tests and an extra aliquot of blood available for HIV antibody testing. All serum samples were tested for antibody to HIV by using the enzyme-linked immunosorbent assay. The specimen was tested again if the initial results were positive. Repeatedly reactive specimens were analyzed by the Western blot test. The treating physician filled out a questionnaire about the patient's illness and risk factors for HIV infection after patient care was completed.

Results.—Two of 100 major trauma patients and 7 of 100 nontrauma patients had HIV antibody. Seropositive rates varied from 0% to 12.5%, according to age and clinical group. The highest rates occurred in nontrauma patients aged 30 to 39 years. The difference in proportions of seropositivity between men and women was nonsignificant. Physicians obtained data on risk factors from 52% of the nontrauma patients and 17% of the trauma patients. None of the 30 trauma patients for whom information was available and 2 of the 100 nontrauma patients had a history of high-risk behavior.

Conclusions.—The prevalence of HIV infection in this non–inner-city ED is comparable to that reported from inner-city EDs. In most cases, physician assessment of risk factors was incomplete. Health care workers in EDs must take maximum precautions to prevent exposure to blood and other body fluids from ED patients.

▶ The prevalence of HIV in the community is of critical importance to emergency center personnel. The demonstrated level confirms the necessity of practicing universal precautions in the emergency center. Exposure to HIV in the emergency center can occur at any time.

The conclusions are justified based on the population. The population studied is more affluent than inner-city populations studied, but its presence within Los Angeles still should lead to classification as a city population. Results from a truly suburban emergency center might differ significantly.

Our inability to predict HIV positivity forces us to use universal precautions whenever exposure to blood or body fluids is possible in the emergency center (see also Abstract 4–7).—J.E. Clinton, M.D.

Evaluation of Two Rapid Screening Assays for the Detection of Human Immunodeficiency Virus-10 Infection in Emergency Department Patients

Kelen GD, Bennecoff TA, Kline R, Green GB, Quinn TC (The Johns Hopkins Univ, Baltimore, Md; Natl Inst Allergy and Infectious Diseases, Bethesda)
Am J Emerg Med 9:416–420, 1991 4–6

Background.—Although ethically controversial, more widespread testing of patients for HIV-1 infection has been advocated. Because emergency departments (EDs) of inner cities have a high rate of seroprevalence of HIV infection and a significant number of patients at risk for HIV-1, they might provide good sites for screening high-risk patients. Screening for HIV-1 at an ED would be more practical if a rapid assay were used because the standard enzyme immunosorbent and Western blot assays can take 1 to 2 weeks for results, thus necessitating return visits for posttest counseling. The sensitivity and specificity of 2 rapid assays for HIV-1 were tested on excess sera collected from unselected ED patients.

Methods.—Four hundred ninety-five sera samples from patients 15 years and older who were treated at the Johns Hopkins Hospital ED in 1988 were tested by standard enzyme-linked immunosorbent assay (EIA), confirmatory Western blots, and 2 rapid assays. The latter were the HIV-1 Genie, an immunoconcentration assay based on the presence of antibodies to the transmembrane glycoprotein gp 41, and the Abbott Testpack HIV-1, a solid-phase "sandwich principle" EIA. Both rapid assays can be used with serum, plasma, or whole blood, are simple to perform, and give results in about 10 minutes.

Sensitivity, Specificity, and Predictive Values of 2 Rapid Assays Compared With Enzyme Immunoassay and Western Blot

	EIA/Western Blot		
	Positive	Negative	Indeterminate
Abbott Testpack HIV-1			
Positive	25	1	1
Negative	0	466	2
Genetic Systems HIV-1 Genie			
Positive	25	1	1
Negative	0	466	2

Note: Sensitivity = 100%; specificity = 99.8%; positive predictive value = 96.2%; negative predictive value = 100%.
(Courtesy of Kalen GD, Bennecoff TA, Kline R, et al: *Am J Emerg Med* 9:416–420, 1991.)

Results.—The seroprevalence of HIV-1 was 5.1%. Four hundred sixty-seven specimens were negative by EIA, 25 were confirmed positive by Western blot, and 3 were indeterminate by Western blot (table). Both rapid assays correctly identified all 25 positive samples and 466 of the EIA-negative samples. The rapid assays on the 3 indeterminate samples yielded negative readings on 2 specimens and a positive or weakly positive reading on a third. The sensitivities of both rapid systems were 100%, the specificities were 99.8, the positive predictive values were 96.2%, and the negative predictive values were 100%.

Conclusions.—Both rapid assays tested were highly sensitive and specific as well as quick and simple to perform and interpret. If screening of ED patients is desired, both of these tests can identify HIV-1-infected patients.

▶ It is comforting to know that rapid reliable testing for those infected with HIV-1 is possible in the emergency center, especially in those instances where the house staff are inadvertently exposed by needlesticks and other accidents while evaluating and treating patients who are seropositive. The value of testing all patients remains problematic since we do not have plans developed and means to follow the results of this testing.—G.V. Anderson, M.D.

The HIV-1 Seroprevalence Rate of Injured Patients Admitted Through California Emergency Departments

Rhee KJ, for the California HIV-1 Emergency Dept Seroprevalence Study Group (Univ of California Med Ctr, Sacramento)

Ann Emerg Med 20:969–972, 1991 4–7

Introduction.—A significant number of patients seen in the emergency department (ED) may be HIV-positive, and those with penetrating injuries may be especially likely to be seropositive.

Objective.—The seroprevalence of HIV-1 was determined at 10 California hospitals, including 3 in areas of high AIDS incidence, 3 in areas of intermediate incidence, and 4 in low-AIDS areas. All adult trauma patients admitted through the ED during a 3-month period were reviewed.

Findings.—Adequate blood samples were obtained from 2,264 patients. The seroprevalence rate was 2.5% at centers with a high incidence of AIDS (more than 40 per 100,000 population); .9% at intermediate-incidence centers; and .5% where the incidence of AIDS was less than 20 cases per 100,000 population.

Conclusion.—There is considerable variation in the seroprevalence of HIV-1 in patients seen in EDs in different areas.

▶ The results of this article are not surprising in that the highest seropositivity occurred in hospitals serving areas of high AIDS incidence. So far, Johns

Hopkins can still claim the lead in the prevalence of HIV infection (1). A more significant issue is the lack of compliance with universal precautions by ED personnel (2). We have found that periodic, department-wide review of videotaped trauma resuscitations is a useful tool to reinforce such compliance.—R.M. McNamara, M.D.

References

1. Kelen GD, et al: *N Engl J Med* 318:1645, 1988.
2. Baraff LJ, et al: *Ann Emerg Med* 18:654, 1989.

Emergencies in AIDS Patients: The Otolaryngologic Perspective

Rothstein SG, Schneider KL, Kohan D, Persky MS, Holliday R (New York Univ Med Ctr, NY)

Otolaryngol Head Neck Surg 104:545–548, 1991 4–8

Background.—Acquired immunodeficiency syndrome can affect every organ system. Otolaryngologic manifestations can take an unexpected, unusual course.

Case Report 1.—A 34-year-old man was seen with a history of intermittent dysphagia and shortness of breath. The symptoms developed after an upper respiratory infection associated with cough, postnasal drip, sore throat, and clogged ears. His voice had also changed. He had been found to be HIV-positive 6 months earlier. His medical history included biopsy-proved Kaposi's sarcoma of the upper extremities. A diagnosis of a supraglottic Kaposi's lesion was made.

Case Report 2.—A 40-year-old woman complained of dysphagia, painful neck swelling, and fever. She was febrile, with an unremarkable oral cavity. Flexible nasolaryngoscopy showed a pale supraglottis with mild edema and a large pale epiglottis. Within several hours, stridor developed. Laryngeal examination with flexible laryngoscopy showed no discernible airway. She was taken emergently to the operating room, and those findings were confirmed. Cultures from the epiglottis yielded a heavy growth of *Streptococcus viridans.*

Case Report 3.—A 26-year-old man had neck pain and swelling. He had injected heroin into his jugular vein about 12 hours earlier. A CT scan showed a greatly enlarged right internal jugular and subclavian vein with the classic "bull's-eye" appearance of a thrombus in the lumen. Internal jugular and subclavian vein thrombophlebitis was diagnosed.

Case Report 4.—A 35-year-old woman had a sudden onset of profuse bilateral epistaxis while on the medical service for treatment of *Pneumocystis* pneumonia. She had had similar bleeding episodes in the past. Examination showed diffuse bleeding from the septum and turbinates bilaterally. The nose was packed on both sides, and the bleeding stopped. A hematology consultant, on noting a coagulation defect, suggested that the patient's low platelet count or an intrinsic platelet defect might be the cause of the epistaxis and recommended platelet transfusion. Before the intranasal packing could be removed, however, the patient began bleeding from all orifices, including the rectum and vagina. She bled to death despite transfusions.

Case Report 5.—A 32-year-old man complained of a sore throat, tender bilateral cervical lymph nodes, malaise, and a fever. Massive facial and cervical edema developed during the next 24 hours. Significant supraglottic edema was discovered. Stridor began to develop, and a tracheotomy was done emergently. No abscess could be identified. The patient's fever persisted over the next 5 days despite changes in antibiotic therapy. All cultures were negative. His pulmonary function deteriorated, and he died.

Conclusion.—Otolaryngologists must be prepared to diagnose and treat the secondary manifestations of AIDS in emergency as well as routine settings. The immune deficiency resulting from the AIDS virus may directly or indirectly result in an unexpected course of illness despite presentations that are initially benign.

▶ This article demonstrates that people with AIDS get severe infections and have devastating comorbidities. It is startling to see how rapidly otolaryngologic infections progress in patients who are immunocompromised, often requiring a surgical airway.—E.J. Reisdorff, M.D.

Needlestick Injuries and Hepatitis B Immunization in Florida Paramedics: A Statewide Survey

Klontz KC, Gunn RA, Caldwell JS (Ctrs for Disease Control, Atlanta, Ga; Florida Dept of Health and Rehabilitative Services, Tallahassee)

Ann Emerg Med 20:1310–1313, 1991 4–9

Introduction.—Emergency medical services personnel are known to have an increased incidence of serologic markers for previous or current infection with hepatitis B virus. This finding may be the result of the frequency of needlestick injuries in emergency medical workers. The incidence of needlestick injury in a group of paramedics was investigated along with the proportion of these paramedics who have been vaccinated with the hepatitis B vaccine.

Methods.—A 41-item questionnaire was sent to a systematic random sample of 500 of the 4,804 paramedics certified to work in Florida in 1987. The paramedics were asked to record the number of needlestick injuries experienced in 1987 and the circumstances surrounding the injury. Completed forms were returned by 60% of the paramedics, 95% of whom were employed full-time as paramedics in 1987.

Results.—A total of 110 needlestick injuries were reported by 69 paramedics. Most (80%) occurred while recapping needles, inserting intravenous catheters, checking or restocking supply kits, or disposing of needles. Almost two thirds of reported injuries could have been prevented by proper needle disposal. The majority (62%) of paramedics reported having had at least 1 dose of the hepatitis B vaccine; 65% of those who were unvaccinated would take the hepatitis B vaccine if it were offered free.

Conclusion.—Needlestick injuries are probably underreported; 25% of respondents told no one of the incident. Many of the injuries could be avoided, although some will occur because of the awkward conditions in which paramedics work. Findings of this study emphasize the need for hepatitis B vaccination programs for paramedics.

▶ This article clearly documents the need for increasing the efforts to educate everyone involved in emergency medical service about infectious disease. New OSHA requirements are mandating increased attention to this area.

I find it interesting that a majority of unvaccinated providers would be vaccinated if it were provided at no cost. I assume that this number is similar in other systems, and this problem must be addressed. Education of providers regarding the potential devastating effects of hepatitis B infection, the efficacy and safety of currently available vaccination, and the lack of employer liability if the vaccination is refused should be all that is necessary to increase the vaccination rate!—D.J. Cionni, M.D.

Emergency Department Screening for Syphilis in Patients With Other Suspected Sexually Transmitted Diseases

Ernst AA, Samuels JD, Winsemius DK (Louisiana State Univ, New Orleans; Univ of Connecticut, Hartford; St Francis Hosp and Med Ctr, Hartford, Conn)

Ann Emerg Med 20:627–630, 1991 4–10

Objective.—The Centers for Disease Control (CDC) reports that new cases of syphilis are being documented at an alarming rate. Because of patient anonymity and the accessibility of emergency departments (EDs), patients who suspect they may have a sexually transmitted disease (STD) may consult an ED rather than a private physician. The value of screening for syphilis among a high-risk group of ED patients was investigated.

Patients.—During a 4-month period, 260 patients suspected of having traditional STDs were screened for otherwise unsuspected syphilis. Twenty-two patients (8%) had reactive rapid plasma reagins. Sixteen of the 22 patients had titers of more than 1:8 and a reactive FTA-ABS and were determined to have syphilis. The cost of detecting 16 cases of syphilis was $1,679, or $104.90 per positive test.

Conclusion.—Patients admitted to the ED with signs of nonsyphilitic STDs can be screened effectively in the ED and at a low cost.

▶ There is a daunting epidemic of syphilis now occurring, but it is not clear that screening ED patients will have any significant effect on the crisis. Without immediate treatment in suspected cases, the likelihood of successful follow-up contact and subsequent treatment is low.

Several recent studies indicate that ceftriaxone is effective for the treatment of primary and secondary syphilis, although a treatment failure has also been reported (1, 2). I think that patients who are being treated for 1 STD, including pelvic inflammatory disease, *gardnerella* vaginitis, venereal warts, pubic lice or crabs, chancroid, lymphogranuloma venereum, urethritis, or epididymitis, should be treated with ceftriaxone, 250 mg intramuscularly, as an effective means of immediate treatment of syphilis to avoid the problematic logistics of post–emergency visit contract (see Abstract 5–24).—W.P. Burdick, M.D.

References

1. Schofer H, et al: *Chemotherapy* 35:140, 1989.
2. Siqueira LM, et al: *J Adolesc Health* 12:459, 1991.

Congenital Syphilis: An Emerging Emergency
Rosenberg NM (Wayne State Univ, Detroit, Mich)
Pediatr Emerg Care 7:171–176, 1991 4–11

Background.—Three infants seen in the emergency room had congenital syphilis, which suggests that this condition is within the purview of pediatric emergency care.

Case Report 1.—A 10-day-old infant boy born at 40 weeks' gestation to a mother who had received prenatal care was brought to the emergency department with jaundice. The baby was admitted for phototherapy. Several hours later, cardiac arrest developed. He was resuscitated and transferred to a children's hospital. Physical examination there showed jaundice with hepatosplenomegaly. The total bilirubin content was 23.9 mg/dL, with a conjugated fraction of 21.2 mg/dL. His platelet count was 30,000. He had a rapid plasma reagin reactive at 1:256. Disseminated intravascular coagulation and respiratory failure developed, and the infant died after 3 weeks.

Case Report 2.—A 25-day-old infant girl was referred from a well-baby clinic. She had lethargy, jaundice, a papular rash on the palms and soles, microencephaly, and hepatosplenomegaly. Radiographs showed metaphysitis. She was treated with intravenously administered penicillin for 10 days. While hospitalized, she had severe metabolic acidosis, disseminated intravascular coagulation, and nephrotic syndrome. She also sustained a humeral fracture. She was discharged after 10 days.

Case Report 3.—A 1-month-old boy was brought to the emergency department because of constant crying. His mother, who had had no prenatal care, admitted to using cocaine during pregnancy. The initial impression was of colic. The baby was fussy but consolable and had no abnormal findings. Rapid plasma reagin was reactive at 1:64, and radiographs showed metaphyseal bands on long bones, cortical destruction, and deossification of all bones. This baby was treated for 10 days with intravenously administered penicillin and discharged in satisfactory condition.

Conclusions.—Congenital syphilis in infants brought to the emergency department may appear as a very fulminant disease or with subtle findings that simulate conditions as benign as infantile colic. Emergency physicians must obtain a history of prenatal care in young, single, urban mothers.

► Some diseases just will not go away. They seem destined to attack us forever. This disease, syphilis, has been around a long time and has affected not only sexual behavior but also world politics. With the advent of antibiotics, it appeared that the treponemal organism was losing, and we could forget about this disease. Then came the sexual revolution, increased use of intravenous drugs, and HIV disease. Add to this the growing number of women who do not receive prenatal care and more uninsured and underinsured families that utilize the emergency department for their health care, and you realize that you need to know a lot more about syphilis in adults and in children. And, as usual, the great masquerading disease continues to keep you on your toes as evidenced by the child with "colic" (case 3). I wish I knew why they obtained a rapid plasma reagin and radiographs of the long bones. They obviously were checking out something else or left out part of the story. This child's irritability was probably related to his parosteitis and osteochondritis. I assume that these children had CSF studies. Ill infants with jaundice may be in a septic state, suffer from an enzyme deficiency, or need to be evaluated for a TORCHS infective process (To = toxoplasmosis, R = rubella, C = cytomegalovirus, H = herpes, S = syphilis).—R.W. Schafermeyer, M.D.

Tracheitis: Outcome of 1,700 Cases Presenting to the Emergency Department During Two Years

Sendi K, Crysdale WS, Yoo J (Hosp for Sick Children; Univ of Toronto, Canada)

J Otolaryngol 21:20–24, 1992 4–12

Introduction.—Tracheitis (laryngotracheobronchitis or "croup") is a common respiratory disorder in both children and adults. It is a viral infection of the respiratory tract mucosa, most often resulting from infection by parainfluenza types 1 and 2 or respiratory syncytial virus. The subglottic region is especially disposed to be inflamed and edematous, and significant airway narrowing can lead to respiratory distress.

Series.—The outcome in 1,533 pediatric patients seen at an emergency department in 2 years with a diagnosis of croup was assessed. Visits totaled 1,727.

Findings.—Many of the children had a history of airway disease, most often an episode of tracheitis. Cough, stridor, and chest wall retractions were the most common findings. The WBC count most often was normal or only slightly elevated. Viral cultures were positive in 30 of 101 attempts.

Management and Outcome.—Aqueous mist was used to treat 39% of the children, and 27% received antipyretics. Asthma medication was given to 10% of the children and racemic epinephrine inhalations to 8%. Only 17 children received parenteral steroids. Twelve children required endotracheal intubation; there were no tracheotomies. A majority of children were hospitalized for less than 3 days. There were no deaths.

Implications.—A majority of children with croup do well with supportive care. The use of endoscopy to rule out a correctable condition, such as a foreign body must be carefully considered because of the risk involved, although modern endoscopic equipment is relatively safe. Presently endotracheal intubation with a small tube is preferred to tracheotomy.

▶ While the data presented by these authors supports conventional teaching as it relates to the *demographics* of croup (age, sex, bacteriology), more recent studies in the literature suggest that it is time for a reappraisal of conventional *therapies.* In a retrospective study of 50 children treated and discharged home following treatment with racemic epinephrine, Kelley and Simon found that none "rebounded" and required intensive therapy (1). Additionally, a meta-analysis performed by Kairys et al. found that the administration of steroids decreased the frequency of intubation and improved clinical parameters in children hospitalized for croup (2). In the summarized article, only 2.5% of patients receiving racemic epinephrine were discharged, and only 4.5% of all patients received steroids. It is hoped that future studies with patient numbers as large as this one will address these newer treatment strategies. It was reassuring to note that only 16% of patients displayed a leukocytosis. This should reinforce the need to make therapeutic decisions based upon the clinical picture and not laboratory data (see also Abstract 4–14).—H.D. Unger, M.D.

References

1. Kelley PB, Simon JE: *Am J Emerg Med* 10:181, 1992.
2. Kairys SW, et al: *Pediatrics* 83:683, 1989.

Immersion Foot: A Problem of the Homeless in the 1990s
Wrenn K (Grady Mem Hosp, Atlanta, Ga)
Arch Intern Med 151:785–788, 1991 4–13

Introduction.—Immersion foot is a nonfreezing injury caused by prolonged exposure of the foot to a moist, occlusive environment. Immersion foot is characterized by white, wrinkled, painful soles and involvement of the dorsum of the foot after more prolonged exposure. This syndrome is increasingly seen among the homeless and indigent population.

Patients.—Two homeless men aged 34 and 38 years and a woman aged 75 years were seen in the emergency department with bilateral swelling of the feet, tender foot soles, and areas of scaling, mild erythema, and discoloration of the feet. One man was an alcoholic, the other man was an intravenous cocaine abuser, and the woman was mildly demented. Two patients had evidence of peripheral neuropathy. Two patients were cigarette smokers, and 1 patient had underlying atherosclerotic peripheral vascular disease.

Treatment.—Two patients were treated conservatively as outpatients, and 1 homeless patient was admitted to the hospital. The 2 patients who were discharged home were instructed to air-dry and elevate the feet and to take ibuprofen. The patient who was admitted was also treated with bed rest, air drying of the feet, and ibuprofen. All 3 patients had improved when seen at follow-up 1 to 14 days later.

Discussion.—Simple immersion foot uncomplicated by infection or ischemic injury will quickly resolve with conservative measures, whereas the more complicated cases may require antibiotic therapy and surgical intervention. Lack of shelter appears to be a major contributing factor to the development of immersion foot. Physicians who care for the homeless should regularly examine the feet of these patients, and even minor complaints should be taken seriously. Elderly, psychotic, debilitated, and immunosuppressed individuals are also at high risk for the development of immersion foot.

▶ The authors call attention to a condition previously relegated to foot soldiers whose feet were exposed to a wet and occlusive environment. Of interest to note is the fact that the condition is due to simple hyperhydration of the stratum corneum without fungal or bacterial involvement. Investigation has shown that the coefficient of permeability of the thicker plantar skin is ten times greater than that of the dorsal aspect of the foot. Consequently, much more water is absorbed, and the condition is predominantly localized to this aspect of the foot. While frostnip and frostbite may occur in individuals who initially have simple immersion problems, the two conditions are separate pathophysiologically. Inner-city emergency physicians, who may be seeing this condition with increasing frequency, may well have the opportunity to initiate and recommend appropriate therapy by simple provision of a dry environment without the addition of antibiotics, a degree of sophistication in therapy probably not extant with many physicians today.—D.K. Wagner, M.D.

Pneumococcal Bacterial Tracheitis

Orenstein JB, Thomsen JR, Baker SB (Children's Natl Med Ctr, Washington,

DC)
Am J Emerg Med 9:243–245, 1991 4–14

Introduction.—Bacterial tracheitis is an uncommon cause of acute respiratory distress that occurs mainly in younger children. Data were reviewed on a child with bacterial tracheitis.

Case Report.—A 6-year-old girl had a 1-day history of a hoarse and barky cough. Acute respiratory distress developed, but it responded dramatically to nebulized racemic epinephrine and oxygen. A chest roentgenogram, which was initially considered to be normal, showed subglottic narrowing and a ragged, intraluminal mass anterior to C5. Because a foreign body was suspected, direct laryngoscopy and bronchoscopy were performed and showed a shaggy and edematous larynx with a thick purulent tracheal exudate. Cultures from the trachea showed *Streptococcus pneumoniae.* The patient improved with intubation and antibiotics.

Conclusion.—Bacterial tracheitis should be considered in older children in whom foreign-body aspiration, croup, and epiglottiditis are suspected. Bacterial tracheitis in older children may resemble croup with a more gradual onset. The presence of subacute respiratory distress and irregular narrowing of the trachea radiographically are important clues to the diagnosis. Airway management should take into account the age of the child and size of the tracheal lumen; intubation may not be necessary in all patients.

▶ Bacterial tracheitis is rare and presents more like epiglottiditis in its course, with more prominent signs of airway obstruction in the younger child. Bronchoscopy and aggressive removal of purulent material and pseudomembranous material may be essential and lifesaving in some children. This case study points to some differences noted in the older child. I, however, would be uncomfortable with a nonintubation approach in most children. Aggressive tracheobronchial suctioning would be facilitated by intubation until antibiotics bring the disease under control.

This article also points out the key findings of bacterial tracheitis on a lateral neck radiograph: that of an irregular shadow in the tracheal air column. However, if I suspected epiglottiditis, the patient should go to the operating room first, not to the radiography suite (1). If in doubt and the patient is not in severe distress, an upright cross-table lateral neck radiograph should be performed in the emergency department with emergency airway equipment at the bedside.—R.W. Schafermeyer, M.D.

Reference

1. National Asthma Education Program: *Guidelines for the Diagnosis and Management of Asthma.* Bethesda, Md., National Heart, Lung and Blood Institute, 1991.

Soft Tissue Infections in the Emergency Department: The Case for the Use of 'Simple' Antibiotics

Powers RD (Univ of Virginia, Charlottesville)

South Med J 84:1313–1315, 1991 4–15

Background.—Informal observation in the emergency department of a teaching hospital suggested that infections of skin and soft tissue are frequently treated with newer, more expensive, broader-spectrum antibiotic agents. Data from a prospective study were analyzed to determine whether this prescribing pattern is appropriate.

Methods.—Seventy-two healthy adult volunteers were randomized to receive a 10-day regimen of either cephalexin (34 patients) or ofloxacin (38 patients). The clinical response was assessed at 2 follow-up visits.

Results.—Pretreatment cultures were positive for aerobic pathogens in 45 patients with abscesses, wound infections, cellulitis, or impetigo. *Staphylococcus aureus* was found in 31 cultures, 5 grew gram-negative rods, and 5 grew streptococcal species. The infections treated had clinical response rates exceeding 95%. Overall, 71 of 72 patients had cure or substantial improvement by the posttreatment visits and required no further therapy. In 1 patient parenteral therapy was initiated when oral therapy did not improve the infection with *S. aureus*. The 27 patients with no pathogen isolated had excellent clinical response rates, comparable to those of the group with identified pathogens.

Conclusions.—The bacteriologic profile and clinical course of uncomplicated soft-tissue infections responded well to a "simple" antibiotic such as cephalexin. The empirical use of a broader-spectrum, often costlier antibiotic for the treatment of mild-to-moderate skin and soft-tissue infections cannot be justified.

▶ Similar studies to this one, with similar results, have been published many times. The study groups are small in this study. If they had been larger, then the more expensive antibiotic may have produced a statistically significant improvement in results.

Statistically, according to this study, using the "cheaper" antibiotic probably makes no difference in outcome. Unfortunately, in private practice, you are dealing with causes on an individual basis. Several "bad" results in a study make no statistical difference, but several "bad" results in a physician's practice can make a lot of difference. Patients often want "the best" antibiotic. Also, if a "cheaper" antibiotic is used and a "bad result" goes to court because of poor outcome, the aggressive attorney may try to prove that you used a "poor" antibiotic. I am not saying that medically I would recommended "the lastest-generation" antibiotic, but in our litiginous society, it is something you have to think about.—G.J. Ordog, M.D.

Malaria in an Urban Emergency Department: Epidemiology and Diagnostic Features of 25 Cases

diMaggio CJ, D'Addesio J (City Hosp Ctr at Elmhurst, Queens, NY)

Am J Emerg Med 9:347–349, 1991 4–16

Background.—Populations of ethnically diverse new immigrants seem to be at high risk of having parasitic infections, probably because of the ease of international travel. Emergency physicians should consider such infections, especially malaria, in febrile patients in multiethnic regions. The epidemiology and diagnostic features of malaria in an urban emergency department (ED) were studied.

Methods and Findings.—Twenty-five patients had malaria in the ED of the City Hospital at Elmhurst in New York City between 1986 and 1989. In this study group, the mean annual case rate of malaria was more than 3 times the national rate. All patients eventually admitted to a history of travel to an area endemic for malaria. Fifty-six percent complained primarily of fever, whereas 12% complained mainly of abdominal pain. Seventy percent of the patients had elevated temperatures, with a mean of 102.9°F. Gender was an important factor in delayed diagnosis. Eighty-three percent of a group requiring multiple ED visits before diagnosis were women.

Conclusions.—Emergency physicians must consider malaria in the diagnosis of patients in ethnically diverse populations. Women appear to be at an increased risk of delayed diagnosis. Physicians should obtain a careful travel history and a peripheral smear to aid with prompt diagnosis.

▶ Malaria must be high on the differential list in patients who have traveled to endemic areas.

This is an interesting review of the presentation of patients from diverse cultures who had a common disease in the emergency center.

Most patients arriving at our center with malaria suspect the diagnosis. The occasional patient who does not suggest the possibility presents a much greater diagnostic challenge.—J.E. Clinton, M.D.

Bites and Stings

Dog Bites in Urban Children

Avner JR, Baker MD (The Children's Hosp of Philadelphia; Univ of Pennsylvania)

Pediatrics 88:55–57, 1991 4–17

Objectives.—Dog bites account for up to 90% of all animal bites in the United States, and the majority occur in children. The epidemiologic characteristics of dog bite injuries seen in an urban pediatric emergency department were evaluated.

Patients.—From January to December 1989, 168 children were seen with dog-bite–related injuries. The mean age of the patients was 8 years, and the male-to-female ratio was 1.5:1.

Clinical Features.—The injuries included lacerations (38%), abrasions (33%), and puncture wounds (29%). Thirteen bites had associated complications, including infection in 9, partial amputation of digits in 2, muscle injury in 1, and tendon rupture in 1. Twelve (7%) children required admission to the hospital. Most of the injuries (61%) occurred in or around the house, and 77% involved dogs known to the patient. The German shepherd and pit bull were the most common breeds of dogs involved in the attacks. Most (54%) of the animals were contained at the time of injury, and 46% were provoked before biting. When compared with injuries from all other breeds, pit bull injuries were significantly associated with unprovoked attacks (94% vs. 43%) and involved freely roaming animals (67% vs. 41%). Children aged 5 years or younger were more likely to be bitten in or around the home and to provoke animals before injury than were older children.

Conclusion.—Measures should be undertaken to identify a potentially dangerous dog early and to restrict ownership, and families with young children should be the target of pet safety education.

▶ Small children and large or unpredictable pets do not mix. For families considering pet ownership, I usually recommend waiting until the children are at least 4 or 5 years of age, a time when they are able to maintain their balance when pushed and can understand the concept of "gentleness" toward pets. Even at that age, care must be taken in the choice of a pet. This study indicates that some dogs, such as pit bulls, German shepherds, and rottweilers, might be poor choices for pets for families with children of any age. In addition, the authors' final statement bears repeating: "infants and young children should never be left unsupervised around any dog, no matter how well known the dog is, or how friendly the dog may appear".—R.M. Rutstein, M.D.

Cat Bite Wounds: Risk Factors for Infection

Dire DJ (Darnall Army Community Hosp, Fort Hood, Tex)

Ann Emerg Med 20:973–979, 1991 4–18

Purpose.—Up to 19% of bite wounds treated by physicians may be inflicted by cats. Most studies of the emergency management of these wounds have considered the controversies of giving prophylactic antibiotics or suturing wounds. This prospective study assessed risk factors for cate bite wound infections.

Methods.—All patients seen in the emergency department (ED) with mammalian bite wounds during a 2-year period were eligible for the study. If they agreed to participate, they were given a standard data form to carry with them until ED discharged. Wound cleaning was done according to a standardized protocol and included high-pressure irrigation. Debridement and suturing were done if indicated. Risk factor analysis included patient age and sex; wound age, type, number, location, and depth; prehospital and ED therapy; and the use of antibiotics.

Results.—Of 1,075 patients entered into the study, 186 patients had a total of 216 cat bites or scratches, a rate of 17.3%. The mean time from the injury until ED treatment was 10.2 hours. The hand was wounded in 45% of cases, the arm was injured in 22%, the head or neck was wounded in 15%, the lower extremity was injured in 13%, and the trunk was wounded in 5%. Fifty-six percent of wounds were punctures, 25% were abrasions, 17% were lacerations, and 1% was avulsions. Seventy-one percent of wounds were partial-thickness wounds. On ED arrival, 12.9% of patients already had evidence of infection, and 2.7% had such signs despite receiving ED treatment. The infection rate for patients with bite wounds was 15.6% vs. 0% for those with only "claw" injuries. Older age, longer time until ED treatment, wounding by a pet cat, attempting wound care at home, a more severe wound, and a deeper wound were all associated with infection. Among patients with no signs of infection on presentation, infection was more likely in those with lower-extremity wounds or puncture who did not have prophylactic, orally administered antibiotics.

Conclusions.—The type and depth of the wound rather than prophylactic antibiotic treatment appear to be the most important factors in determining the likelihood of infection developing in patients with cat bite wounds. Randomized studies of these injuries are needed.

▶ This contribution to our understanding of the perennial cat bite wound problem and the decision whether or not to administer antibiotics suffers from the same problems as its predecessors: nonrandomized treatment groups, an unknown denominator of total bite wounds in the community, and numbers of infections too small to reach statistical significance.

Some cat bite wounds become infected, often with *Pasteurella multocida,* but the actual percentage is unknown. The author found that only 5% of wounds that were uninfected initially later developed infection, which suggests that the infection rate is much lower than the 30% to 50% sometimes quoted. The total infection rate the author reports, 16%, is deceiving: it lumps together patients who came to the ED within a few hours of their bite and those who came days later once an infection had developed. One must suspect that many people were bitten, never saw a doctor, and never became infected.

The wounds that were treated with antibiotics had a lower rate of infection (2%) than those untreated (6%), but because of the very small number of infections, this difference did not reach statistical significance. As the author notes, we badly need a large-scale study randomized as to treatment. A meta-analysis of the existing studies might also help to clarify the issues.

The author's conclusion that bite type and depth are more important determinants of wound infection than antibiotic use may be correct, but this is not supported by his data.—J. Schoffstall, M.D.

Portuguese Man-of-War Envenomation

Kaufman MB (Massachusetts College of Pharmacy and Allied Health Sciences, Boston)

Pediatr Emerg Care 8:27–28, 1992 4–19

Background.—Portuguese man-of-war and jellyfish stings are common in the coastal waters of the southern United States.

Case Report.—A 14-year-old girl was wading in the ocean off the Florida coast when she suddenly felt intense burning and pain on her right knee and ankle. This was quickly followed by numbness and paralysis of the lower part of her right leg. She became disoriented and complained of nausea, chills, diffuse pruritus, and paresthesia in her leg. A lifeguard applied 70% isopropyl alcohol and removed a 12-cm tentacle from the girl's knee. Her knee was swollen, with linear erythematous streaks at the site of the tentacle contact. On her arrival in the emergency department, her blood pressure was 95/60 mm Hg; pulse rate, 110 per minute; respiratory rate, 22 breaths per minute; and temperature, 37.8°C. She was oriented to place but not time. She had a loss of proprioception in the toes of her right foot, reduced sensation in the affected lower portion of her leg, and decreased strength in all muscle groups of the anterior and posterior tibial compartments. The diagnosis was *Physalia* (Portuguese man-of-war) envenomation, which was supported by the lifeguard's report that several man-of-wars had been seen on the beach in previous weeks. The girl was kept in the emergency department for observation for 6 hours. Her symptoms did not worsen, and she was discharged with her parents. She was advised to keep the right leg elevated and immobilized. Subsequently, all pain, swelling, and numbness resolved.

Conclusions.—Reaction to Portuguese man-of-war envenomation are commonly localized and consist of pain, paresthesia, and intense burning. A linear, red, papular eruption or urticaria is usually seen at the contact site. The signs and symptoms of such envenomation typically appear immediately after the sting but may be delayed for several hours. Patients may have the systemic signs of nausea, myalgia, headache, chills, or pallor. Some patients have suffered cardiovascular collapse and died. The venom can be inactivated with dilute acetic acid, proteolytic meat tenderizer, or baking soda. Tentacle debris needs to be extracted. Typically, symptoms resolve within 72 hours with no sequelae.

Marine Envenomations. Part 2: Invertebrates
McGoldrick J, Marx JA (Denver Gen Hosp, Colo)
J Emerg Med 10:71–77, 1992 4–20

Background.—With more people traveling to the oceans for diving and other water sports, there has been an increase in the incidence of marine envenomations. The varying marine envenomations, their clinical presentation, and recommended treatment were reviewed for emergency medicine physicians.

Treatment of Marine Invertebrate Envenomations.—For patients stung by hydroids, fire coral, Portuguese man-of-war, sea nettles, box jellyfish, and anenomes, detoxification consists of irrigation with seawater and topical 5% acetic acid, or vinegar. The affected area should be shaved. In addition to this treatment, patients stung by a Portuguese man-of-war and box jellyfish need the invertebrate's tentacles removed with forceps. Emergency department treatment consists of topical corticosteroid cream for dermatitis and, in the case of Portuguese man-of-war and sea nettle stings, observation of patients with systemic symptoms for 8 hours. Severe systemic symptoms require hospitalization and supportive care. Patients with box jellyfish stings should be given chironex antivenin and supportive care for hypotension and respiratory depression. Patients with blue-ringed octopus envenomation need a pressure immobilization bandage and supportive care for respiratory depression. For cases of cone shell contact, treatment consists of hot water, pressure immobilization bandages, and supportive care for hypotension and respiratory depression. Starfish stings require irrigation with fresh water, removal of the spines, and topical corticosteroid for dermatitis. For sea urchin envenomations, treatment consists of hot water and removal of any spines or pedicellariae. Detoxification for patients with sea cucumber contacts involves the application of topical 5% acetic acid, and emergency department care includes topical corticosteroid for dermatitis.

Conclusions.—The general principles of emergency medicine apply when treating a marine envenomation or wound. Sometimes envenomations are accompanied by allergic reactions, which require treatment for anaphylaxis.

▶ These two papers (Abstracts 4–19 and 4–20) are very interesting reading to a landlubber like me. My learnings are that if I am envenomated by marine fauna, I hope there are experts in my midst who can recognize and then appropriately render first aid. For instance, in Abstract 4–20, McGoldrick and Mark, for octopus envenomation, advise "the pressure immobilization technique that has been popularized in Australia" and provide a reference that I am sure I will not be able to find in the lifeguard's library! (This refers to elastic bandage wrapping and elevating the extremity.) For box jellyfish, they advise chironex vaccine produced by an Australian laboratory. To my relief, I read that box jellyfish are found in Northern Australia and the "Indo-Pacific" region. It is interesting that while the review of McGoldrick and Marx does not recommend isopropanol (because it has been suggested that it may increase nematode discharge), the lifeguard in southern Florida in Kaufman's paper (Abstract 4–19) used it. In fact, many experts do not subscribe to the increased nematode discharge theory and indeed recommend isopropanol as an alternative if vinegar is not available. My local expert advises that vinegar may be effectively used for all marine envenomations except for the Chesapeake Bay sea nettle, where baking soda is preferred.—S. Wason, M.D.

Fire Ants: The Death March

Schwartz MP (Med Coll of Georgia, Augusta)
J Fam Pract 33:406–410, 1991 4–21

Introduction.—Fire ants are virtually indestructible insects that wreak havoc on everything from human and animal life to highway systems and farm machinery. Two species of the fire ant, the black and the red fire ant, were introduced into the United States by ship some time early in this century. Fire ants now cover between 160 and 250 million acres in 13 southern states. Fire ant bites may cause a range of symptoms from an annoying burning sensation to anaphylaxis and death. A case report is presented.

Case Report.—A 31-year-old man came to the emergency department 30 minutes after having been bitten by a fire ant on the right thumb. He reported that 2 to 3 minutes after the bite he noted a metallic taste in his mouth and the sudden onset of a severe headache. Subsequently he developed shakiness, paresthesia, and tachycardia. The patient had no known hypersensitivities and was in good health before the bite. Physical and neurologic examinations were normal. A CT scan of the head was within normal limits. Respiratory or cardiac support was not needed. The patient was observed in the hospital overnight and discharged. Intradermal allergy testing for fire ant sensitivity performed 4 weeks later showed that he reacted at 1:1 million for fire ant whole-body extract. He then underwent desensitization and maintenance therapy. The patient suffered another bite approximately 1 year after the initial bite but suffered only local erythema requiring no treatment.

Discussion.—Between 17% and 56% of all patients bitten by fire ants have large, local reactions at the sting site. It is estimated that anaphylaxis occurs in .6% to 4% of bites. Anaphylaxis to imported fire ant stings is treated as are other types of anaphylaxis, with respiratory and cardiac support as needed. The natural history of sensitivity to imported fire ants is unknown. Thus, indications for immunotherapy to prevent bite-related anaphylaxis are unclear. Because it is impossible for sensitized persons living in infested areas to completely avoid fire ants, desensitization is commonly used.

▶ Help—another vicious alien on the attack! Perhaps we could entice Sigourney Weaver to help us in fending off this new menace. Apparently, fire ants have the same spectrum of potential problems as hymenoptera stings, with a particular concern regarding the .6% to 4% incidence of anaphylaxis—be on the lookout.—F.M. Henretig, M.D.

Psychiatric Emergencies

The Misdiagnosis of Conversion Disorder in a Psychiatric Emergency Service

Fishbain DA, Goldberg M (Univ of Miami, Fla)
Gen Hosp Psychiatry 13:177–181, 1991 4–22

Introduction.—Conversion disorder, an alteration in physical functioning that is an expression of a psychological conflict, classically appears as neurologic disease. Although psychiatric emergency services are common in hospitals, the incidence of conversion disorder is not known. A study was done to determine the incidence of a specific type of this disorder: conversion paresis and/or paralysis.

Methods.—A retrospective review was conducted of the 8,400 psychiatric emergency room visits at the study institution during 1982. The review identified 3 patients with the conversion symptom of limb paresis and/or paralysis. Each met *Diagnostic and Statistical Manual of Mental Disorders,* ed III (DSM-III), criteria.

Case Report.—A 32-year-old black woman had severe bilateral headaches that began after an argument with her husband. While waiting in the emergency room, she began to complain of bilateral leg weakness and give-away weakness. Because of the patient's argument with her husband and a history of intravenous drug use, the neurologist diagnosed hysteria and referred the woman to the psychiatric emergency service. An hour later the woman complained of increasing paralysis, had a disturbance of consciousness, and died. Postmortem examination revealed a massive subarachnoid hemorrhage from a ruptured mycotic aneurysm in the circle of Willis.

Conclusion.—The other 2 illnesses were similarly misdiagnosed as conversion disorder, although the symptoms resulted from organic disease. Conversion disorder seems to have an extremely low incidence. Furthermore, the reliability and validity of the DMS-III-R criteria are unproved. Psychiatrists must demand adequate medical evaluation of patients because of the serious medical and legal consequences of misdiagnosis.

▶ Due to declining resources for outpatient mental health care, emergency physicians and their colleagues in psychiatry are evaluating an increasing number of patients with mental illness in the acute-care setting. This article deals with a select group of such patients, namely, those with a conversion disorder. Conversion disorder is defined as "an alteration in physical functioning that suggests physical disease, but instead is apparently an expression of a psychological conflict or need." Conversion symptoms usually suggest neurologic disease and include paresis/paralysis, blindness, paresthesias, and akinesia to name a few. Two previous studies have addressed the incidence of conversion disorders in the setting of psychiatric emergency care. The combined incidence of the various types of conversion disorders/symptoms was .23% in one study and 1% in the other. The report by Fishbain and Goldberg is unique in that only the incidence of the conversion symptom of paralysis/paresis was evaluated. From a population of 4,220 nonduplicate visits in a 1-year period, 3 patients were given diagnoses of paralysis/paresis resulting from a conversion disorder (incidence, .07%). All 3 patients were later given diagnoses of organic disease (true incidence, 0%; 100% false-positive rate). The message here is that paralysis/paresis is rarely a conversion symptom, and when encountered, organic illness should be suspected and aggressively pursued with an appropriate workup. This article points out the medicolegal ramifications of not doing so.—J.T. Niemann, M.D.

Droperidol Versus Haloperidol for Chemical Restraint of Agitated and Combative Patients

Thomas H Jr, Schwartz E, Petrilli R (Wake Forest Univ, Winston-Salem, NC)
Ann Emerg Med 21:407–413, 1992 4–23

Background.—Emergency physicians commonly provide care for patients who are acutely violent and agitated. Diagnosis is difficult in such patients, and they are a threat to themselves, other patients, and health care personnel. The efficacies of haloperidol and droperidol for chemical restraint of violent and agitated patients were compared.

Methods.—Sixty-eight combative adults were entered into the randomized, double-blind, prospective trial. In all cases, the attending physician believed that chemical restraint would protect the patient and staff and expedite assessment. Twenty-one patients were given haloperidol, 5 mg intramuscularly; 26, droperidol, 5 mg intramuscularly; 12, haloperidol intravenously; and 9, droperidol intravenously. Patients were rated on a 5-point scale of combativeness 5, 10, 15, 30, and 60 minutes after the drug was administered. Vital signs were also noted at those intervals.

Results.—Intramuscular droperidol reduced combativeness significantly more than intramuscular haloperidol at 10, 15, and 30 minutes. Drug effects did not differ significantly when the drugs were given intravenously. Only 1 adverse reaction occurred. One patient given haloperidol intramuscularly returned 18 hours later with an acute dystonic reaction that was treated easily.

Conclusions.—Intramuscular administration of droperidol, 5 mg, is more rapidly effective in controlling agitated and combative patients in the emergency department than an equal dose of haloperidol given intramuscularly. Adverse effects resulting from such treatment are minimal and manageable.

▶ Sedation should be used to control violent or combative patients. Haloperidol, 5 mg intramuscularly (IM), or droperidol, 5 mg, may be used initially, followed by either drug, 5 mg IM every 30 minutes until the patient is controlled (rapid neuroleptization or psychotolysis). In the elderly, use 1 to 2 mg IM. The literature supports the use of intravenous (IV) haloperidol. However, at this time, haloperidol is not approved for IV use by the Food and Drug Administration (FDA). Droperidol is presently approved for IV use by the FDA. The problem with the use of these butyrophenones is that these drugs have both an α-blocking effect and an anticholinergic effect. The α-blocking effect can produce hypotension. When IV butyrophenones are used, careful monitoring is mandatory. Poorly monitored patients have died in the emergency department following the administration of butyrophenones. The anticholinergic effects of butyrophenones can cause patients to become hot. Combative phencyclidine- or cocaine-intoxicated patients may have a fever. Haloperidol or droperidol given to patients with a fever can induce the malignant neuroleptic syndrome.—J. Wasserberger, M.D.

Repeated Use of Psychiatric Emergency Services by Children

Cole W, Turgay A, Mouldey G (Royal Ottawa Hosp, Ont; Wayne State Univ, Detroit, Mich; Children's Hosp of Eastern Ontario, Ottawa, Canada)

Can J Psychiatry 36:739–742, 1991 4–24

Background.—Little is known about the use and abuse of psychiatric emergency services by children and adolescents. The Canadian system of universally available medical services enabled such a study.

Methods.—At 1 Canadian hospital, 556 children and adolescents were referred to the psychiatric emergency service during the study period. Data on presenting problems and diagnosis were obtained at the first visit. Repeat visits to the emergency department (ED) and compliance with follow-up treatment were documented.

Findings.—Children and adolescents making repeat visits to the emergency service were more likely to threaten to harm others; to have a diagnosis of adjustment disorder, conduct, or oppositional disorder; and to be under the care of a child welfare agency. Also, repeat users were significantly more likely than 1-time patients to be less compliant with outpatient follow-up, to be admitted to the hospital more often, to need more social support, and to have more difficulty remaining in a residential treatment setting. Emergency department intervention appeared to have no effect on how repeat users used the emergency services.

Conclusions.—Repeat users of psychiatric emergency services in Canada represent a significant proportion of child psychiatric emergencies seen in EDs. Such patients more frequently have chronic behavior problems with aggression that is more likely to evoke a sense of urgency and crisis necessitating immediate resolution.

▶ It is not surprising that children with an adjustment reaction tend not to be repeat ED users, while those with chronic behavior problems who threaten others (usually after 5 P.M.) are repeatedly brought to the ED for acute intervention. Some of the findings may not be generalizable. The authors state that it is the policy of many child welfare agencies in Canada to require any child who is acting up to be taken to an ED. This may explain why younger children with chronic behavior problems under the care of a child welfare agency were among the repeat users.—K.N. Shaw, M.D.

Functional Upper Airway Obstruction: Psychogenic Pharyngeal Constriction

Nagai A, Yamaguchi E, Sakamoto K, Takahashi E (Tokyo Women's Med College, Japan)

Chest 101:1460–1461, 1992 4–25

Background.—Most cases of inspiratory airway obstruction are caused by organic abnormalities such as inflammation, trauma, edema, and tumors. Abnormal motion of the vocal cords is an uncommon cause of reversible airway obstruction. A patient was seen with inspiratory airflow obstruction and stridor caused by pharyngeal constriction, a previously unreported cause.

Case Report.—A 15-year-old boy was hospitalized with severe shortness of breath of several hours' duration. He was known to have asthma. He had marked inspiratory stridor on physical examination, but rhonchi were not durable anywhere in the chest on auscultation. Spirometry showed a reduced airflow and a plateau configuration with a wave at the inspiratory portion. However, the loop at the expiratory portion was nearly normal and indicated extrathoracic airway obstruction. Bronchofiberscopy was done during the stridor, and marked narrowing in the hypopharynx with an abnormally shaped tremulous epiglottis was found during the inspiratory phase. The glottis, vocal cords, and trachea were normal. An acute respiratory alkalosis with a normal PaO_2 was indicated on arterial blood gas analysis. The patient's condition did not respond to treatment with aminophylline and steroid injection, inhalation of β_2-adrenoceptor agonists, anticholinergic agents, or gargling with atropine sulfate and lidocaine. The stridor suddenly stopped 30 minutes after an intramuscular injection of 10 mg of diazepam. After 2 days in the hospital the patient was discharged, thereafter requiring frequent emergency treatment with sedatives for stridor attacks. A psychiatric assessment during the initial hospitalization suggested that he was depressed. He is currently undergoing psychotherapy, and the frequency of his stridor attacks is diminishing.

Conclusions.—In this case, spirometry indicated extrathoracic airway obstruction, and bronchofiberscopy assessment revealed hypopharyngeal narrowing. The boy's stridor disappeared suddenly after sedatives were administered. Psychogenic pharyngeal constriction may have been responsible for the upper airway obstruction with respiratory distress.

▶ Direct visualization of the anatomy is invaluable in determining the cause of stridor in a patient with suspected upper airway obstruction.

I think that this is an interesting case report, but ruling out trauma, allergic reaction, neoplasm, inflammation, a foreign body, and neurologic etiologies must be done before entertaining this uncommon cause of reversible airway obstruction.—J.J. Kelly, D.O., F.A.C.E.P.

Domestic Violence: Risk Factors and Outcome

Berrios DC, Grady D (Univ of California, San Francisco)

West J Med 155:133–135, 1991 4–26

Introduction.—Domestic violence is a frequently unrecognized cause of acute and chronic illness among women and may occur each year in as many as 16% of relationships. Injuries caused by domestic violence account for 20% of all emergency room visits by women and 29% of women's suicide attempts.

Methods.—To determine the risk factors for and outcomes of domestic violence, data on 218 women who sought medical care at an emergency room were reviewed. Since 1983, 492 women who had injuries caused by domestic violence or who reported that they were victims of domestic violence were interviewed by the staff of a social service agency for victims of domestic violence. Interviewers completed standardized data forms describing the victim, the batterer, the victim's children, and the injuries. When questionnaires were not complete, the individual was excluded from the study.

Results.—The 218 evaluated women were aged 16 to 66 years (median age, 29 years). They were ethnically heterogeneous. One third were employed, and only 7% were dependent solely on their attacker for financial support. In 93% of cases, the batterer was a current or former spouse or boyfriend, and 67% of the victims were presently living with the batterer. Previous episodes of abuse were reported by 86% of the women, with 40% reporting previous abuse requiring medical attention and 13% reporting previous abuse requiring hospitalization. Children lived in about half of the households where the violence occurred and witnessed the abuse in 35% of the episodes. Major surgery was performed in 13% of the women; 28% were admitted to the hospital. The most frequent injury was bruises (70%), followed by lacerations (39%), choking or strangulation (23%), musculoskeletal injuries (25%), and internal injuries (13%). Permanent injury resulted from the episode in 5%

of the women. The face, skull, eyes, upper part of the trunk, and extremities were the most frequently assaulted parts of the body. Weapons were involved in one third of the episodes.

Conclusion.—Domestic violence is a recurrent problem. If physicians were more aware of its prevalence, severity, frequency, and typical presentation, diagnostic sensitivity could be improved and lead to referral of victims to appropriate agencies.

▶ As evidenced by recent editorials in the *Journal of the American Medical Association,* violence against women of all ages is pervasive in our society and might be unrecognized in the emergency department or the primary-care physician's office. Some time should be spent trying to ascertain the true mechanism of injury. There is a strong possibility of recurrent battering if no intervention occurs. A good working relationship with the local Battered Women Society can help provide additional counseling or shelter to prevent future abuse. However, none of this is possible if the true pathology is not recognized at the time of treatment (see also Abstract 2–7).—J.T. Amsterdam, M.D.

Pregnancy-Related

New Options For Diagnosis and Treatment of Ectopic Pregnancy
Ory SJ (Mayo Clinic and Found, Rochester, Minn)
JAMA 267:534–537, 1992 4–27

Introduction.—Since 1970, the incidence of ectopic pregnancy has increased fivefold in the United States, from 4.5 in 1970 to 16.8 per 1,000 pregnancies in 1987. Paradoxically, the case-fatality rate decreased 90% from 35.5 to 3.4 per 10,000 ectopic pregnancies during this time.

Discussion.—The origin of this epidemic of ectopic pregnancies is not clear. Several risk factors contribute to this rate of increase, including the application of conservative tubal surgery to treat ectopic pregnancy and the use of intrauterine devices and ovulation-inducing drugs. However, diagnostic advances during the same period have contributed to an earlier and more consistent diagnosis. The availability of a highly specific radioimmunoassay for human chorionic gonadotropin (HCG), the development of high-resolution ultrasonography, and the more frequent use of laparoscopy have contributed to improved diagnostic accuracy.

Serum HCG radioimmunoassays are more than 99% sensitive in detecting ectopic pregnancy; radioimmunoassays can detect the presence of HCG as early as 1 week before expected menses. The HCG–doubling time concept is a useful test for screening early suspected pregnancies. The availability of high-resolution ultrasonography and vaginal transducers has permitted the discriminatory zone, an HCG range above which a gestational sac could be reliably seen, to be redefined to a lower level. A discriminatory zone with an HCG range of 1,200 to 1,500 IU/L permits the diagnosis of tubal pregnancy as early as 1 week after the expected menses. The new generation of vaginal transducers and the advent of color-flow Doppler technology may permit the discriminatory zone to be further reduced and possibly allow the identification of a gestational sac in the adnexa. Vaginal transducers can visualize gestational sacs within a tube in more advanced ectopic pregnancies.

Conclusion.—Advances in treatment, including tubal-conserving operations, laparoscopic approaches, and medical treatment with methotrexate, are safe and effective. The remaining principal challenge is to improve future fertility.

▶ This review article should be common knowledge to every emergency physician. Nothing new is stated. Almost every emergency physician deals with this problem many times on a daily basis. Vaginal ultrasonography should be available in every emergency department.—G.J. Ordog, M.D.

Ruptured Ectopic Pregnancy in a Patient With a Recent Intrauterine Abortion

Nugent PJ (Bethesda Hosp, Cincinnati, Ohio)

Ann Emerg Med 21:97–99, 1992 4–28

Introduction.—Combined intrauterine and extrauterine pregnancy is rare, with an estimated incidence of 1 in 30,000 patients. The diagnosis of this condition is often difficult but must be considered under the right clinical circumstances.

Case Report.—A 33-year-old woman had lower abdominal pain. She had a successful elective intrauterine abortion 2 weeks earlier at about week 8 of pregnancy. Physical examination revealed diffuse abdominal tenderness without rebound and bilateral adnexal and cervical motion tenderness. Laboratory examinations revealed increasing WBC counts and neutrophils but a decreasing hematocrit. Pelvic inflammatory disease was suspected. A urinary pregnancy test result was positive. The patient became hypotensive, and a ruptured tubal pregnancy was evident at surgery.

Conclusion.—The possibility of combined intrauterine and extrauterine pregnancy should be considered in a patient with a previous history of pelvic inflammatory disease, ovulation-inducing treatment, and in vitro fertilization with embryo transfer. Only about 10% of all intrauterine and extrauterine pregnancies are diagnosed by clinical evidence alone. In the presence of appropriate symptoms, a high level of suspicion should be maintained for combined intrauterine and extrauterine pregnancy.

▶ This case report demonstrates a catastrophic, albeit rare condition. This case clearly supports the liberal use of serum pregnancy tests and implies the helpfulness of obtaining quantitative human chorionic gonadotropin (HCG) levels. Had a quantitative HCG test been done in this case to better define the author's concern about retained placental fetal tissue, an ectopic pregnancy may have been more rapidly diagnosed (see also Abstract 4–27).—E.J. Reisdorff, M.D.

Blunt Trauma During Pregnancy: Factors Affecting Fetal Outcome

Scorpio RJ, Esposito TJ, Smith LG, Gens DR (Univ of Maryland, Baltimore)

J Trauma 32:213–216, 1992 4–29

Introduction.—Seventy-six pregnant women seen in a 9½-year period who were admitted to a level I trauma center were studied. The fetal outcome was determined in 59 instances, and 8 of these women had elective abortion, which left 51 cases for analysis.

Outcome.—Successful delivery took place in 46% of the entire group. The rate of fetal loss was 21%. The Injury Severity Score and the serum bicarbonate level at admission correlated most closely with the fetal outcome. A low serum bicarbonate level reflected maternal hypoperfusion and hypoxia, which may otherwise be masked by the physiologic changes expected in pregnancy. Surgery was done in 27 cases, and 16 patients underwent diagnostic peritoneal lavage.

Discussion.—Both the severity of injury and the degree of tissue hypoperfusion and hypoxia predict the fetal outcome in women who incur blunt trauma while pregnant. It does not appear to be justified to withhold peritoneal lavage or surgery for fear of increasing the risk of fetal loss.

► In the introduction, the authors of this paper point out that while much has been written about factors concerning maternal physiologic changes during pregnancy and the resuscitation of pregnant mothers, little has been written about the factors that affect or predict fetal outcome. They also note that the physiologic changes of pregnancy may mask maternal hypoperfusion and hypoxia.

The message to remember here is get arterial blood gas determinations early in the course of care. Maternal hypoperfusion and hypoxia, as reflected by a low serum bicarbonate level, are best detected and addressed early in the resuscitation (see also Abstracts 4–30 and 4–31).—E.H. Taliaferro, M.D.

Trauma: The Leading Cause of Maternal Death

Fildes J, Reed L, Jones N, Martin M, Barrett J (Cook County Hosp; Univ of Illinois at Chicago; Cook County Med Examiners Office, Chicago)

J Trauma 32:643–645, 1992 4–30

Background.—In the past 60 years the leading causes of maternal death have changed markedly. Seven percent of pregnant women sustain trauma, with the rate of fatal injury remaining almost constant. As the

Causes of Maternal Death

Causes of Death	Number of Deaths	Percentage of Total Deaths
Maternal		
Direct	18	18.9
Indirect	12	12.6
Nonmaternal		
Traumatic	44	46.3
Nontraumatic	21	22.1

(Courtesy of Fildes J, Reed L, Jones N, et al: *J Trauma* 32:643–645, 1992.)

rate of preventable pregnancy-related deaths decreases, the rate of injury-related deaths should be considered.

Methods and Findings.—The Cook County Medical Examiner records were reviewed. Ninety-five maternal deaths were identified between 1986 and 1989. The causes of death were classified as direct maternal, indirect maternal, or nonmaternal. Direct maternal causes of death, accounting for 18.9%, resulted from complications of pregnancy, labor, delivery, or its management. Indirect maternal causes of death, accounting for 12.6%, occurred when pregnancy exacerbated pre-existing health problems. Nonmaternal causes of death were further categorized as traumatic or nontraumatic. The 46.3% dying of traumatic causes were victims of homicide in 57% of the cases and suicide in 9%. Other mechanisms of injury were gunshot wounds in 22.7%, motor vehicle accidents in 20.5%, stab wounds in 13.6%, strangulation in 13.6%, blunt head injuries in 9.1%, burns in 6.8%, falls in 4.5%, toxic exposure in 4.5%, drowning in 2.3%, and iatrogenic injury in 2.3% (table).

Conclusion.—Trauma is the leading cause of maternal death in Cook County, Illinois, a finding not predicted by traditional methods of defining and reporting maternal death. Unanimity in the definition of maternal death and improvement in the way that cases are reported need to be adopted. In addition, comprehensive prenatal care must include programs aimed at preventing injury.

▶ This sad fact presented by the trauma surgeons and forensic pathologists in Cook County, Chicago, reflects another segment of Americans at risk for death from trauma. Over 80% of the victims in this study were young black females of inner-city Chicago. From this paper, it would seem that the urban black male is not the only gender at risk for traumatic death in the inner city. I would like to see a study from the whole state, which may reflect a more accurate profile of the risk of traumatic death in pregnant patients.

Since 50% of these reported maternal deaths were due to gunshot, stabbing, or stangulation injuries, an injury prevention program that concentrates on domestic violence would be a start.—J.J. Kelly, D.O., F.A.C.E.P.

Maternal Predictors of Fetal Demise in Trauma During Pregnancy

Hoff WS, D'Amelio LF, Tinkoff GH, Lucke JF, Rhodes M, et al (Lehigh Valley Hosp Ctr, Allentown, Pa)

Surg Gynecol Obstet 172:175–180, 1991 4–31

Introduction.—An accidental injury occurs in 6% to 7% of otherwise normal pregnancies; the incidence of fetal death because of maternal injury is much lower. The physiologic and anatomic maternal characteristics that might predict fetal demise in maternal trauma were examined.

Methods and Findings.—The records of 73 pregnant patients admitted to 4 level 1 trauma centers with a combined registry base of 30,000 patients were evaluated. The analysis focused on fetal demise as a function of 21 maternal characteristics assessed during the initial 24-hour resuscitation period. Nine of the fetuses died. Associations were seen between fetal death and increasing Injury Severity Score (means of 10 for fetal survival and 21 for fetal demise), increasing Abbreviated Injury Scale for the face and abdomen, increasing fluid requirements, and maternal acidosis and hypoxia. None of the standard laboratory and physiologic indices—including hematocrit and hemoglobin, oxygen and hemoglobin saturation, partial pressure of carbon dioxide, systolic blood pressure, and heart rate—were significant predictors. In contrast to the Injury Severity Score, the Trauma Score was not predictive.

Conclusions.—In pregnant trauma victims, the severity of injury is significantly correlated with the occurrence of fetal death. Significant predictors include the presence of shock, as reflected by the need for fluids; the need for blood component therapy, as observed with hypoxia and acidosis; and the mechanical force of the injury, as reflected in abdominal and facial injuries.

▶ This is a typical trauma study where the results provide the profound wisdom that more severely injured patients die more often. Trauma in pregnancy should cue several responses in emergency physicians, including (1) in hypotension, get the uterus off the inferior vena cava; (2) monitor the fetus after even minor abdominal trauma; and (3) if you ever need to do a peri-omortem cesarean-section, do it within 5 minutes of maternal arrest.—R.M. McNamara, M.D.

CA 125 Levels in Abruptio Placentae

Witt BR, Miles R, Wolf GC, Koulianos GT, Thorneycroft IH (Tulane Univ, New

Orleans, La)
Am J Obstet Gynecol 164:1225–1228, 1991 4–32

Background.—Diagnosing abruptio placentae is often difficult despite ultrasonography. Additional diagnostic parameters would be useful. CA 125 may be increased in pregnancies complicated by abruptio placentae.

Methods.—Serum CA 125 levels were measured in 27 patients past 20 weeks' gestation who were first seen with vaginal bleeding. Seventeen other women at similar gestational stages and labor status were assessed for comparison.

Results.—Mean CA 125 levels were higher in patients with abruptio placentae than in those with different sources of bleeding and control subjects. The means in these 3 groups were 105.9, 13.7, and 18.2 units/mL, respectively. The mean serum CA 125 levels in 7 control subjects within 6 hours after birth were higher than in patients first seen with abruptio placentae. The sensitivity of CA 125 for abruptio placentae was 70% and its specificity was 94%.

Conclusions.—These findings are consistent with a decidual source for CA 125. Further study of the usefulness of CA 125 as a diagnostic test for abruptio placentae or as a marker for monitoring premature patients with mild abruptio placentae under expectant management is warranted.

▶ This preliminary study indicates that the CA 125 antigen as a marker of abruptio placentae could be very helpful to the emergency physician's evaluation of the pregnant patient. It could be particularly helpful in the pregnant trauma patient.

The study size is very small. Results need to be confirmed by a larger study.

Abruptio placentae is of particular concern in the third-trimester patient who has sustained blunt abdominal trauma. The availability of a sensitive screening test with a low false-negative level could avoid some unnecessary observation periods in these patients.—J.E. Clinton, M.D.

Ocular

Airbag-Mediated Corneal Injury
Larkin GL (William Beaumont Hosp, Royal Oak, Mich)
Am J Emerg Med 9:444–446, 1991 4–33

Background.—Automobile airbags are effective in providing protection in frontal collisions and are now standard equipment in many new cars. No previous reports have documented any possible detriment of their use by passengers. Airbag use was associated with facial and corneal abrasions and blurred vision in 1 patient.

Case Report.—A 29-year-old man was admitted to the emergency department after a tangential automobile collision in which his airbag activated and struck his right eye and face. He complained of decreased vision, epiphora, and pain with foreign-body sensation in the right eye. His vital signs were normal, and he appeared healthy and alert. He demonstrated marked photophobia and lacrimation from his right eye and multiple abrasions on the right side of his face, with an edematous right upper lid resulting in an ipsilateral ptosis. The visual acuity in the right eye was 20/50, and in the left eye it was 20/20. A +2 ciliar flush of the conjunctiva and a full-thickness epithelial defect of the central corneal surface were seen with slit-lamp biomicroscopy. Mild edema was found in the corneal stroma, and the anterior chamber was cell free but has a +2 proteinaceous flare. No foreign bodies were found. After the diagnosis of corneal and facial abrasions with traumatic iritis was made, treatment with homatropine 2% cycloplegia, sulfa eye ointment, and a patch were instituted. By 10 days after the accident, the corneal abrasion and iritis were healed, and all medication use was discontinued. At 16 days after the accident, visual acuity in the right eye was 20/25, and the patient complained of blurred near vision. Slit-lamp examination showed an irregularly healing corneal epithelium, and corrective lenses were prescribed. The patient continues to wear them.

Conclusions.—The corneal abrasion resulting from the airbag activation was large and had delayed healing because of the extent of epithelial involvement. Because large traumatic corneal abrasions may be complicated by prolonged or permanent loss of vision, continued follow-up and ophthalmologic referral of these patients should occur. The abrasion may have been the result of a seam in the airbag. Although it is unknown how much damage a seat-belted patient would have sustained in the accident if an airbag had not been present, a seat-belted passenger without an airbag in the front seat of the car during the accident sustained no injuries. Physicians should monitor and report airbag-associated injuries to determine whether design alterations are necessary.

▶ This article emphasizes the importance of the recognition and reporting by emergency physicians of an injury associated with a new device—in this case, automobile airbags. The Centers for Disease Control have identified injury control as a major effort for the 1990s. Our specialty can surely offer significant input to this effort by reporting all such injuries.—E.J. Lucid, M.D.

Eye Injuries With Metal Missiles Presenting to an Emergency Center: A Three Year Study

Schwartz JG, Somerset JS, Harrison JM, Garriott JC, Castorena JL (Univ of Texas Health Science Ctr; Bexar County Medical Examiner's Office, San Antonio)

Am J Emerg Med 9:313–317, 1991 4–34

Introduction.—During the past 3 years, a slight increase in the number of patients seen in the emergency department (ED) with eye injuries caused by metal missiles has been noted. In most cases, only the cornea

Moving?

I'd like to receive my ***Year Book of Emergency Medicine*** without interruption.

Please note the following change of address, effective: ______________________

Name: ______________________

New Address: ______________________

____

City: ______________________ State: __________ Zip: __________

Old Address: ______________________

____

City: ______________________ State: __________ Zip: __________

Reservation Card

Yes, I would like my own copy of the ***Year Book of Emergency Medicine***. Please begin my subscription with the current edition according to the terms described below.* I understand that I will have 30 days to examine each annual edition. If satisfied, I will pay just $59.95 plus sales tax, postage and handling (price subject to change without notice).

Name: ______________________

Address: ______________________

City: ______________________ State: __________ Zip: __________

Method of Payment

❏ Visa ❏ Mastercard ❏ AmEx ❏ Bill me ❏ Check (in US dollars, payable to Mosby-Year Book, Inc.)

Card number ______________________ Exp date ______________________

Signature ______________________

LS-0907

*Your *Year Book* Service Guarantee:

When you subscribe to the ***Year Book***, we'll send you an advance notice of future volumes about two months before they publish. This automatic notice system is designed to take up as little of your time as possible. If you do not want the ***Year Book***, the advance notice makes it quick and easy for you to let us know your decision; and you will always have at least 20 days to decide. If we don't hear from you, we'll send you the new volume as soon as it's available. And, of course, the ***Year Book*** is yours to examine free of charge for 30 days (postage, handling and applicable sales tax are added to each shipment).

NO POSTAGE
NECESSARY
IF MAILED
IN THE
UNITED STATES

BUSINESS REPLY MAIL
FIRST CLASS MAIL PERMIT No. 762 CHICAGO, IL

POSTAGE WILL BE PAID BY ADDRESSEE

Chris Hughes
Mosby-Year Book, Inc.
200 N. LaSalle Street
Suite 2600
Chicago, IL 60601-9981

NO POSTAGE
NECESSARY
IF MAILED
IN THE
UNITED STATES

BUSINESS REPLY MAIL
FIRST CLASS MAIL PERMIT No. 762 CHICAGO, IL

POSTAGE WILL BE PAID BY ADDRESSEE

Chris Hughes
Mosby-Year Book, Inc.
200 N. LaSalle Street
Suite 2600
Chicago, IL 60601-9981

is involved, and the metal fragment can be removed with a needle or cotton swab. However, when an intraocular metal fragment is retained, the problem is much more complex because many factors need to be considered.

Patients.—During the 3-year period, 31 men with a mean age of 30.3 years came to the ED with 33 eye injuries involving metal missiles. Twenty-five injuries involved only the cornea, and the metal fragment was completely removed with a syringe needle. Rust rings were seen in 15 eyes. The metal content of fragments obtained from 2 patients was analyzed by atomic absorption spectrophotometry. Both fragments contained copper and lead. Only 3 injuries involved intraocular metallic foreign bodies. Nine injuries occurred when patients were grinding metal and 6 when patients were working on a car. Four injuries were caused by shotgun pellets, BBs, or darts.

Outcome.—Eight patients did well after their injury; 1 had a corneal scar, 1 had a mild infection of the conjunctiva, and 1 had corneal ulcers. No follow-up information was available for 21 of the 33 injuries.

Discussion.—The removal of metallic foreign bodies from the eye is a very complex problem. A multitude of diagnostic and therapeutic factors must be considered, including infection, age of the injury, and the existence of acute glaucoma, traumatic cataract, and retinal detachment. The solubility of the metal is an important parameter of its toxicity since the rate of metal ion release into the tissue will affect the development of metallosis and its clinical manifestations. The electroretinogram (ERG) is an important tool in the management of intraocular metal foreign-body injuries because alterations of the ERG are often the first signs of the insidious onset of widespread metallosis resulting from dissemination of the metal ions. There is some evidence that the ERG also has some prognostic value.

▶ The authors present an interesting review of metal ocular injuries. The emergency physician must be able to separate those metallic objects that are superficially based from those that are deeply embedded. With corneal injuries, metallic objects superficial to the deep corneal membrane represent an entirely different problem from those that penetrate or are deep to this barrier. In a similar fashion, scleral foreign objects represent significantly more complex problems when global penetration has occurred. Removal of superficially based metallic foreign bodies commonly can safely occur in the emergency center. Deeply embedded objects are always the immediate purview of the ophthalmologist.—D.K. Wagner, M.D.

Geriatric

Prediction of Electrolyte Abnormalities in Elderly Emergency Patients

Singal BM, Hedges JR, Succop PA (Wright State Univ, Dayton, Ohio; Oregon Health Sciences Univ, Portland; Univ of Cincinnati, Ohio)

Ann Emerg Med 20:964–968, 1991 4–35

Background.—Lowe et al. have created a criteria set for ordering the stat serum electrolyte panel. It included 10 clinical features that individually discriminate between patients with and without clinically significant electrolyte abnormalities (CSEAs) with a sensitivity of .99 and a specificity of .3. A cross-sectional study was conducted to cross-validate Lowe's criteria and identify factors from the history and physical examination that may be predictive of CSEAs in older emergency patients.

Methods.—A total of 1,766 patients aged 55 years and older (average, 68 years) who were seen in an urban university hospital emergency department were studied. The physicians were interviewed to determine the presence or absence of 20 dichotomous clinical variables, 10 of which constituted Lowe's criteria. The patients were followed by chart review and/or telephone interview.

Results.—A serum electrolyte panel was ordered on 800 (45%) patients at the index visit. Of these, 126 (16%) resulted in a CSEA (Fig 4–1). Lowe's criteria had a sensitivity of .95 (95% confidence intervals .89 to .98) and a specificity of .10 (95% confidence intervals) .07 to .12) for predicting CSEAs in this older population. Logistic regression analysis showed that impaired ability to communicate, acute seizures, vomiting, and a history of abnormal electrolytes were independent predictors of CSEA.

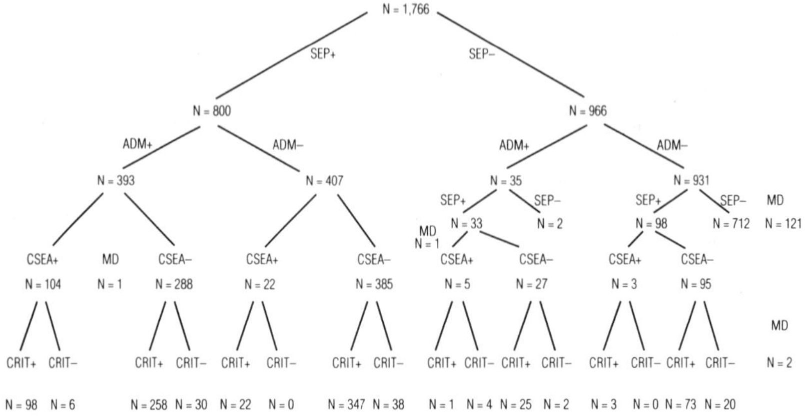

Fig 4–1.—Patients, aged 55 years or older, in an emergency department. (Courtesy of Singal BM, Hedges JR, Succop PA: *Ann Emerg Med* 20:964–968, 1991.)

Implications.—For the older patient seen in the emergency department, Lowe's criteria for ordering a serum electrolyte panel has a useful sensitivity but poor specificity. Lowe's criteria may be used to encourage selective test ordering by physicians when a low pretest probability for CSEA exists and as part of an algorithm for emergency nurses who order tests to expedite patient care.

► This article verifies that CSEAs are uncommon (8%) but not rare in the adult emergency department population 55 years of age or older. Historical criteria can help guide serum electrolyte studies in adults. However, most of the historical criteria are only weakly associated with a CSEA. This forces the clinician to choose between schemes that are either highly sensitive and poorly specific or are poorly sensitive and highly specific. Most emergency physicians seek to maximize their diagnostic sensitivity and are liberal in the ordering of serum electrolyte panels in this age group. The downside of this practice is that the clinician must at times chase an irrelevant laboratory abnormality.—J.R. Hedges, M.D.

Social and Functional Impact of Minor Fractures in Elderly People

Nankhonya JM, Turnbull CJ, Newton JT (Arrowe Park Hosp, Wirral; Salford Univ, England)

BMJ 303:1514–1515, 1991 4–36

Introduction.—Illnesses and fractures form part of the social milieu of elderly persons. Minor fractures, although they do not require hospitalization, can exert influence over the daily life of the older person, but no evidence exists about how bothersome these breakages can be. The impact of the frequent small fractures that afflict the older population on their social interactions and how today's established support programs can help the older person heal were measured.

Methods.—Subjects included patients aged 70 years or older with minor breakages that had not required hospitalization. Of the 105 patients included, 93 were women and 12 were men. The study population had a mean age of 77 years.

Results.—Eleven patients had received aid for home services that arrived after a median waiting period of 8 days. Four subjects had received a visit by a district nurse, whereas 3 others received "meals on wheels." Some 44 individuals used the help of family and friends, with 6 of these 44 moving in with the caretaker temporarily. Nine patients employed the services of housekeepers, and 1 had a cook come in during the healing of the minor fracture. Of the total 105 patients, 65 said that they had needed extra home aid after the fracture, particularly during the first 2 to 4 weeks after the injury. Fifteen patients were classified as severely disabled.

Conclusions.—Although the elderly patient can be discharged from emergency services after the initial treatment for a minor fracture, many have to deal with the adverse effects of the fracture during their everyday lives. It appears that the present social services do not adequately help those individuals who seem to require minimum care but actually experience severe disruptions of their daily life. An immediate revamping of patient services is recommended so that they become more structured and efficient. Social workers should inform the emergency hospital staff about the availability of such services.

▶ Minor fractures in young patients are an inconvenience, but in the elderly, these same injuries may be totally debilitating. When fractures occur in the elderly, many do not have the social structures available to them to handle it at home initially. For this reason, we have found that many elderly patients with a minor fracture require short-term hospitalization until Social Services can arrange for the appropriate nursing care or home help. These admissions are often required for social reasons, and because of this, the resource management and insurance companies often complain. However, it would be malpractice to send a patient home who would not even be able to perform vital functions by himself.

Another topic that was not covered in this article is "elder abuse." As with "child abuse," only the tip of the "iceberg" has been discovered and reported. Legally, any suspected elder abuse must be documented and reported. Failure to do so could result in criminal and civic prosecution, both of which, by the way, would probably be covered under your liability insurance!!—G.J. Ordog, M.D.

Foreign Bodies

Foreign Bodies in the Esophagus. A Study of Causative Factors

Tibbling L, Stenquist M (Linköping and Uppsala Univ Hosps, Sweden)
Dysphagia 6:224–227, 1991 4–37

Introduction.—It is generally thought that foreign bodies remain in the esophagus because they are too large and the patient has poor peristalsis or because an esophageal stenosis is present. Thus, these impactions are generally treated by extraction with rigid or fiber-optic endoscopy. To understand why foreign bodies become impacted in the esophagus, the authors studied a series of 229 affected patients.

Patients.—The patients (mean age of 62 years) were admitted as emergency cases during a 5-year period. Of the 29 patients with strictures, 52% had been hospitalized for foreign-body impaction more than once. This was so for only 8.5% of the rest of the sample. For patients up to 15 years of age, the foreign body was located in the hypopharynx, whereas this location was extremely uncommon in adults. Solid foreign bodies were common in children but rare in adults (Fig 4–2). More than one third of the patients had spontaneous disimpaction, which became

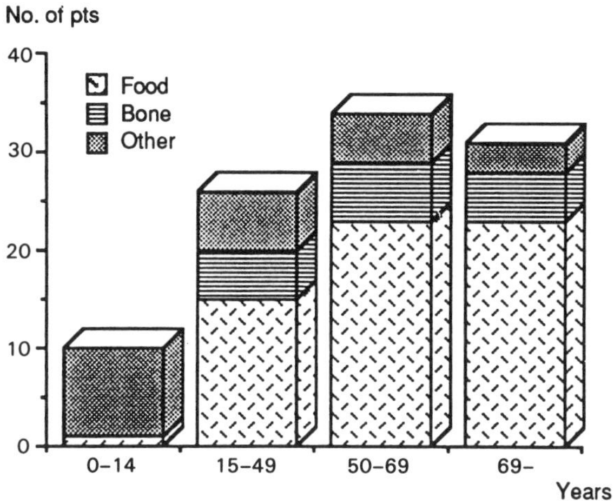

Fig 4–2.—Number of patients with foreign bodies according to age. (Courtesy of Tibbling L, Stenquist M: *Dysphagia* 6:224–227, 1991.)

more common as time went on. Sixteen patients were given spasmolytic drugs, and 63% of these had spontaneous disimpaction. In half of the cases, the foreign body was located in the proximal portion of the esophagus, distal to the narrower passage of the upper esophageal sphincter. Eighty-six percent of the patients had never had the problem before. All of these findings supported the hypothesis that in patients without a stricture, the obstruction occurred because of spasm distal to the foreign body.

Conclusions.—Spasm of the esophageal smooth muscle is responsible for food impaction in adult patients without stricture whose foreign body does not consist of sharp bones. These patients should be treated with spasmolytic or analgesic therapy before endoscopy is performed. Endoscopy is needed when the presence of sharp bones is suspected or when a patient with documented stricture swallows a bone.

▶ It makes sense that foreign bodies in children most often lodge at the cricopharyngeus, which is the narrowest spot in the gastrointestinal tract. Foreign bodies lower in the esophagus get more notice because they erode and cause more complications. It is heartening to learn that in adults without stricture, many foreign bodies are held up by spasm and eventually spontaneously disimpact. How often is glucagon a placebo? None of this information, however, changes the emergency department strategy. We still need to hasten disimpaction and find underlying pathology.—T. Stair, M.D.

Permanently Imbedded Subcutaneous Acupuncture Needles: Radiographic Appearance

Hollander JE, Dewitz A, Bowers S (Albert Einstein College of Medicine, Bronx, NY)

Ann Emerg Med 20:1025–1026, 1991 4–38

Introduction.—Acupuncture is usually not an issue for the emergency physician, but the placement of acupuncture needles can produce potentially confusing radiographic appearances in a patient seen in the emergency department.

Case Report.—A 26-year-old man was seen after an automobile accident with lacerations in the frontal and temporoparietal regions. Radiographs showed radiopaque foreign bodies posteriorly along the neck, chest, abdomen, and pelvis. No foreign bodies were embedded in the skin. The patient described having received acupuncture treatment in Korea 5 years earlier for lower back pain.

Discussion.—There are 3 previous reports of gold acupuncture needles being permanently placed subcutaneously. The needles are typically 1 mm in diameter and 3 to 15 mm long, with a straight, curved, or semicircular configuration. It is important not to confuse these needles with other opaque foreign bodies, surgical wires, or parasitic infection.

▶ Was it Confucious who said, "a picture is worth a thousand words"? This is one of the most bizarre pelvic radiographs I have ever seen—a very interesting case report, to say the least.—J.J. Kelly, D.O., F.A.C.E.P.

Environmental

Comparison of Three Methods of Rewarming From Hypothermia: Advantages of Extracorporeal Blood Warming

Gregory JS, Bergstein JM, Aprahamian C, Wittmann DH, Quebbeman EJ (Med College of Wisconsin, Milwaukee)

J Trauma 31:1247–1252, 1991 4–39

Background.—Many methods of rewarming from hypothermia have been examined, but all have disadvantages. The physicians of this report have been treating severe hypothermia with extracorporeal warming and recirculation of blood and intravenous fluids. This and other rewarming techniques were studied.

Methods.—During a 3-year period, 32 patients underwent active rewarming. Hypothermia resulted from traumatic causes in 21 cases, accidental causes in 6, and iatrogenic causes in 5. Fifteen patients were rewarmed with standard techniques, including warming blankets, heated ventilator circuits, warmed intravenous fluids, and lavage; 14 had extracorporeal venovenous rewarming (EVR); and 3 had cardiopulmonary bypass. These 3 groups had no significant differences in demographic

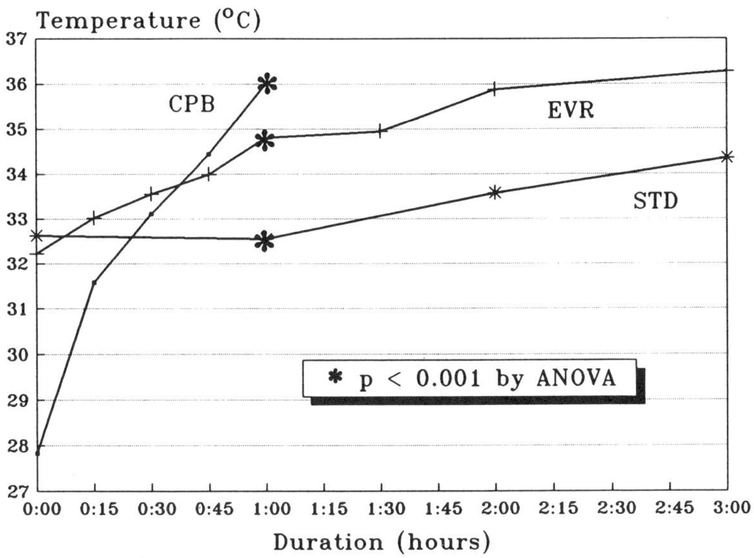

Fig 4–3.—Rewarming curves. Average temperature vs. duration of rewarming. *Abbreviations: CPB,* cardiopulmonary bypass; *EVR,* extracorporeal venovenous rewarmer; *STD,* all other (standard) techniques. Change in temperature at 1 hour significantly different between all groups by analysis of variance (ANOVA), $P < .001$. (Courtesy of Gregory JS, Bergstein JM, Aprahamian C, et al: *J Trauma* 31:1247–1252, 1991.)

characteristics or severity scores, although the bypass group had lower initial core temperatures.

Results.—Rewarming rates were 6.9°C/hr for bypass, 2.1°C/hr for EVR, and .8°C/hr for standard techniques (Fig 4–3). Rewarming times were 1.4, 2.3, and 5.9 hours, respectively. With EVR, blood, blood products, and crystalloids could be warmed to 40°C at a rate of 150 to 400 mL/min; 1 patient survived from a core temperature as low as 31.1°C. EVR also facilitated rapid warm transfusion.

Discussion.—The use of EVR as a treatment for hypothermia was evaluated. It appears to be most appropriate for patients with multisystem trauma and for rapid correction for hypovolemia, coagulopathy, and arrhythmia. For severe hypothermia with cardiac arrest, cardiopulmonary bypass should be done if available. For patients who do not have these immediately life-threatening conditions, standard techniques can be used.

▶ Although I have never used this device, it sounds like a good idea. It makes sense to remove the blood, warm it, and return it in a warm state. One can add just so much warm saline before the possibility of fluid overload occurs. The other common methods of external warming really are not very effective or rapid.—W.H. Spivey, M.D.

Continuous Arteriovenous Rewarming: Rapid Reversal of Hypothermia in Critically Ill Patients

Gentilello LM, Cobean RA, Offner PJ, Soderberg RW, Jurkovich GJ (Univ of Washington, Seattle)

J Trauma 32:316–327, 1992 4–40

Background.—Critically ill patients with hypothermia can be difficult to treat with standard rewarming (SR) methods. A rewarming method that is significantly faster than SR was developed and assessed.

Methods.—Thirty-four patients with hypothermia were treated in one 10-month period. Percutaneously placed femoral arterial and venous catheters were connected to the inflow and outflow side of a countercurrent fluid warmer. This created a fistula through the heating mechanism. Eighteen patients were treated with SR only; in the remaining 16 patients, continuous arteriovenous rewarming (CAVR) was added to SR.

Findings.—The 2 treatment groups had comparable APACHE II, Injury Severity, and Acute Physiology scores. Prewarming blood and fluid requirements and the incidence of coagulopathy were also similar. Hypothermia resolved in 3.23 hours in the patients treated with SR only vs. 39 minutes in patients treated with both CAVR and SR. The faster resolution of hypothermia was associated with an improved survival rate in patients with moderately severe injuries and with a significant decrease in blood and fluid requirements, organ failure, and length of stay in the intensive care unit.

Conclusions.—In this series, CAVR was associated with improved survival rates after moderately severe injuries and a significant reduction in blood and fluid requirements, the number of organ failures, and intensive care unit length of stay. The increased mortality rate among victims of hypothermia seems to be directly attributable to the effects of altered body temperature rather than underlying injury. Further research is needed to define the patient population that would benefit most from CAVR.

▶ This is an interesting study with a small number of patients enrolled in each group. All of these patients exhibited "mild" hypothermia (32 to 35°C) since the average prewarming temperature in the SR group was 33.2°C and the average prewarming temperature in the CAVR group was 33.5°C.

Traditionally, mild hypothermia is treated with passive rewarming when hypothermia is an isolated problem. However, hypothermia in critically ill or injured patients is a serious problem that does not respond well to traditional treatment strategies. In addition, a temperature below 32°C is highly predictive of postinjury death.

Because the patient outcomes were definitely better in the CAVR group, the point to remember is to get the surgical consultants alerted and involved as early as possible in these patients.—E.H. Taliaferro, M.D.

Efficacy and Safety of Prehospital Rewarming Techniques to Treat Accidental Hypothermia

Sterba JA (Navy Experimental Diving Unit, Panama City, Fla)

Ann Emerg Med 20:896–901, 1991 4–41

Objective.—There is ongoing debate over the benefit of external vs. internal active rewarming as a prehospital treatment in accidental hypothermia victims. A human experimentation study examined the efficacy and safety of adding inhalation rewarming, peripheral rewarming, or both to reduce the body core temperature afterdrop and accelerate the rewarming rate in hypothermic victims in a rescue sleeping bag.

Methods.—Eighty healthy U.S. Navy divers with a mean age of 31.8 years volunteered for the study. All experiments were carried out in a physiology laboratory in a windy, cold air environment. Each diver was cooled in ice water in a 1-man immersion tank to mild clinical hypothermia as measured by esophageal or rectal temperatures (Te or Tr). A portable device that delivers humidified heated air by face mask was used for active inhalation rewarming. A charcoal-fueled heat generator was placed in the rescue sleeping bag for active peripheral rewarming. Afterdrop was defined as the duration to minimum Tr and Te plus recovery time to Tr and Te values at the onset of rewarming.

Results.—Neither inhalation rewarming nor peripheral rewarming when used alone or in combination as an adjunct to rewarming in a rescue sleeping bag significantly affected the afterdrop duration, afterdrop recovery, or rewarming rates in subjects cooled to a minimum body core temperature ethically allowed for human experimentation. In addition, numerous unsafe characteristics of the inhalation rewarming device were observed. The ignition of a propane canister caused an explosion that burned the arms of 3 operators. The inhalation temperature was difficult to control and caused a mild first-degree burn on the face of 1 volunteer despite constant monitoring in the laboratory. All 8 volunteers complained of dyspnea because of water from condensation that restricted the airflow in the breathing tubes.

Conclusions.—Inhalation rewarming and peripheral rewarming for the prehospital treatment of hypothermia victims are ineffective and unsafe and cannot be recommended.

► Alas, the controversy surrounding the prehospital treatment of accidental hypothermia continues. The authors demonstrate no benefit to active inhalation or peripheral rewarming in 8 healthy divers cooled to 35°C, the upper limit of mild hypothermia. Unfortunately, these findings may not be relevant in treating the elderly, alcoholic, or severely hypothermic and hemodynamically unstable patients more commonly encountered in the field. These are the patients who would most likely benefit from aggressive prehospital rewarming.

Of significance to prehospital providers is the potential for harm to the patient and the operator when certain rewarming devices are used. In this study, 3 operators and 1 volunteer were burned during the use of an inhalation rewarming device. The risk of exposure to toxic levels of carbon monoxide is present with both inhalation and peripheral rewarming devices marketed for prehospital use.

Most would agree that an otherwise healthy victim of mild hypothermia does not require active rewarming techniques in the field. However, hypothermic patients with persistent hypotension or life-threatening arrhythmias need to be rewarmed rapidly. Therefore, inhalation or peripheral rewarming devices may still have a place in the prehospital treatment of these patients; however, their benefit should be weighed against the time spent in initiating this therapy. In urban and suburban environments, early and expeditious transport may be preferable.—Carol A. Hart, M.D., EMS Fellow, Medical College of Pennsylvania, with S.J. Davidson, M.D.

5 Emergency Procedures, Techniques, and Instrumentation

Airway Control

Manual Resuscitators and Spontaneous Ventilation: An Evaluation
Mills PJ, Baptiste J, Preston J, Barnas GM (Univ of Maryland, Baltimore)
Crit Care Med 19:1425–1431, 1991 5–1

Background.—Manual resuscitation units are sometimes beneficial for patients who are breathing spontaneously, but there have been few studies regarding their performance in such situations. Such patients' ability to breathe through manual resuscitator units in the clinical range of tidal volume and respiratory frequency was studied. Recommendations as to the best unit design for this purpose were made.

Methods.—Thirteen commonly used manual resuscitator units were studied, 6 with a single "duck-bill" valve, 4 with a combination of disks, and 3 with various combinations of duck-bills and disks. A piston pump was used to simulate spontaneous ventilation, and a function generator was used to adjust the respiratory frequency and tidal volume. Mass spectrometry was used to measure the concentration of delivered oxygen. In addition, resistive pressure was measured during simulated ventilation and at a constant inspiratory flow rate of 50 L/min.

Results.—The concentration of delivered oxygen, which varied from 25% to 100% at a minute ventilation of 2.5 L, was affected by the oxygen supply, tidal volume, and reservoir volume. However, valve design was the most important factor. Oxygen delivery was most efficient in valve designs incorporating a disk that prevented entrainment of air from the expiratory port. Designs with a duck-bill only did not prevent air entrainment and showed great variability in the concentration of delivered oxygen. High resistive pressure occurred in only 2 of the tested units.

Conclusions.—In spontaneously breathing patients, high oxygen concentrations are best delivered with a low-resistance manual resuscitator with a disk design to prevent air entrainment. Manufacturers of these units should provide information on the degree to which their product prevents resistance and delivers oxygen to such patients.

▶ This article emphasizes that not every manual resuscitator, i.e., "Get me the Ambu Bag!" is the same, especially when used in a spontaneously breathing patient. Bags with *both* the "duck-bill" and a compliant, flexible disk to prevent air entrainment are recommended by the authors based on their research. It is important for all manufacturers to include a description of the components of their bag; both the physician and respiratory therapist (or emergency medical technician) should be familiar with the bag's operation. In addition, airway equipment should be standardized in the hospital so that the staff can become familiar with its operation.—J.T. Amsterdam, M.D.

Reliability of Capnography in Identifying Esophageal Intubation With Carbonated Beverage or Antacid in the Stomach

Ping STS, Mehta MP, Symreng T (Univ of Iowa College of Medicine, Iowa City)

Anesth Analg 73:333–337, 1991 5–2

Introduction.—Unidentified esophageal intubation is an avoidable cause of morbidity and mortality from attempted endotracheal intubation. Capnography is a widespread method for ensuring correct tube placement, but there is evidence that similar CO_2 waveforms may be recorded when the end-expired CO_2 is as high as 2%.

Objective.—The amounts of CO_2 released from various carbonated beverages and antacids were determined on a simulated stomach, a rubber breathing bag placed in a water bath. End-expired CO_2 levels were then measured in swine with carbonated beverage in the stomach.

Findings.—All carbonated beverages tested (including Pepsi, Diet Coke, and Diet 7-Up) consistently produced CO_2 levels of about 20%. Comparable levels were produced by sodium bicarbonate, but Maalox produced only 2% CO_2, and sodium citrate produced none. Carbon dioxide waveforms were recorded during esophageal ventilation in 5 of 6 swine after the intragastric administration of Diet Coke. Two animals had an end-expired CO_2 content of 2.5% or higher; the highest measured level was 5.3%.

Conclusions.—Capnography is an effective and convenient means of identifying esophageal intubation, but it is far from an ideal monitor. The use of a capnograph rather than a capnometer is suggested. Waveforms should be observed for at least 1 minute after tube placement.

▶ Confirmation of endotracheal intubation should be based on direct visualization of the tube through the vocal cords, equal breath sounds in the upper part of the chest, and absent sounds over the stomach. Measurement of end-tidal CO_2 is frequently a reassuring adjunct to these standard methods, but as this study points out, it can also occasionally be misleading.—W.P. Burdick, M.D.

Percutaneous Tracheostomy After Trauma and Critical Illness
Ivatury R, Siegel JH, Stahl WM, Simon R, Scorpio R, et al (Univ of Maryland, Baltimore; Lincoln Hosp, New York, NY)
J Trauma 32:133–140, 1992 5–3

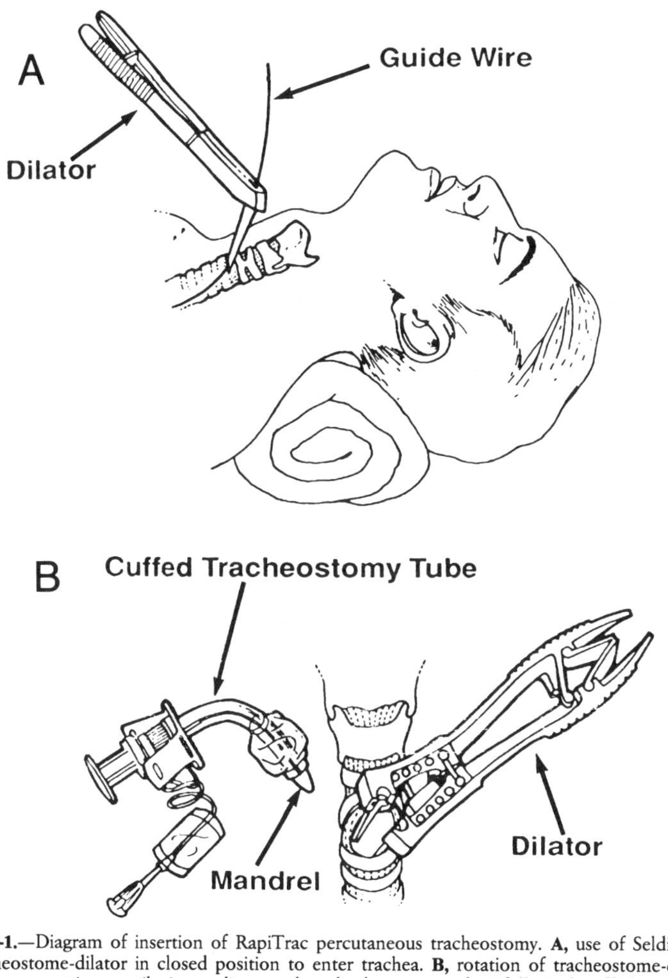

Fig 5–1.—Diagram of insertion of RapiTrac percutaneous tracheostomy. **A,** use of Seldinger wire and tracheostome-dilator in closed position to enter trachea. **B,** rotation of tracheostome-dilator 90 degrees to convert intracartilaginous slit to oval tracheal stoma to admit full-sized, cuffed tracheostomy tube with stiffening mandrel inserted. After tube insertion, mandrel is withdrawn and balloon cuff is inflated. (Courtesy of Ivatury R, Siegel JH, Stahl WM, et al: *J Trauma* 32:133–140, 1992.)

Introduction.—Many techniques for rapid cricothyroidotomy or emergency percutaneous intubation of the trachea have been studied. Most, however, do not allow placement of a tracheostomy tube large enough to handle copious secretions or a tube with a balloon cuff. The RapiTrac device for percutaneous tracheostomy (PT) was tested in a population of predominantly young trauma patients.

Methods.—In this method, based on a Seldinger technique, a hollow needle is placed percutaneously through an intercartilaginous membrane. An intratracheal guidewire is introduced, and the operative tracheostome is inserted along it. This tracheostome is then used to split the intercartilaginous membrane in speculum-like fashion to allow placement of a standard cuffed endotracheal tube (Fig 5–1). The device was evaluated in 61 critically ill or injured patients with a mean age of 38.5 years. Fifty-four had sustained trauma, 65% of these to the brain, 33% to the face or jaw, 15% to the lungs, and 14% to the cervical spinal cord. Coma was the most common indication for PT, followed by pneumonitis, sepsis, facial or jaw injury, and adult respiratory distress syndrome. In 51% of the patients, PT was done specifically to manage pulmonary secretions. It was done on an elective basis in 77% of the cases.

Results.—Ninety percent of PTs were successful. In 8% of the cases, the PT attempt was converted to a surgical tracheostomy. The technique was performed at the bedside in 46% of the cases, the operating room in 46%, and the emergency department in 7%. In each patient, a #6 to #8 tracheostomy tube was inserted, which was optimal or larger than needed in 87% of the cases. Most complications were minor, although 1 patient died of bronchospasm and cardiac arrest, 1 had severe bradycardia, and 1 had significant bleeding from the trachea. Ninety-five percent of patients had excellent healing, and 97% of physicians stated that they would use the device again.

Conclusions.—The RapiTrac PT technique is easy and quick when compared with conventional tracheostomy. It should continue to be used for urgent and semielective tracheostomy in critically ill or injured patients. Contraindications include pathologic obesity or a very large, thick neck; significant burns of the head and neck; some cases of severe respiratory distress with prolonged high airway pressures; and coagulation abnormalities.

▶ My only response to this paper is, why? Why do the authors feel they need to perform cricothyroidotomy so frequently? We have completely gone away from tracheostomy to in-line stabilization of the neck with oral intubation. It is rare that a tracheostomy has to be performed, and usually the few times they are, it is a disaster. In fact, I can't remember the last time I saw a rapid, efficient tracheostomy. Furthermore, there is absolutely no doubt in my mind that in-line traction with stabilization is a safe and effective way of stabilizing the neck for oral intubation.—W.H. Spivey, M.D.

Emergency Percutaneous Dilatational Cricothyroidostomy: Use of Modified Nasal Speculum

Ciaglias P, Brady C, Graniero KD (St Elizabeth Hosp, Utica, NY)
Am J Emerg Med 10:152–155, 1992 5–4

Background.—An emergency percutaneous airway should be safe, quick, and simple. Disadvantages accompany most previously proposed techniques. A percutaneous dilational tracheostomy method is proposed that is safe and quick for physicians and nonphysicians alike.

Technique.—The technique uses a modified nasal speculum, 1 blade of which is attached to a tapered J-tipped dilator-catheter, which is straightened by a needle (Fig 5–2). The cricothyroid membrane or cartilage is located and a single 1 cm incision made. The speculum is inserted just above the cricoid cartilage. The covered needle is directed posteriorly and somewhat caudad. When free airflow is obtained, a small amount of lidocaine is instilled. When the blades of the speculum traverse the tissues, it is turned and forced through the cricothyroid ligament with a slight twisting motion to penetrate about 2 cm. The speculum is then opened by dilating first in a transverse and then in a vertical direction. The 6-mm tracheostomy tube, well lubricated and with the cuff deflated, is then inserted as the speculum is held open. The speculum is removed, and active suctioning and ventilation can begin.

Discussion.—This percutaneous dilational cricothyroidostomy technique has worked well in mannequins and cadavers. It is simple and quick and provides unique safety features. An experience of 165 tra-

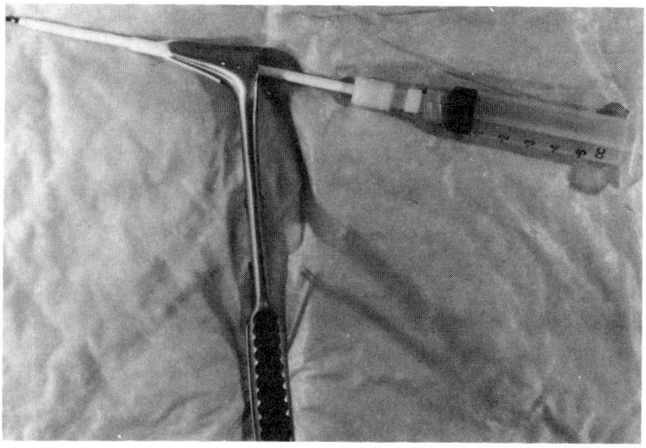

Fig 5–2.—Instrument closed and J-tipped cannula straightened. (Courtesy of Ciaglias P, Brady C, Graniero KD: *Am J Emerg Med* 10:152–155, 1992.)

cheostomies is in press, and a pilot study with trained emergency medical technicians, paramedics, and physicians is planned.

▶ Beware of special equipment that must be used for the first time during a disaster. It may not be found quickly and is likely to be used badly. You are better off to press into service familiar tools. Nonetheless, after losing their first lost-airway lawsuit, many ambulances, recovery rooms, and emergency departments may buy a supply of cricothyroidostomy devices as misguided risk management. This device looks better thought out than some others already on the market, especially since the patient winds up with a standard tracheostomy tube in place. Have the authors tried it in any actual patient resuscitations yet?—T. Stair, M.D.

Accuracy of the FEF CO_2 Detector in the Assessment of Endotracheal Tube Placement

Ping STS, Mehta MP, Symreng T (Univ of Iowa, Iowa City)

Anesth Analg 74:415–419, 1992 5–5

Background.—Unidentified esophageal intubation can cause morbidity and mortality in anesthesia. The finding of carbon dioxide (CO_2) in the expired gas is a convenient, reliable way to detect esophageal intubation. However, capnography requires electronic equipment. The new forced expiratory flow (FEF) CO_2 detector, a small disposable device, involves no electronic equipment. The sensitivity and reliability of the FED end-tidal CO_2 detector were studied to determine its suitability in assessing the correct placement of an endotracheal tube.

Methods.—Eight volunteers observed the color change in the FEF detector after the administration of different volumes and varying CO_2 concentrations of a gas mixture. Color changes were also evaluated during esophageal ventilations before and after the administration of carbonated beverage into the stomach of swine and during CPR of the animals.

Findings.—The observers showed an interpersonal variation in the color matching. Different colors were observed when the volume and CO_2 concentrations of gas mixture were the same. During esophageal ventilations before and after carbonated beverage was administered, the FEF detector was neither accurate nor rapid in identifying esophageal placement of the tube. In 1 swine, the "C" color was displayed during the initial 6 ventilations, an indication that esophageal intubation would have been missed. The FEF detector identified 1 of 6 correctly intubated swine during CPR.

Conclusion.—The performance of the FEF detector in detecting CO_2 levels semiquantitatively was unsatisfactory because of the interpersonal variation in colors observed. Most important, the FEF detector was not able to detect an esophageal intubation or confirm correct intubation under adverse conditions.

▶ Demonstrating failure under extreme conditions does not disprove the clinical value of the FEF end-tidal CO_2, detector; it only shows its limitations. I am not surprised that carbonated water in the stomach can produce CO_2 in the esophagus. I am surprised that some users could not match indicator colors with the attached scale for accurate readings. (By the way, "C" is yellow, 2.5% CO_2; "B" is tan, .5% to 2%; "A" is purple, .03 to .5%, or room air.) No one test should be trusted to guarantee an airway. The physician must keep rechecking various clinical parameters. A tube verified as being in the trachea can then slide out. A tube in the esophagus with an erroneously high CO_2 concentration can be discovered soon by other means.—T. Stair, M.D.

Multicenter Study of a Portable, Hand-Size, Colorimetric End-Tidal Carbon Dioxide Detection Device

Ornato JP, Shipley JB, Racht EM, Slovis CM, Wrenn KD, et al (Virginia Commonwealth Univ, Richmond; Strong Mem Hosp, Rochester, NY; Baylor College of Medicine, Houston, Tex; City of Houston Emergency Med Services; San Mateo Emergency Med Services Agency, San Mateo, Calif)

Ann Emerg Med 21:518–523, 1992 5–6

Background.—Monitoring of end-tidal carbon dioxide tension ($PETCO_2$) during shock or cardiac arrest provides useful data about the adequacy of circulatory flow and may have prognostic value during the resuscitation. Semiquantitative evaluation of $PETCO_2$ can now be achieved with a portable colorimetric device. A multicenter study was done to assess the value of continuous $PETCO_2$ monitoring by prehospital and emergency department (ED) personnel to confirm endotracheal tube placement and to evaluate the prognosis and blood flow during CPR.

Methods.—The study included 227 patients who had an endotracheal tube inserted by prehospital personnel or an emergency physician for cardiac or respiratory arrest, respiratory insufficiency, or airway protection. One hundred forty-four patients had cardiopulmonary arrest. The portable colorimetric $PETCO_2$ detector was attached to the tube after each attempt at insertion. The user noted the color of the detector membrane at the seventh breath after intubation and again if spontaneous circulation returned immediately before and after conversion from manual to mechanical CPR. The prognostic importance of the initial read was evaluated by survival to hospital admission.

Results.—A reading of more than .5% $PETCO_2$ was 100% sensitive and 93% specific in detecting proper tube placement in patients who were not in cardiopulmonary arrest. Its specificity reached 100% with the endotracheal tube cuff inflated. In the cardiac arrest patients, the same reading was 69% sensitive and 100% specific. An apparent association was found between a longer period of arrest and a lower PETCO[2] detector reading. In the arrest group, all patients who survived to admission had an initial reading after proper tube placement of more than 0.5% $PETCO_2$. Most of the time, $PETCO_2$ improved with the return of spontaneous circulation. With mechanical CPR, $PETCO_2$ was always at least as high as that with manual CPR.

Conclusions.—The portable colorimetric $PETCO_2$ monitoring device seems to accurately confirm endotracheal tube position in patients without cardiopulmonary arrest. In patients with arrest, a $PETCO_2$ reading over .5% confirms correct tube placement, whereas a lower reading during resuscitation indicates a problem. Such problems can include esophageal intubation, inadequate circulation, prolonged downtime interval, hypothermia, or ventilation/perfusion mismatch.

▶ It looks as though the measurement of end-tidal carbon dioxide with a handy portable colorimetric device will be a useful adjunct in determining endotracheal tube placement in the field by prehospital care providers, as well as potentially providing some prognostic information for patients who have been in cardiac arrest and who have endotracheal tube placement confirmed by a variety of other clinical and/or laboratory variables. The study was done entirely on adult patients, and I can only wonder whether it would be possible to replicate it in the pediatric-aged population since there is probably even more difficulty with early recognition of esophageal tube placement in children.—F.M. Henretig, M.D.

Confirmation of Endotracheal Tube Placement: A Miniaturized Infrared Qualitative CO_2 Detector

Vukmir RB, Heller MB, Stein KL (Presbyterian-Univ Hosp, Pittsburgh; Univ of Pittsburgh, Pa)

Ann Emerg Med 20:726–729, 1991 5–7

Background.—The most catastrophic complication of endotracheal intubation is unrecognized esophageal intubation. Current methods to confirm placement may not be able to distinguish endotracheal from esophageal intubation even with the greatest care. Detection of end-tidal CO_2 was used under rigorous conditions to confirm endotracheal tube placement in airway emergencies.

Methods.—A miniaturized qualitative capnometer was used to confirm tube position by detecting end-tidal CO_2. One hundred cases of emergency intubation in 88 patients were studied in a 6-month period. The device was not used in every emergency intubation, but every recorded use was included in the analysis. Physicians rated the difficulty of intubation and confirmation on a linear scale of 0 to 10, lowest to highest.

Results.—Intubation was urgent in 79% of the cases and was done in cardiac or traumatic arrest in 21%. The mean required number of intubations was 1.83. The difficulty of intubation was rated at 6.48, and the difficulty in confirmation was rated at 7.75. Intratracheal intubation was demonstrated in 96% of cases and esophageal intubation in 4%. In all cases, placement was confirmed by direct visualization or radiography. Endotracheal tube localization had a sensitivity and specificity of 100%.

Conclusions.—A hand-held infrared capnometer reliably confirms endotracheal tube placement under emergency conditions. False-positive results in 4 cases of esophageal intubation did not complicate the minimal sensitivity for CO_2 detection. The device is not recommended for use in the field.

▶ The catastrophic results of an unrecognized esophageal intubation can be devastating. The availability of portable, reliable, and inexpensive end-tidal CO_2 indicators should prevent such an event from occurring. The infrared indicator described in this study appears to be accurate and easy to use. While its small size may be considered an attribute by some, we have seen pulse oximeters and electronic thermometers of the same dimensions mysteriously disappear from our emergency center. In my department, we utilize colorimetric end-tidal CO_2 indicators. While they do have some limitations during the arrest/low-perfusion state, they are otherwise accurate, inexpensive, easy to store, and easy to use. Regardless of the specific system chosen, I think it is clear that anyone performing an intubation should have available to them a CO_2 indicator of some sort.—H.D. Unger, M.D.

Vascular/Intraosseous/Volume Replacement

Emergency Central Venous Catheterization During Resuscitation of Trauma Patients

Pappas P, Brathwaite CEM, Ross SE (Camden Cooper Hosp/Univ Med Ctr, Camden, NJ)

Am Surg 58:108–111, 1992 5–8

Background.—Authors continue to debate the value of central venous catheterization during resuscitation of trauma victims. The largest series to date of emergently placed percutaneous central venous catheters in such patients was evaluated.

Patients and Outcomes.—All catheterizations done at 1 center in 1988 and 1989 were reviewed. Two hundred sixty-nine catheters were inserted by the Seldinger technique. Attending traumatologists or emergency medicine and surgical staff under direct attending supervision placed the catheters through the internal jugular or subclavian veins. The 238 patients ranged in age from 6 to 90 years; 156 were male. The mean Trauma Score was 9, and the mean Injury Severity Score, 30. Thirty of 161 patients undergoing CPR or in shock during resuscitation died in the resuscitation area. The rest of this group, with 150 catheterizations, had 12 complications, which included pneumothorax, hemothorax, and malposition. Seventy-seven patients were not in shock. Those patients had 80 catheterizations and 6 complications, including pneumothorax, hematoma, and malposition. Resuscitation survivors had a complication rate of 7.8%. No one died of catheter-related causes.

Conclusions.—Emergency central venous catheterization performed by experienced physicians during the resuscitation of trauma victims appears to be safe. In addition, central catheterization is useful for resuscitating patients in hemorrhagic shock.

▶ Hypotensive or hemodynamically unstable patients may require immediate surgical exploration. Hence, when indicated, transport to the operating room (OR) should be expedited. Inserting central venous pressure (CVP) catheters may serve as a guide to fluid therapy, but not if it delays getting critical patients to the OR. While facilitating transport of the patient to the OR., such patients should receive 3 to 5 L of fluid intravenously at a rapid rate. In more stable patients, fluids should be administered to maintain a CVP of 16 to 18 cm H_2O to optimize tissue perfusion. If the CVP increases to 20 cm or higher and hypotension persists, consider the possibility of pericardial tamponade, tension pneumothorax, or a spuriously elevated CVP reading from inflated military antishock trousers. Ultimately, trying to manage shock without a CVP catheter is like driving on a freeway at night with your parking lights on.—J. Wasserberger, M.D.

Comparison of Intravenous and Endotracheal Administration of Midazolam and the Effect on Pulmonary Function and Histology in the Lamb Model

Jaimovich DG, Osborne JS III, Shabino CL (Bronson Methodist Hosp, Kalamazoo, Mich)

Ann Emerg Med 21:480–485, 1992 5–9

Background.—Initially, stabilizing, obtaining vascular access in, and managing small children with generalized tonic-clonic seizures can be very difficult. Midazolam is a rapid-onset anticonvulsant given intravenously and intramuscularly in adult epileptics. No one has studied its endotracheal administration. The effect of endotracheal administration of midazolam on pulmonary function and histology in lambs was studied.

Methods.—Twenty lambs weighing 10 to 20 kg were included in this prospective, randomized, controlled study, Two groups received endotracheal midazolam, 0.1 and 0.2 mg/kg, and 2 received intravenous midazolam, 0.1 and 0.2 mg/kg. In the endotracheal group, midazolam was injected rapidly through the catheter, followed by a 2-mL normal saline flush. After 2 rapid insufflations, the lambs were returned to the ventilator.

Findings.—The endotracheal and intravenous groups did not differ statistically or clinically in pulmonary function. At 24, 28, and 120 hours after endotracheal midazolam administration, histologic assessment of the lungs showed no pathologic changes. Acceptable midazolam levels were attained by the endotracheal route without clinically deleterious effects.

Conclusions.—Midazolam can reach acceptable levels without significantly deleterious effects on pulmonary function or histology when given endotracheally. The authors do not recommend that midazolam be used alone to control seizures or that the endotracheal route be the route of choice. Further clinical research is needed before this alternative method can be recommended for the treatment of humans.

▶ The 'V' in the NAVEL mnemonic for drugs that can be administered endotracheally has been under a cloud for the last several years since it was reported that endotracheal diazepam (Valium) causes significant pneumonitis (1), possibly due to its propylene glycol vehicle. There has been speculation that midazolam, packaged in an aqueous vehicle, would be a better choice, and this article supports that idea. Blood levels differed from those achieved when midazolam was administered intravenously, and an appropriate dose has yet to be determined.

The NAVEL mnemonic has become rather tattered of late, with new research suggesting that the 'E' should not be there as well (2). If a human study confirms Jaimovich and associates' results, perhaps we can at least put the V back in.—J. Schoffstall, M.D.

References

1. Rusli M, et al: *Ann Emerg Med* 16:314, 1987.
2. Crespo SG, et al: *Ann Emerg Med* 20:230, 1991.

Typing and Screening of Blood From Intraosseous Access

Brickman KR, Krupp K, Rega P, Alexander J, Guinness M (Toledo Hosp, Ohio)

Ann Emerg Med 21:414–417, 1992 5–10

Purpose.—In pediatric emergencies, intraosseous (IO) infusion provides a noncollapsible route for fluid resuscitation when hypovolemia makes peripheral intravenous line placement impossible. This route has been successfully used for blood transfusion. If blood from the bone marrow aspirate could be used for typing and screening, evaluation of blood compatibility could begin while IO volume expansion was underway. The use of blood from bone marrow aspirate for typing and screening was prospectively assessed.

Methods.—The subjects were 28 adults at a mean age of 55.48 years who were admitted to the hematology/oncology service. Bone marrow aspirate from the posterior superior iliac crest and a peripheral venous sample were tested in parallel for typing and screening according to blood bank protocol, including ABO and Rh typing. The presence of human leukocyte activity was assessed by evaluating reaction strength between the 2 samples.

Results.—None of the paired samples showed a visually significant difference in the strength of reaction for ABO and Rh typing. When the blood sample was less than 3 mL, use of a filter sampler provided a larger volume of plasma for typing and screening. One patient had cross-reactivity to a previously documented human leukocyte antibody in both the marrow and venous blood samples.

Conclusions.—Blood from bone marrow aspirate appears to be suitable for blood screening and typing in adults. When venous blood cannot be obtained, blood typing can proceed during IO volume expansion, followed by easier placement of a peripheral intravenous line and transfusion of compatible blood products. To allow complete typing and screening from these samples, saline displacement or the use of a special filter may be necessary. Studies in children are called for.

▶ As we gain more experience with the IO infusion route, we find additional advantages to the technique and relatively few disadvantages. The report by Brickman and colleagues proves the utility of the route for obtaining samples for blood typing. Other investigators have shown good correlation between blood gases in bone marrow samples and those in a venous samples. The only problem is in obtaining a specimen. Unlike the experience reported in 28 male patients getting bone marrow aspirates from the iliac crest, we are coping with infants in shock who have tibial lines. Often, it is impossible to aspirate back any blood or bone marrow. Perhaps the IO needles of the future will be constructed with sampling ports that will make aspiration as easy as infusion.—S. Ludwig, M.D.

Bilateral Lower Extremity Compartment Syndromes Secondary to Intraosseous Fluid Resuscitation

Galpin RD, Kronick JB, Willis RB, Frewen TC (Children's Hosp of Western Ontario, London, Canada)

J Pediatr Orthop 11:773–776, 1991 5–11

Background.—Intraosseous infusions are used in life-threatening hypovolemic or cardiogenic shock when intravenous access cannot be established readily. Minor fluid extravasation is commonly associated with this technique. There have been no reports of a fully established compartment syndrome, however. A child had severe compartment syndromes of both lower extremities complicating the use of intraosseous fluid resuscitation.

Case Report.—A 3-year, 9-month-old girl was brought to an emergency department in shock. Her history was complex, including congenital adrenal hyperplasia, functional short-gut syndrome, previous ileostomy, total colonic Hirschsprung's disease, and many episodes of hypovolemic dehydration. She was in profound hypovolemic shock with a heart rate of 210 beats per minute and poor peripheral perfusion. An intraosseous infusion into the right proximal tibia with a 16-gauge bone marrow needle was begun as a lifesaving measure. A 5% dextrose-in-normal saline infusion was begun. After about 20 minutes, her leg was noted to be swollen and discolored, and the infusion was stopped. About 350 mL of crystalloid had been infused. A similar intraosseous line was then established in the left proximal tibia at an infusion rate of 750 mL/hr. Intravenous access became possible after about 1.5 L of fluid was infused. At this time, her left leg was also swelling, and the intraosseous needle was removed. Her legs became tenser and more swollen during the next 12 hours. Examination at 16 hours showed very tense swelling and firmness to palpation over the anterior, lateral, and posterior compartments of both legs. The left foot was also involved. Blistering began to appear. Deep pressure elicited a painful withdrawal response. Compartment pressures were between 65 and 70 mm Hg. Immediate fasciotomy was done, at which time a standard 4-compartment decompression of both legs was performed through separate medial and lateral incisions. The patient subsequently made a full recovery.

Conclusions.—Intraosseous drug and fluid infusion is a useful technique for emergency resuscitation, especially in children in whom intravenous access may be difficult. Such patients should be monitored carefully for the development of swelling in the extremities. Compartment pressures greater than 30 to 35 mm Hg accompanied by the clinical signs of compartment syndrome necessitate immediate fasciotomy of all compartments involved.

▶ The increased use of intraosseous fluid infusions has become a well-established adjunct to the treatment of life-threatening hypovolemic shock in the pediatric patient, and this paper simply reminds us that like any worthwhile advance in emergency procedures and techniques, there will inevitably be some complications observed as the procedure is used more frequently. This patient developed a bilateral compartment syndrome that was recognized promptly and treated by bilteral fasciotomies. Additional complications are undoubtedly going to appear with increased use of intraosseous infusion (see Abstract 5–12). In the future, I will carefully follow lower-leg perfusion and look for evidence of swelling after an intraosseous infusion.—F.M. Henretig, M.D.

Skin Necrosis Complicating Intraosseous Infusion

Christensen DW, Vernon DD, Banner W Jr, Dean JM (Univ of Utah, Salt Lake City)

Pediatr Emerg Care 7:289–290, 1991 — 5–12

Background.—Intraosseous (IO) infusion is a useful technique for gaining rapid vascular access in the prehospital or emergency department (ED) setting. This technique commonly causes minor complications, but major ones are infrequent. Two children had local skin necrosis after IO infusion.

Case 1.—A 3-month-old boy with failure to thrive, chronic diarrhea, and gastroesophageal reflux was found with apnea and asystole. On arrival at the ED, the child was intubated, and resuscitative fluids and drugs were given by a right tibial IO line. A second cardiac arrest occurred, and the child was successfully resuscitated. He was transferred for further stabilization. After central venous access was obtained and the IO line removed, purple skin with irregular margins around the right tibial IO site was noted. No change in this condition had occurred when he died of anoxic encephalopathy the following day.

Case 2.—An 11-month-old boy was found trapped under a chest of drawers. He was cold, blue, and bradycardic when his parents began CPR. Paramedics intubated the patient and inserted a right tibial IO line through which they administered fluids and drugs en route to the ED. Infiltration of fluid around the IO site was noted in the ED, and a right femoral IO needle was inserted after unsuccessful attempts to gain peripheral vascular access. Epinephrine was administered, and a pulse was found. The patient was later transferred and venous access was obtained; his condition stabilized over a 2-day period. A purple discoloration measuring 12 × 8 cm with irregular, erythematous margins was noted around the tibial IO site; it was most severe on hospital day 2. The skin improved without treatment over a period of 9 days. Skin around the femoral IO site was normal.

Conclusions.—Local skin necrosis may occur in children undergoing IO infusion. To prevent this complication, placement should be verified before fluids are given; fluids and drugs should be infused gently, with careful monitoring for infiltration, and the needle should be promptly removed when intravenous access is established or if infiltration occurs.

▶ Surprise—even more IO complications! These authors describe 2 children with skin necrosis after IO infusions of fluids and catecholamines. As previously noted in the paper by Galfin et al. (see Abstract 5–11), IO infusion is a lifesaving technique that represents a real advance in modern pediatric emergency medicine, but as such, will undoubtedly be associated with occasional complications. Patients who undergo IO infusion should be monitored for such complications, including necrosis of skin, decreased perfusion, swelling, and evidence of early compartment syndrome, and obviously undergo appropriate therapy for such complications as they arise. It is also mandatory to switch to alternative sites of intravenous access as soon as feasible.—F.M. Henretig, M.D.

Long-Term Local Effects of Intraosseous Infusion on Tibial Bone Marrow in the Weanling Pig Model

Pollack CV Jr, Pender ES, Woodall BN, Tubbs RC, Iyer RV, et al (Univ of Mis-

sissippi, Jackson; Mississippi State Univ, Mississippi State)
Am J Emerg Med 10:27–31, 1992 5–13

Background.—Rapid, reliable access to the intravascular space is often difficult to achieve in infants and young children in hypodynamic cardiovascular states. The intraosseous route has become the access method of choice in many centers. The potential long-term injury to marrow after bolus injection or continuous intraosseous infusion of resuscitation fluid and drugs at standard dosages was assessed.

Methods.—Eighteen pigs 4 weeks of age were used. By random assignment, the pigs were treated with 1 of 6 intraosseous treatments: bolus sodium bicarbonate; 10% sodium bicarbonate infusion at a maintenance rate for 1 hour; bolus 1:10,000 epinephrine; 1:10,000 epinephrine solution infusion; 1 μg/kg/min for 1 hour; dopamine infusion; or a normal saline bolus. Treatments were administered through the left tibia. The pigs were monitored for 3 months, at which time the marrow from the same space and peripheral blood were studied. Marrow from the right tibia of each animal and untreated historical controls was used for comparison.

Results.—Marrow assessment showed normal cell differentials in all limbs in all groups. The overall cellularity was reduced somewhat in the experimental limbs of animals treated with a normal saline bolus vs. their own control limbs. Peripheral blood counts and differentials in all the pigs were normal.

Conclusions.—These findings provide some assurance that the intraosseous administration of commonly used resuscitative drugs does not significantly adversely affect tibial bone marrow. A pressure effect from rapid bolus fluid administration may reduce cellularity locally but apparently does not otherwise affect marrow development.

► The revival of intraosseous access for resuscitation of babies and young children has been a "godsend" to practicing emergency physicians. The authors provide an extensive review of the clinical and experimental experience with the intraosseous technique from the 1940s until the present that illustrates its safety.

However, this study does not have the power to add much to this literature. Within each study group of 3 pigs, it is neither reassuring that 5 groups found no change in the marrow (0/3 or a 95% confidence interval CI of 0% to 71%) nor worrisome that a high-volume bolus of normal saline did cause changes (2/2 or 95% CI of 16% to 100%).—K.N. Shaw, M.D.

Intraosseous Administration of Antibiotics: Same-Dose Comparison With Intravenous Administration in the Weanling Pig

Pollack CV Jr, Pender ES, Woodall BN, Parks BR (Univ of Mississippi Med Ctr, Jackson)

Ann Emerg Med 20:772–776, 1991 5–14

Introduction.—Peripheral access to the intravascular space is difficult or impossible in infants and young children in shock states and cardiac arrest. The intraosseous (IO) route is found to be a safe and reliable alternative. In a pediatric animal model, the administration of antibiotics by IO and peripheral intravenous routes were compared.

Methods.—Twelve weanling pigs were used in the study. Each anesthetized animal received, through a proximal tibial IO catheter, 50 mg/kg of ceftriaxone, 50 mg/kg of cefotaxime, or 300 mg/kg of ampicillin followed immediately by 2.5 mg/kg of gentamicin. To assess serum levels of the antibiotics, venous blood was obtained at 15, 30, 45, 60, and 90 minutes after IO injection. The protocol was repeated 1 week later by using a peripheral intravenous route.

Results.—At each time interval, the levels of ceftriaxone were significantly lower with IO dosing than with intravenous administration. Cefotaxime and ampicillin levels were significantly lower after IO administration at 15 and 30 minutes, but they were indistinguishable thereafter from levels achieved by the intravenous route. The levels of gentamicin were similar after IO and intravenous dosing throughout the sampling period.

Conclusion.—The IO line has been advocated for initial management in young children who are hemodynamically unstable and presumed to be in a septic condition thereby avoiding the delay of traditional intravenous access. The findings in this animal model suggest that comparable serum levels of these 4 antibiotics are achieved with the IO and intravenous routes. Because there may be a high degree of immediate, local protein binding of ceftriaxone in the marrow, this antibiotic may have to be given at its highest recommended IO loading dose.

▶ With this study, it is apparent that most medication required in an emergency setting may be administered by the IO route. Emergency center staff should not hesitate, therefore, in giving needed parental therapy for lack of intraveous access. As the emergency center staff proceeds in working with an ill patient in shock, the first round of medications, including antibiotics, may be given through an IO line. It is hoped that after fluid resuscitation, cardiac medications, and antibiotics, the child's cardiovascular system may then be stable and intravenous access attainable. The authors note that with the exception of using a loading dose for ceftriaxone, the usual recommended doses of common antibiotics will deliver adequate plasma levels.—R.M. Rutstein, M.D.

Serum Glucose After Intraperitoneal Infusion of 5% Dextrose Solution

McNamara RM, Schoffstall JM, Fuerst RS (The Med College of Pennsylvania, Philadelphia)

Ann Emerg Med 20:777–781, 1991 5–15

Background.—When oral or venous glucose administration is not possible, safe and effective alternatives to glucagon treatment for the emergency treatment of hypoglycemia are needed. The use of intraperitoneal (IP) glucose infusion as a treatment for hypoglycemia was explored.

Methods.—Seven female New Zealand White rabbits with a mean weight of 3.7 kg were used in a randomized, placebo-controlled, crossover study. Each animal, serving as her own control, was subjected to 3 experiments separated by a 4- to 7-day period. The interventions were the control, with no treatment given; the placebo, with 10 mL/kg of .9% normal saline solution IP; and the treatment; consisting of 10 mL/kg of 5% dextrose solution IP.

Results.—The mean absolute serum glucose value associated with the treatment was significantly higher than with the control and placebo groups beginning 10 minutes after intervention and continuing until the study was concluded at 30 minutes. The mean increase in serum glucose

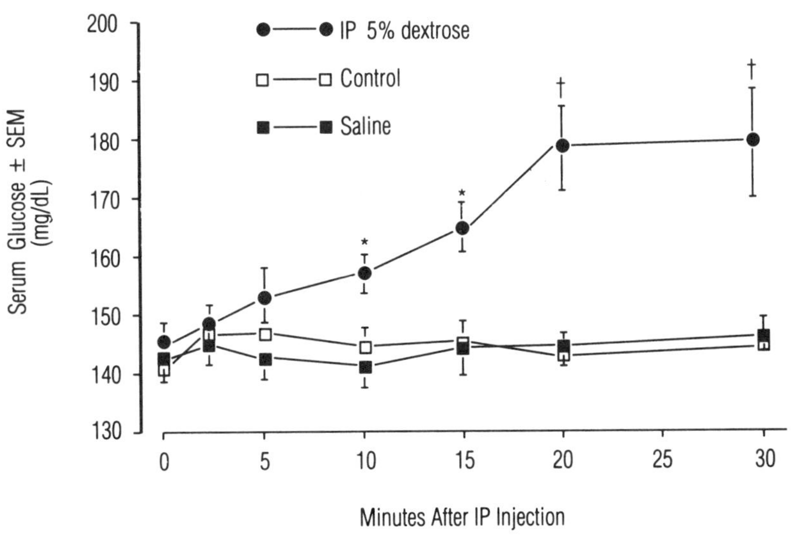

*$P < .01$ vs saline and vs control.

†$P < .001$ vs saline and vs control.

Fig 5–3.—Mean serum glucose levels of treatment and control groups. (Courtesy of McNamara RM, Schoffstall JM, Fuerst RS: *Ann Emerg Med* 20:777–781, 1991.)

levels of the treatment group vs. the control group was 15.5 mg/dL at 10 minutes, 20.6 mg/dL at 15 minutes, 36.5 mg/dL at 20 minutes, and 34.7 mg/dL at 30 minutes (Fig 5–3).

Conclusions.—Glucose instilled into the peritoneal cavity of euglycemic rabbits is rapidly absorbed into the animals' systemic circulation. Further research in a hypoglycemic model or in human beings would now be useful.

▶ Intramuscular glucagon and intraoral glucose jelly are still widely used. A subsequent study should compare all three in hypoglycemic humans.—T. Stair, M.D.

Conscious Sedation/Analgesia

Midazolam Use in the Emergency Department

Ramoska EA, Linkenheimer R, Glasgow C (Thomas Jefferson Univ Hosp; Methodist Hosp; Frankford Hosp, Philadelphia, Pa)
J Emerg Med 9:247–251, 1991 5–16

Purpose.—Midazolam is a new imidazobenzodiazepine derivative that is 2 to 3 times as potent as diazepam. It has a rapid onset and short duration of action and produces profound antegrade amnesia. These features make it an ideal drug for outpatient sedation. The usefulness of midazolam in a general emergency department (ED) was evaluated by a retrospective chart review.

Patients.—During a 1-year period, midazolam was used in 71 men and 49 women with an average age of 46 years. The most common use of midazolam was to provide sedation for painful, uncomfortable procedures such as fracture reduction, intubation, and wound care. Small doses of midazolam were used to calm agitated or severely anxious patients. In addition, midazolam was often used as a chemical restraint to quiet patients who were violent or psychotic after ingesting hallucinogenic drugs. The average total dose was 3.4 mg with a range of 1 to 10 mg. All doses were administered intravenously. Sixty-nine patients (57%) also received other drugs, mostly opiates.

Results.—Midazolam was not effective in achieving adequate sedation in only 2 patients. There were 4 adverse reactions, including urinary retention, vomiting, and prolonged somnolence, but none of those were serious. None of the patients had cardiovascular or respiratory problems, and none were admitted because of complications. Forty-eight patients were eventually discharged from the ED, and 72 were admitted to the hospital.

Conclusion.—Midazolam has the potential to become an extremely useful ED drug.

▶ A number of other uses of midazolam are emerging since this study of its use during 1988. Among these new uses are continuous infusion for the treatment of status epilepticus (1). In addition, other routes of administration including oral (2), nasal (3), rectal (4), and intramuscular routes are being used routinely in some children's hospitals. The oral route, mixed with juice and dosed at .5 to .75 mg/kg, may be an excellent way to sedate a child before intravenous cannulation, laceration repair, spinal tap, or other painful procedures. Intramuscular administration (.3 mg/kg) may be a more reliable route for delivering the prescribed dose to an agitated patient. I expect the use of midazolam to increase significantly in the next several years.—W.P. Burdick, M.D.

References

1. Kumar A, Bleck, TP: *Crit Care Med* 20:483, 1992.
2. Feld LH, et al: *Anesthesiology* 73:831, 1990.
3. Rice TL, Kyff JV: *Burns* 16:307, 1990.
4. Spear RM, et al: *Anesthesiology* 74:670, 1991.

The Efficacy and Safety of Methohexital in the Emergency Department

Zink BJ, Darfler K, Salluzzo RF, Reilly KM (Albany Med College, Albany, NY)
Ann Emerg Med 20:1293–1298, 1991 5–17

Background.—Methohexital sodium (MTX), an ultrashort-acting barbiturate, is used in the emergency department (ED) for a variety of surgical and nonsurgical procedures. It would appear to be ideal for use in the ED, but its use in the ED has not been addressed in the literature.

Methods.—Over a 1-year period, 102 patients received MTX in a university hospital ED. The drug was given by emergency physicians trained in its use. The attending physician and nurse completed a form addressing dosage and response, indications, final diagnosis, hemodynamic and respiratory parameters, and an efficacy survey. There were 66 male patients and 36 female patients with an average age of 28 years; 30 patients were younger than 20 years of age.

Findings.—The average cumulative MTX dose was 1.6 mg/kg, with an average duration of action per dose of 7.6 minutes. The most common indication was orthopedic procedures, 54 cases, followed by endotracheal intubation, 18 cases; head CT, 10 cases; and wound care, 8 cases. Only minimal hemodynamic changes were noted, with an average change in systolic blood pressure of −1.8 mm Hg 5 minutes after the drug was given and an average change in heart rate of 3 beats. The average degree of respiratory depression was 17%, but this was not correlated with dose. In 92 cases, MTX was given along with narcotics and/or benzodiazepines; there was no increased respiratory depression in those patients. No major complications could be attributed to the use of MTX.

Conclusions.—Methohexital sodium appears to be safe and effective for use in the ED when given by trained practitioners according to an established protocol. It has minimal effects on the respiratory and cardiovascular systems and few complications. It does not appear to be ideal for assisting in intubation.

▶ Methohexital has been around for a long time, but its use in the ED has not "caught on." While the authors found it useful and safe for sedation in orthopedic procedures, wound care, and CT scanning, I would like to see a comparison to other agents. Is there any benefit to using MTX over others? For example, I have successfully used patient-administered nitrous oxide/oxygen mixtures for orthopedic procedures, abscess drainage, and large abrasion debridement. One patient with recurrent shoulder dislocations found it markedly superior to previous regimens of meperidine and diazepam.

Since the duration of action is short (< 10 minutes), the authors point out that multiple doses of MTX were required in the majority of cases. I would question the use of this agent for CT sedation since, in most instances, this would necessitate redosing at the CT scanner. The agent was not useful in assisting intubation.

MTX probably has a place on the list of ED sedative agents. The authors show that adverse cardiorespiratory effects are limited and, therefore, the drug is relatively safe. I would reserve its use for very brief procedures.—J.M. Mitchell-Savinsky, M.D.

Conscious Sedation in the Emergency Department: The Value of Capnography and Pulse Oximetry

Wright SW (Vanderbilt Univ, Nashville, Tenn)

Ann Emerg Med 21:551–555, 1992 5–18

Background.—Emergency department patients often need sedation for painful procedures. Accurate, continuous measurement of oxygen saturation and the partial pressure of expired CO_2 (P_{ETCO_2}) would be useful for monitoring heavily sedated patients. An observational study was done to describe the use of pulse oximetry and nasal capnography in monitoring heavily sedated, nonintubated patients undergoing painful procedures in the emergency department.

Methods.—Twenty-seven patients were studied in a prospective, nonblinded, nonrandomized, uncontrolled clinical trial. All patients required sedation with benzodiazepines and/or narcotics for painful procedures. Ventilatory status was monitored with a capnometer by nasal cannula and with a pulse oximeter before, during, and after the sedatives were administered.

Results.—The mean $PETCO_2$ increased from 35.9 to 42.1 mm Hg during the procedure. The mean oxygen saturation dropped from 98% to 94.3%. In 1 patient, clinically significant apnea after the procedure was detected by the apnea alarm. Eight other patients had clinically silent hypoxemia and increased $PETCO_2$ during the procedure.

Conclusions.—Pulse oximetry was recommended for detecting unrecognized hypoxemia during conscious sedation in the emergency department. Capnography by nasal cannula is apparently also useful in monitoring during conscious sedation, but more research and clinical experience are needed before this modality can be recommended for routine use.

► Emergency physicians' use of conscious sedation is steadily becoming more sophisticated in the drugs we use, in our ability to titrate and reverse them, and in the intensity with which we monitor the patient (1). Intensive cardiovascular and respiratory monitoring has evolved partly because of the development of very effective, but also potentially dangerous, sedative drugs (e.g., the fentanyl/midazolam combination) and partly because of an increasingly hostile legal climate.

This noncontrolled, nonrandomized study is basically a report of the author's experiences with pulse oximetry and expired CO_2 monitoring during the use of a variety of conscious sedation protocols. He liked these monitoring techniques. I like them, too, and I use pulse oximetry routinely in managing patients with conscious sedation, but I recognize that hard data to support their use are lacking. To get a good picture of the strengths, weaknesses, and costs of these techniques would require a much larger study with better control of variables.—J. Schoffstall, M.D.

Reference

1. Hennes HM, et al: *Ann Emerg Med* 19:1006, 1990.

Emergency Department Analgesia Without Narcotics for Adults With Acute Sickle Cell Pain Crisis: Case Reports and Review of Crisis Management

Pollack CV Jr, Sanders DY, Severance HW Jr (Univ of Mississippi Med Ctr, Jackson)

J Emerg Med 9:445–452, 1991 5–19

Background.—Patients with vaso-occlusive pain crisis of sickle cell disease commonly go to the emergency department (ED). Treatment is not standardized but usually includes parenteral narcotic analgesics and intravenous hydration. A new regimen of analgesia in the ED for adults with sickle cell pain crisis (SCPC) has recently proved successful.

Case Report.—A 38-year-old black woman who was known to have hemoglobin S-S disease came to the ED with a 3-day history of bilateral upper- and lower-extremity pain. She had been to the ED 20 days before, at which time she was treated with intramuscular administration of meperidine and promethazine. Her temperature was 37.4°C; pulse, 110 per minute; and blood pressure 128/76 mm Hg. Her WBC count was 18,500 with 75% polymorphonuclear cells, 1% band forms, and a 26% hematocrit. An intravenous line of half-normal saline, 125 cc/hr, was begun, and the patient was given ketorolac, 60 mg intramuscularly, and amitriptyline, 60 mg orally. Fluids were continued while the patient rested for 6 hours, and she requested discharge when she awoke. She was sent home with a prescription for oxycodone; her next SCPC was 16 days later.

Discussion.—A parenteral nonsteroidal anti-inflammatory drug and an oral antidepressant were used in 4 cases of SCPC. There is no preventive treatment for this frustrating problem. Recent advances such as peroral morphine sulfate, injectable nonsteroidal anti-inflammatory drugs, and patient-controlled analgesia may eventually allow standardized treatment for SCPC.

▶ The authors present 4 cases of SCPC managed with keterolac and promethazine in 1 and ketorolac and amitriptyline in 3. The first patient (ketorolac/promethazine) subsequently required meperidine. The case reports are then followed by a good review of the evaluation/management of SCPC and an introduction to their prospective study of the use of ketorolac and amitriptyline.

It would be beneficial to emergency practitioners to find a treatment regimen for these patients that *works* and does not require repeated doses of narcotics. While the incidence of addicted sickle cell patients is reportedly small, it is often the addicted patients we see repeatedly in the ED. We frequently get caught up in bartering over narcotics. Sickle cell patients are potentially seriously ill and can succumb to infection, stroke, aplastic crisis, and other complications. I always tell my students that one of our hardest tasks is distinguishing the drug seeker from the truly ill. If we can find a nonaddictive effective management protocol for SCPC, this task will be lessened. I wish the authors success in their prospective study.—J.M. Mitchell-Savinsky, M.D.

Taking the 'Sting' Out of Local Anesthetics

Long CC, Motley RJ, Holt PJ (Univ Hosp of Wales, Cardiff)

Br J Dermatol 125:452–455, 1991 5–20

Background.—Lidocaine is widely used as a local anesthetic because of its rapid onset and prolonged duration of action. However, injections of lidocaine are associated with a burning sensation. Several factors such as the needle gauge, site, and speed of injection may influence the discomfort from injections of local anesthetics. The acidity of lidocaine has been targeted as the major cause of the burning sensation, and some have advocated the addition of sodium bicarbonate to lessen discomfort. The characteristics of lidocaine preparations that may be responsible for the discomfort after injection were examined.

Methods.—A randomized, double-blind comparison of paired injections of 2% plain lidocaine, .5% plain lidocaine, and .5% lidocaine with 1:200,000 epinephrine was made in 32 patients. A .5-mL syringe with a 27-gauge needle was used in all cases.

Findings.—The concentration of lidocaine was a major factor—the discomfort after injection. All 32 subjects found 2% lidocaine more painful than .5%. The addition of epinephrine or sodium metabisulfite to plain .5% lidocaine made the injection more painful. Neutralization of acidic .5% lidocaine reduced the discomfort in 44% of the patients, but the difference was not statistically significant.

Conclusions.—The concentration of lidocaine and the presence of epinephrine or sodium metabisulfite in lidocaine were the major factors in the discomfort after injection. Increasing the pH of lidocaine reduced discomfort, but the difference was not significant. An initial injection of .5% lidocaine followed by an injection of stronger lidocaine or lidocaine with epinephrine into the already anesthetized skin minimizes patient discomfort.

▶ Lidocaine injections are always going to be painful. The use of TAC, with or without lidocaine injection, works well in many patients when lessening the discomfort of the injection is desired, especially in children (see also Abstract 5–21).—G.J. Ordog, M.D.

Buffered Lidocaine as a Local Anesthetic: An Investigation of Shelf Life

Bartfield JM, Homer PJ, Ford DT, Sternklar P (Albany Med College, NY)

Ann Emerg Med 21:16–19, 1992 5–21

Introduction.—Buffered lidocaine appears to be less painful during administration than commercially supplied lidocaine, but preparing the solution just before use may limit its application in emergency settings. The shelf life of buffered lidocaine was examined to determine whether this solution could be prepared safely in advance.

Methods.—Three solutions of buffered lidocaine were compared: 7 days old, 1 day old, and freshly prepared. A control solution of plain lidocaine was also tested. The 24 adult volunteers received .5 mL intradermal injections of each solution. For each forearm injection, the pain of infiltration was rated by using a previously validated visual-analogue pain scale. The extent and duration of anesthesia were also recorded.

Results.—All 3 buffered solutions were significantly less painful than the control solution. The mean maximum diameter of anesthesia and the mean duration of anesthesia were similar for the 4 solutions. When contacted 2 to 4 days later, none of the volunteers reported signs of infection at the injection sites. Although the lidocaine concentration of the buffered solution decreased approximately 10% after 7 days of storage, this change was not clinically relevant.

Conclusion.—Buffered lidocaine can be stored at room temperature for up to 7 days without loss of its effectiveness. This finding should enable buffered solutions to be used more widely in emergency settings.

▶ Now that it has clearly been shown that buffered lidocaine is less painful and that its shelf life can be extended, it remains for some company to develop a way to prolong its shelf life even beyond that noted in the article. Prepackaged preparations are always more convenient in a busy emergency department.—E.J. Lucid, M.D.

The Reversal of the Ischemic Effects of Epinephrine on a Finger With Local Injections of Phentolamine

Markovchick V, Burkhart KK (Denver Gen Hosp; Rocky Mountain Poison & Drug Ctr, Denver, Colo)

J Emerg Med 9:323–324, 1991 5–22

Introduction.—Individuals at high risk of life-threatening anaphylactic reactions are commonly prescribed automatic epinephrine injection syringes. The automatic triggering device may lead to accidental injection. In 1 patient, the ischemic effects of accidentally injected epinephrine were reversed by phentolamine.

Case Report.—A 30-year-old female nurse punctured her right thumb with an automatic syringe while cleaning out a drawer. The needle penetrated to the bone at the mid tuft and injected the entire contents of the syringe (0.3 mL of 1:1000 epinephrine). Within a few minutes, the area began to blanch, and the woman noted an increase in her heart rate. In the emergency room, 2.5 mg of phentolamine diluted in 2.5 cc of normal saline was injected along the course of the digital arteries of the thumb. Sensation and capillary filling began to return in 10 minutes. When intense blanching and anesthesia remained in the area about 1 hour later, an additional 1 mg of phentolamine was injected. Sensation gradually returned, her pulse slowly decreased, and the woman recovered well.

Conclusion.—Ischemic necrosis may lead to infection, sepsis, or loss of the digit. Previous studies have reported the success of phentolamine in preventing necrosis after dopamine and norepinephrine infiltrations. The α-blocking qualities of phentolamine, first used as a digital block and then injected directly into the affected area, reversed the ischemic effects of epinephrine.

▶ In addition to being cognizant of therapy for this complication of the epinephrine auto-injector, the emergency physician can offer preventive guidance. When prescribing these devices, the patient should be carefully instructed in their safe storage as well as their usage. The patient also should be cautioned to seek medical attention in the event of an accidental discharge into the digits (or elsewhere, if systemic findings of catecholamine toxicity develop). The overall risk-benefit of these devices remains to be determined. Their prescription should be reserved for those patients with documented life-threatening systemic reactions to insect stings and for those who also demonstrate the physical and mental capacity to use the device correctly.—J.R. Hedges, M.D.

Emergency Diagnostic Imaging/Ultrasound

Bedside Ultrasound in Decision Making for Emergency Surgery: Its Role in Medical Intensive Care Patients

Lerch MM, Riehl J, Buechsel R, Kierdorf H, Winkeltau G, et al (Medizinische Fakultaet der Rheinisch-Westfaelischen Technischen Hochschule, Aachen, Germany)

Am J Emerg Med 10:35–38, 1992 5–23

Background.—Portable ultrasound has proven to be of great value in intensive care units for postoperative monitoring of surgical patients and for facilitating invasive bedside procedures. The role of abdominal ultrasound in surgical decision making under critical care conditions was assessed.

Methods.—For 18 months, 1,024 patients referred to a general medical intensive care unit were followed. Seven percent of these patients had emergency surgery at some point in their hospitalization. Patients for whom the pathologic result of sonography was considered sufficient to perform surgery without additional imaging procedures were identified.

Findings.—Abdominal ultrasound provided a definitive diagnosis for 18 of 71 patients with surgical emergencies. In this 25%, the decision to operate was made without delaying for further or more invasive diagnostic procedures. The sonographic diagnosis was confirmed during surgery in all cases. Patients most likely to benefit from the bedside ultrasound in a surgical emergency were those with hemorrhage of unknown origin which occurred in 44% or septicemia from an undetected focus which occurred in 39%. In cases in which ultrasound was considered diagnostic, the most common site of surgery was the urinary tract, especially in emergencies after renal transplantation.

Conclusions.—Abdominal ultrasound has particular value in critical care settings. Ultrasound can provide a definite diagnosis in as many as one fourth of the patients with surgical emergencies, and the decision to operate can be made without delay caused by further or more invasive imaging procedures.

▶ And just when you were so proud of yourself that you could pretty much reach those late-night CT scans. Now get ready for the ultrasound generation: save those hardearned bucks for ultrasound training. This is just one more article pointing to a future that is trying to crowd into today. Ultrasound is coming and will soon be a featured and standard diagnostic tool in your emergency center.

Should you doubt, should you think that we can wiggle out of this dire prediction by astutely pointing out that the title of this article clearly states that the study occurred in the intensive care unit, simply pull the article. Note the very first sentence of the article: "Abdominal ultrasound has become a diagnostic procedure of increasing importance in many emergency departments."—E.H. Taliaferro, M.D.

Visualization of Ingested Medications in the Stomach by Ultrasound

Amitai Y, Silver B, Leikin JB, Frischer H (Rush-Presbyterian St Luke's Med Ctr, Chicago, Ill)

Am J Emerg Med 10:18–23, 1992 5–24

Background.—Patients with a drug overdose may be unable or unwilling to provide information on the ingested medication. Because plain radiography will not detect most capsules or tablets in the gastrointestinal tract, the capability of ultrasound to physically image pills in the stomach was investigated.

Methods.—Thirty commonly ingested medications were selected for the study. In an in vitro experiment, ultrasound was compared with plain radiography in the detection of pills. Ultrasound was then examined in vivo following ingestion of pills by human volunteers and by patients with drug overdoses. Pills used in the in vivo study were chosen for their relative safety. Four of these pills had a slow disintegration time and 2 had a fast disintegration time.

Results.—The grading score for the detectability of pills was significantly higher with ultrasound than with plain radiography. Ultrasound clearly detected all 4 pills in the stomach with slow disintegration times. One of the immediate release pills was not detected, but the other was visible 3 minutes after its ingestion. Ultrasound detected pills in the stomach in 1 of 4 patients who had intentionally ingested multiple pills. The 3 patients who had no evidence of pills on ultrasound had arrived at the emergency department 1 to 6 hours after taking immediate-release medications.

Conclusion.—Ultrasound is able to image ingested medication in the stomach, provided that the pills are enteric-coated or sustained-release preparations. The size of the pill does not appear to limit the use of ultrasound; pills detected in this study ranged in size from 7.1 to 16 mm (diameter of round tablets or the long axis of capsules).

► With the increased use of bedside ultrasonography by emergency physicians, the concept described in this article may become more applicable. The actual clinical benefits of ultrasound to evaluate a drug overdoes is not well defined yet, but its use seems limited to only slow-release medications. In a suspected overdose, a negative ultrasound should not be used to withhold standard methods of therapy or gastrointestinal decontamination. One uncommon scenario where ultrasound may be useful would be in patients with increasing drug levels (such as theophylline, salicylates, lithium) or in the setting of prolonged or fluctuating coma when a persistent drug mass, concretion, or medication bezoar is suspected. Gastroscopy is currently suggested for these indications, but ultrasound is certainly easier to obtain and much less invasive.—J.R. Roberts, M.D.

Magnetic Resonance Imaging for Calf Deep Venous Thrombophlebitis

Vukov LF, Berquist TH, King BF (Mayo Clinic and Found, Rochester, Minn)
Ann Emerg Med 20:497–499, 1991 5–25

Background.—Clinical signs and symptoms are frequently not an accurate indicator of deep venous thrombophlebitis (DVT) in the calf. Ascending venography is an invasive and costly procedure, and noninvasive methods are not usually helpful in diagnosing DVT below the popliteal vein level. Scanning with ^{125}I-fibrinogen has many practical limitations.

Objective.—A pilot study was undertaken to evaluate MR-I in 10 consecutive patients seen with clinical features suggesting DVT of the calf.

Methods.—Magnetic resonance imaging with both axial spin-echo and axial gradient-recalled acquisition in a steady state as performed on prone patients. Venography was also carried out, and the MRI studies and venograms were examined blindly by 2 experienced radiologists.

Findings.—Magnetic resonance images demonstrated a definite clot in the calf veins in 4 of the 5 patients having positive venograms. All 5 patients with negative venograms had MRI findings of a patent deep venous system. Calf muscle hematoma was demonstrated in 2 of these patients as the cause of calf swelling and warmth.

Conclusion.—Magnetic resonance imaging might replace ascending venography as the standard diagnostic measure when DVT of the calf is suspected.

► A patient with possible DVT in the ED makes for a difficult diagnostic challenge for all of us. Impedance plethysmography, color flow Doppler ultrasound, and venography are the usual diagnostic media to make the diagnosis; however, each modality has as many pros as cons. Magnetic resonance imaging has recently been reported to be a promising diagnostic modality for thigh and deep pelvic vein thrombosis, and now these authors attempt to promote MRI for the diagnosis of calf DVT in a pilot study of 10 patients.

As the diagnostic test for this very tough-to-pin-down clinical entity evolves into standards of care, open-mindedness along with open discussion with radiology colleagues will be the common thread connecting us to the best patient outcome. It may all boil down to what resources are available in a particular radiology department and what the level of experience is for the operator doing the diagnostic study and attempting to interpret the information from that study (see Abstract 5–27).—J.J. Kelly, D.O., F.A.C.E.P.

Emergency Center Arteriography

Itani KMF, Burch JM, Spjut-Patrinely V, Richardson R, Martin RR, Mattox KL (Ben Taub Gen Hosp, Houston, Tex)

J Trauma 32:302–307, 1992 5–26

Background.—Indications for emergency arteriography in assessing patients with suspected peripheral vascular injuries are changing. The sensitivity and specificity of emergency center arteriography (ECA) in patients with possible peripheral vascular injuries were determined.

Methods and Findings.—Between 1983 and 1989, 1,882 ECA procedures were done on 1,802 patients. The most common indication was the proximity of an injury to a major vascular structure, which was the only indication in 91% of the cases. The sensitivity and specificity of ECA were 95.5% and 97.7%, respectively. Fifty-seven arteriograms were equivocal or inadequate technically. Further patient assessment revealed another 11 vascular injuries. Surgery was needed for 64.3% of the injuries detected by ECA. One hundred nine injuries were considered minor and were not repaired. Ninety-one patients with minor vascular injuries were available for follow-up a mean of 12 months later; none of those patients had any complications. One thousand forty-eight patients with negative arteriograms were followed for a mean of 18 months; none of those patients had any vascular complications either.

Conclusions.—Emergency center arteriography is a sensitive, accurate, and safe way to assess patients with possible peripheral vascular injuries. The advantages of ECA include speed and low cost in comparison to formal arteriography. In addition, ECA's ability to detect minor arterial lesions is a clear advantage over noninvasive vascular testing and physical examination.

▶ This article includes an analysis of an impressive number of arteriograms. One question that always arises in treating a patient with no physical findings of vascular injury and a wound that is in the "proximity" of a vessel is when to perform angiography. A definition of proximity is never given in these articles. We have just completed a review of 33,000 gunshot wound cases, one of the purposes of which was to define proximity. We now use the following for proximity and therefore indication for arteriography (or duplex Doppler ultrasonography, which will be discussed below):

1. Low velocity handguns—within 1 in. of the zone of obvious cavitation as visualized radiographically or clinically and as described in 1.
2. Shotgun wounds—within 1 in. of the vessel's course of any pellet or pellet tract, as described above.

It is interesting to note that CT scanning often shows a missile tract well, even when the metallic fragments are not obvious radiologically. The way of the future may involve ultrafast CT angiography, which is noninvasive, and further research in this area is ongoing.

The current study also focused on duplex Doppler ultrasonography, before or in place of formal angiography. If duplex Doppler findings of a vessel at the missile tract site are normal, then arteriography may not be required. Because this is a noninvasive test, there is no morbidity or mortality as in formal angiography. Studies have shown that the results are just as reliable in asymptomatic patients.

At the King/Drew Medical Center, we see 6 patients a day who have asymptomatic vascular proximity gunshot wounds. Our current protocol for potential vascular injuries is as follows:

1. With physical findings of vascular injury or unstable patients go directly to surgery and perform intraoperative angiography.
2. With physical findings of vascular injury and a stable patient the patient has angiography and then surgery, depending on the findings.
3. With proximity only and no physical findings (as defined above), perform duplex Doppler ultrasonography. If the results are negative, the patient may be discharged; if positive, perform angiography.—G.J. Ordog, M.D.

Real-Time Ultrasound for the Detection of Deep Venous Thrombosis

Chance JF, Abbitt PL, Tegtmeyer CJ, Powers RD (Univ of Virginia, Charlottesville)

Ann Emerg Med 20:494–496, 1991 5–27

Introduction.—Accurately diagnosing deep venous thrombosis (DVT) remains a problem because the clinical features are unreliable, plethysmography is not always available, and venography is an invasive and costly method. The value of ultrasonography was therefore examined in a prospective series of adult patients in the emergency department who were clinically suspected of having DVT.

Methods.—Ultrasonography was first performed, and the patient then had contrast venography of the same extremity by a physician blinded to the ultrasound findings.

Findings.—Twenty of 70 patients had positive venographic findings. Fourteen of them had proximal DVT, whereas 6 had isolated calf-vein DVT. Four of 18 initially positive ultrasound studies were negative on the final reading. Six of 52 patients with negative ultrasound findings for proximal DVT had calf-vein thrombosis on venography. Initial ultrasonographic readings were 100% sensitive and 93% specific for proximal DVT.

Conclusions.—A negative real-time B-mode ultrasound study reliably rules out proximal DVT. A positive study, however, detects proximal thrombosis only when done by an experienced operator.

▶ Real-time ultrasound, which essentially examines the compressibility of the proximal leg veins, is replacing impedance plethysmography as the noninvasive test of choice for the emergency department patient with suspected DVT. This study is rapidly performed and, in the hands of the right operator, will effectively rule out a proximal DVT (see Abstract 5–25).—R.M. McNamara, M.D.

Procedures/Instrumentation

Direct Mechanical Ventricular Actuation for Cardiac Arrest in Humans: A Clinical Feasibility Trial

Anstadt MP, Bartlett RL, Malone JP, Brown GR, Martin S, Nolan DJ, Oberheu KH, Anstadt GL (Wright State Univ, Dayton, Ohio; Richland Mem Hosp, Columbia, SC)

Chest 100:86–92, 1991 5–28

Background.—Conventional CPR is limited because of the low flow state generated. Low cerebral blood flow is a particular problem. Direct mechanical ventricular actuation is a non blood-contact approach to biventricular cardiac massage that can be expeditiously applied after refractory cardiac arrest.

Method.—The direct mechanical ventricular actuation device uses a contoured cup that is pneumatically driven to actuate the ventricular myocardium. The myocardium is "pushed" into a systolic configuration and "pulled" into a diastolic one. Direct mechanical ventricular actuation is applied via a left anterior thoracotomy.

Series.—Direct mechanical ventricular actuation was applied to 22 patients, in 12 of whom it was possible to place catheters for hemo-dynamic monitoring. Ten of these patients were seen in the emergency room in cardiac arrest, whereas 2 had refractory cardiac arrests while hospitalized.

Outcome.—The mean cardiac output during nearly 4 hours of circulatory support was 3.1 L/min. The device was sometimes removed for 2 to 3 minutes for open-chest cardiac massage. The arterial pH increased during the time the device was in place, and the serum lactate level declined. Four patients were successfully defibrillated, but 2 of them died within an hour, and the other 2 died later of heart failure and respiratory insufficiency. Another patient underwent emergency coronary artery bypass graft surgery but died of myocardial infarction. One patient incurred an epicardial laceration during pericardiotomy, and another had a ventricular tear during open-chest cardiac massage.

Conclusions.—Direct mechanical ventricular actuation is a feasible means of stabilizing cardiac function during cardiac arrest. It is rapidly applied and can markedly improve hemodynamics. The device may provide a way of bridging to more involved methods of circulatory support.

▶ Standard CPR with external chest compression has yielded disappointing results over the years. While the technique can deliver a palpable pulse to the carotid and femoral arteries (and thus a delusion of comfort to the resuscitator), it is now realized that coronary artery and cerebral blood flow are quite poor. Coronary artery flow, in particular, is dependent on an effective gradient between aortic pressure at the coronary artery ostium and pressure in the right atrium, into which the coronary circulation empties. Since closed-chest massage generates equivalent pressure throughout the thorax during each phase of the compression cycle, aortic and right atrial pressures are not much different. Hence, coronary artery blood flow is exceedingly unimpressive. While a satisfying pulse can thus be obtained with a standard CPR, the one organ most crucial to successful resuscitation benefits minimally, if at all.

Because of this fact, some authorities have advocated a return to open-chest cardiac massage. With this technique, an aortic/right atrial gradient is generated, and myocardial circulation is improved. The problems with open-chest massage include a lack of familiarity or comfort with so invasive a procedure, potential perforation of the heart by a finger, and if resuscitation is prolonged, eventual resuscitator fatigue.

The technique of "direct mechanical ventricular actuation" described in this article is thus an attempt to utilize the advantages of open-chest over closed-chest massage while minimizing the disadvantages. The results are promising. In a small number of patients, cardiac output was increased 190%, systolic pressure 59%, and diastolic pressure 65% by mechanical actuation as compared with standard open-chest massage. No statistics were attempted. While there were no survivals to hospital discharge, the average time of arrest prior to application of the device (which required only about 2 minutes to perform) was 81 ± 9 minutes. Results might be improved considerably if the device were applied sooner after arrest.

The authors claim that this technique is a "non blood-contacting method." In comparison to intravascular modalities, I suppose it is. However, there are those who would nevertheless consider open thoracotomy a somewhat invasive procedure.

Recently, a very similar, yet completely noninvasive method of cardiac massage has been described (1). It is rumored that the technique was originally performed by an adolescent boy who successfully resuscitated his own father with the rather low-tech device commonly known as a toilet plunger. A modified toilet plunger has now been developed and tested on patients.

The device is basically a suction cup applied to the chest wall. The physiology of the compression phase (systole) is similar to that of standard closed-chest massage. However, the diastolic phase employed active suction generating a significant negative intrathoracic pressure in comparison to the passive "relaxation" phase of standard CRP. Because of the aortic valve, blood does not flow retrogradely during "diastole" and is actually sucked into the coronary circulation. The external suction device is thus physiologically similar to the device described in this article but does not require thoracotomy.

There has been a plethora of research involving various attempts to increase coronary circulation during CPR, thereby providing some meaning to the letters "C" and "R." The technique described here, as well as its closed-chest analogue referred to above, both show promise and merit further investigation.—M.J. Bresler, M.D.

Reference

1. Cohen T J, et al: *JAMA* 26:21, 1992.

Esophageal Electrodes Allow Precise Assessment of Cardiac Output by Bioimpedance

Balestra B, Malacrida R, Leonardi L, Suter P, Marone C (Univ of Geneva, Switzerland)

Crit Care Med 20:62–67, 1992 5–29

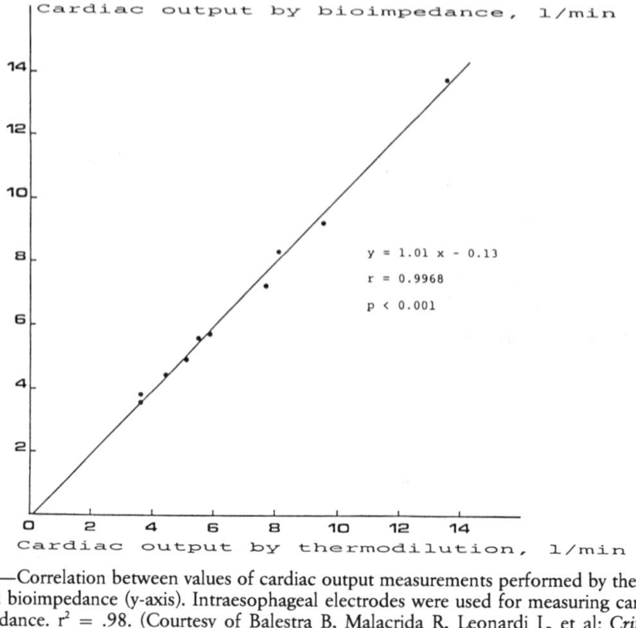

Fig 5–4.—Correlation between values of cardiac output measurements performed by thermodilution (x-axis) and bioimpedance (y-axis). Intraesophageal electrodes were used for measuring cardiac output by bioimpedance. r^2 = .98. (Courtesy of Balestra B, Malacrida R, Leonardi L, et al: *Crit Care Med* 20:62–67, 1992.)

Purpose.—Measurements of cardiac output by thermodilution and bioelectric impedance may vary widely, partly because of the position of the electrodes. To test this hypothesis, the effect of the position of external thoracic electrodes on cardiac output as measured by bioimpedance was compared with the results oubtained by thermodilution in critically ill patients.

Study Design.—In an open, prospective, comparative trial, cardiac output was measured by bioimpedance at rest and after physical activity in 20 healthy volunteers and after changing the neck or xiphoid electrodes. Comparisons of cardiac output obtained by thermodilution and bioimpedance through internal and external electrodes were performed in 10 critically ill patients.

Results.—The mean cardiac output increased significantly from 6.7 L/min at rest to 10.8 L/min after exercise. While the position of the neck electrodes did not affect cardiac output, there was a linear relationship between the position of the xiphoid voltage-sensing electrodes and measured cardiac output. Displacing the xiphoid electrodes 3 cm in the caudal direction significantly decreased cardiac output, and displacing the xiphoid electrodes 3 and 6 cm cranially significantly increased cardiac output. In critically ill patients, measurements of cardiac output by thermodilution and by bioimpedance through internal esophageal electrodes were highly correlated (Fig 5–4). Cardiac output measured by bioimpedance with external electrodes was significantly lower than that measured by thermodilution in 9 of 10 critically ill patients.

Conclusion.—If confirmed in a larger patient population, bioimpedance using internal esophageal electrodes to measure cardiac output could be a good alternative to the more invasive thermodilution technique. Measurements of cardiac output by bioimpedance through external thoracic electrodes are dependent on the position of the xiphoid electrodes.

▶ Emergency physicians have long sought an accurate and simple means of noninvasively estimating cardiac output. Bioimpedance with surface electrodes has been disappointingly inaccurate. As shown by this study, the deficiency may, in part, be related to electrode placement. The authors found a surprisingly high correlation of thermodilution cardiac output measurements and bioimpedance values obtained with internal (esophageal) leads in critically ill patients. While this report is promising, the esophageal lead was precisely placed with radiographic confirmation prior to measurements. We do not know how sensitive the bioimpedance cardiac output measurements are to esophageal lead movement. Nonetheless, this technique warrants further investigation in the critical care unit and the emergency department. —J.R. Hedges, M.D.

Incidence of Loss of Consciousness During Automatic Implantable Cardioverter-Defibrillator Shocks

Kou WH, Calkins H, Lewis RR, Bolling SF, Kirsch MM, et al (VA Med Ctr, Ann Arbor, Mich)

Ann Intern Med 115:942–945, 1991 5–30

Background.—An automatic implantable cardioverter-defibrillator (AICD) can terminate arrhythmias, although not prevent them, in patients with life-threatening arrhythmias who cannot take anti-arrhythmic drugs. It is unknown, however, whether it is safe for patients who have had AICD implantation to drive. For this reason, the incidence and predictors of loss of consciousness in association with AICD shocks were studied.

Methods.—The subjects were 180 patients who had undergone AICD implantation for ventricular tachycardia or ventricular fibrillation. Most had coronary artery disease. The pulse generators used were capable of delivering high-energy shocks only. Patients were followed for a mean of 16 months to assess the incidence of loss of consciousness in association with spontaneous AICD shocks. Various clinical factors were studied to identify predictors of loss of consciousness.

Findings.—During follow-up, 59% of the patients experienced AICD shocks, with a mean of 11 shocks per patient. Loss of consciousness occurred in 16 patients, or 9%. Of these, 13 had syncope, and 3 died suddenly. An absence of syncope during shocks could not be predicted by a previous absence of syncope. None of the variables investigated could predict syncope.

Conclusions.—Patients with implanted AICDs that deliver only high-energy shocks are at moderate risk of loss of consciousness during shocks. Syncope cannot be predicted by any clinical variable. For patients who have these implants, it is therefore not safe to assume that they can drive or engage in other activities requiring extra vigilance.

▶ Patients with diabetes and epilepsy have been shown to have an increased risk for traffic accidents (1). This study suggests that patients who have an AICD should be considered another population at increased risk, especially if the AICD delivers only high-energy shocks. Newer AICDs deliver lower-energy shocks and are also capable of delivering antitachycardia and bradycardia pacing, and the risk of syncope with AICD discharge may be less with these newer models. Of note, the time to the first shock after AICD implantation in the syncope and nonsyncope groups averaged 6 months. It might be reasonable to consider restricting driving for 1 year after implantation to determine the likelihood of syncope with AICD discharge. One issue not addressed in this study is the incidence of syncope in patients with life-threatening arrhythmias who are taking anti-arrhythmics but who have not been treated with an AICD. This represents a substantially larger population at risk for syncope.—J.T. Niemann, M.D.

Reference

1. Hansotia P, Broste SK: *N Engl J Med* 324:22, 1991.

Unsuccessful Emergency Medical Resuscitation—Are Continued Efforts in the Emergency Department Justified?

Gray WA, Capone RJ, Most AS (Rhode Island Hosp, Providence; Univ of Rochester, NY)

N Engl J Med 325:1393–1398, 1991 5–31

Background.—It is not usually possible to resuscitate victims of prehospital cardiac arrest; they often undergo further efforts at resuscitation after transportation to the hospital. The efficacy and cost-effectiveness of this practice were studied by evaluating 185 patients who could not be resuscitated before arrival at the hospital.

Methods.—The patients were identified by examination of patient logs for a 21-month period. All patients had unsuccessful but ongoing attempts at resuscitation for prehospital arrest by an emergency medical team. Advanced cardiac life support was begun after the patients arrived in the emergency department. Prehospital and in-hospital characteristics of the resuscitative efforts and the patients' eventual outcome in the emergency department were evaluated. For patients who were revived in the emergency department, the hospital course and costs were studied.

Findings.—The mean age was 67 years; 66% were men, and 34% had pre-existing coronary artery disease. Seventy-four perent of emergency medical units arrived at the scene within 5 minutes of receiving the call for help and 62% of the patients received advanced cardiac life support. Only 16 patients, or 9%, were successfully resuscitated and admitted to the hospital. The only factor that improved emergency department outcome was shorter duration of prehospital resuscitation. None of the successfully resuscitated patients survived until hospital discharge, and only 1 patient regained consciousness before death. They stayed in the hospital for a mean of 12.6 days and in the intensive care unit for an average of 2.3 days; the total hospital cost for all 16 patients was $180,908.

Conclusions.—Patients who cannot be resuscitated from cardiopulmonary arrest during transport to the emergency department are not commonly resuscitated in the hospital, and those who are subsequently revived have a poor outcome. These patients consume significant resources with little justification. Protocols to cease prolonged, unsuccessful resuscitation at the arrest scene should be considered.

▶ The results of this study are hardly surprising. It is now well accepted that immediate defibrillation is the best treatment for ventricular fibrillation. For those found in asystole or electrical mechanical dissociation, the prognosis is grim regardless of the resuscitation effort.

In this study, of the patients unsuccessfully resuscitated in the field, only 62% were treated by emergency medical service (EMS) units capable of advanced cardiac life support (ACLS). Of those patients whose initial cardiac rhythms could be determined by prehospital care providers, 60% demonstrated either ventricular fibrillation or ventricular tachycardia. By the time of arrival in the emergency department (ED), however, these rhythms were seen in only 32% of these patients, thus reflecting continued deterioration prior to ED arrival despite ACLS.

While no patients in this study survived to leave the hospital, the factor that was associated with improved outcome in the ED was total field time (on scene plus transport) of less than 15 minutes.

The authors conclude that money would be best spent in providing communities with a sufficient number and distribution of EMS teams capable of rapid defibrillation and that prolonged ED resuscitation is not useful for the patient unsuccessfully resusciated in the field.—M.J. Bresler, M.D.

Pseudometabolic Acidosis Caused by Underfill of Vacutainer® Tubes

Herr RD, Swanson T (Univ of Utah Med Ctr, Salt Lake City)

Ann Emerg Med 21:177–180, 1992 5–32

Introduction.—A previous study showed that serum bicarbonate levels are lower in samples aspirated into a syringe than those directly aspirated into Vacutainer tubes. Because 1 effect of the syringe is to inadvertently underfill the Vacutainer tube, a study was conducted to determine how serum bicarbonate levels and the anion gap are affected by sample size in a 10-mL red-top (clot) Vacutainer tube at the fixed sample volumes of 10, 3, and 1 mL.

Methods.—A single Vacutainer venous phlebotomy was performed on 30 consecutive patients in the emergency department, with 3 tubes drawn in random order and filled with 10, 3, and 1 mL of blood. The first 20 patients had unvented tubes, and the last 10 patients had the tubes vented within 1 minute of the draw.

Results.—Mean bicarbonate levels in unvented tubes decreased significantly from 21.7 mmo1/L in the 10-mL sample, to 19.4 in the 3-mL sample, and to 16.3 mmo/L in the 1-mL sample. The mean anion gap increased significantly from 16.7 in the 10-mL sample to 17.5 in the 3-mL sample, and to 19.1 in the 1-mL sample. Venting of Vacutainer tubes did not significantly affect these values.

Conclusion.—Underfill of 10-mL Vacutainer tubes results in a significant decline in bicarbonate levels and an increase in the anion gap that may be mistaken for a metabolic acidosis. To correct for these effects, bicarbonate should be increased by .5 to .6 mmo1/L and the anion gap decreased by .2 to .3 mmo1/L for each milliliter of air above the sample in a 10-mL Vacutainer tube. Simply venting the underfilled tubes does not correct the defect. To avoid these effects, all tubes should be completely filled, or small blood samples should be collected in smaller tubes.

▶ The authors elaborately demonstrate a potential source of laboratory error. Despite the findings of the authors, I have never known pseudo-metabolic acidosis caused by underfill to be a clinically significant problem that interferes with the emergent management of ill and injured patients.—E.J. Reisdorff, M.D.

Emergency Department Stat Test Turnaround Times: A College of American Pathologists' Q-Probes Study for Potassium and Hemoglobin

Howanitz PJ, Steindel SJ, Cembrowski GS, Long TA (Univ of California, Los Angeles; Automated Design Systems Inc, Atlanta, Ga; Park Nicolett Med Ctr, Minneapolis, Minn; College of American Pathologists, Northfield, Ill)

Arch Pathol Lab Med 116:122–128, 1992 5–33

Background.—Although stat laboratory testing makes up a high percentage of the work load in the clinical laboratory and is usually required by very ill patients, there have been few studies of turnaround times (TATs) for these tests. Turnaround times for stat tests of potassium and hemoglobin in patients in the emergency department were studied, from phlebotomy to reporting of results.

Methods.—The study was part of the College of American Pathologists' Q-Probes program, which included 722 institutions at the time of the current study. Program participants collected 1 specimen per shift per day for a 4-week period. Thus, data on a total of 28 specimens per shift were analyzed, for a total of 39,105 potassium and 42, 922 hemoglobin specimens.

Findings.—Median TATs were 35 minutes for potassium and 25 minutes for hemoglobin. There was no significant variation by shift, weekday, or weekend. Significant factors affecting TATs included the type of personnel collecting the specimen, method of transport to the laboratory, specimen type, and estimate of transit time. About one third of the total TAT was specimen transit time; however, for couriers transporting hemoglobin specimens, the median transit time was equivalent to the median intralaboratory test TAT.

Discussion.—Turnaround times for stat potassium and hemoglobin tests are examined. Median TATs do not appear to vary by shift. The intralaboratory TAT is quickest in emergency department laboratories. Specimen transport is fastest when done by clinical staff, followed by mechanical transport systems and couriers; transport times are quickest in smaller institutions. Laboratory phlebotomists are associated with the quickest TATs.

▶ No surprises here. This is good information to have available when competing for good laboratory services.—E. Ruiz, M.D.

Rapid Quantitative Determination of Blood Alcohol Concentration in the Emergency Department Using an Electrochemical Method

Wax PM, Hoffman RS, Goldfrank LR (Bellevue Hosp Ctr, NY; New York City Poison Control Ctr)

Ann Emerg Med 21:254–259, 1992 5–34

Background.—The rapid determination of blood alcohol concentration (BAC) may facilitate the initial assessment of patients coming to the emergency department with altered mental status and suspected ethanol intoxication. The accuracy and reliability of measuring BAC with an alcohol meter developed by MediSense were tested.

Methods.—Three hundred eighty-three consecutive patients with altered mental status or suspected alcohol intoxication in the emergency department of a municipal hospital were enrolled in the prospective study. Meter data were compared with immunoassay and gas chromatography criterion standards. The alcohol meter performs an electrochemical quantitative assay of alcohol on venous or capillary blook within 60 seconds.

Results.—Sixty percent of the patients had a detectable BAC by both meter and immunoassay. Meter BAC measurements correlated highly with immunoassay and gas chromatography determinations.

Conclusions.—The MediSense alcohol meter provides rapid, reliable bedside BAC determinations. Unlike other rapid methods that are limited to measuring ethanol in the breath or saliva, this device assays actual blood alcohol levels. In initial resuscitation of patients with altered mental status, the use of this device may provide valuable information and help guide early diagnosis and treatment interventions.

▶ Patients with subdural hematomas are often intoxicated.—J. Wasserberger, M.D.

Lipase/Amylase Ratio: A New Index That Distinguishes Acute Episodes of Alcoholic From Nonalcoholic Acute Pancreatitis

Gumaste VV, Dave PB, Weissman D, Messer J (Mount Sinai Services–City Hosp Ctr at Elmhurst, NY; Mount Sinai School of Medicine, City Univ of New York)

Gastroenterology 101:1361–1366, 1991 5–35

Background.—Prompted by observations that patients with acute alcoholic pancreatitis have high lipase levels and relatively low amylase levels in contrast to patients with nonalcoholic pancreatitis, a prospective study was conducted to determine whether the ratio of serum lipase to serum amylase would distinguish between episodes of alcoholic and nonalcoholic pancreatitis.

Study Design.—In phase 1, 30 patients with acute pancreatitis were divided into 2 groups: group A included 20 patients in whom the etiology of the pancreatitis was alcohol, and group B consisted of 10 patients with nonalcoholic pancreatitis, mainly due to gallstones. Patients with renal failure were excluded. Serum lipase and serum amylase levels were measured on admission. The lipase/amylase (L/A) ratio was calculated by using the amylase and lipase levels expressed as multiples of the upper limit of normal in each patient. The L/A ratios were then applied prospectively in phase 2, which included an unselected population of 21 consecutive patients with acute pancreatitis.

Findings.—Initial amylase values ranged from 104 to 2,985 units/L (median, 331 in group A and from 423 to 13,000 units/L (median, 1,187) in group B. The differences were significant, but there was considerable overlap in the values between the 2 groups. Serum lipase levels did not differ significantly between groups and ranged from 492 to 25,706 units/L (median, 3,433) in group A and from 711 to 31,153 units/L (median, 1,260) in group B. The L/A ratio ranged from 2.2 to 14.8 (median, 4.65) in group A and from 0.31 to 1.93 (median, 0.92) in group B; the differences were significant.

When applied prospectively in 21 patients with acute pancreatitis, an L/A ratio greater than 2 was observed in 11 of 13 patients with pancreatitis caused by alcohol abuse, whereas only 1 of 8 patients with an L/A ratio of less than 2 had acute alcoholic pancreatitis; these differences were significant. An L/A ratio greater than 2 as an indication of alcoholic pancreatitis had a sensitivity of 91%, a specificity of 78%, and a positive predictive value of 85%.

Conclusion.—The L/A ratio, calculated from serum amylase and lipase levels at initial presentation, appears to be a promising discriminatory index between alcoholic and nonalcoholic pancreatitis.

▶ The diagnosis of pancreatitis in this study was based upon clinical features, amylase levels, and pancreatic-imaging methods (ultrasound and/or abdominal CT). The diagnosis of biliary disease was confirmed in a similar fashion. Does the measurement of an L/A ratio add to our diagnostic regimen? Although this study reports an interesting observation, it is unlikely to alter current evaluation methods or therapy.—J.T. Niemann, M.D.

How Does Computer-Aided Diagnosis Improve the Management of Acute Abdominal Pain?

Wellwood J, Johannessen S, Spiegelhalter DJ (Whipps Cross Hosp, London; MRC Biostatistics Univ, Cambridge, England)

Ann R Coll Surg Engl 74:40–46, 1992 5–36

Background.—Diagnosis and management of acute abdominal pain have been improved by the use of standardized data forms and computer-aided diagnosis. However, there is disagreement as to how these benefits are gained. Data were analyzed on 5,193 patients from 1 hospital to address this controversy.

Methods.—Data were gathered during several years and included patients with acute abdominal pain who were treated by 1 of 40 senior house officers in the hospital accident and emergency department. At various times during the data collection period, these physicians standardized data collection forms with or without computer assistance or used neither diagnostic aid. A final or discharge diagnosis was obtained in each case after surgery or at discharge.

Findings.—The final diagnosis was nonspecific abdominal pain (NSAP) in 70% of the cases and appendicitis in 6%. Fifteen percent of patients had diagnoses that the computer could not have diagnosed correctly. Compliance was 65% for data collection forms and 50% for computer use. The computer's diagnostic reliability was less than 50% for any diagnosis other than NSAP. Only 74% of diagnoses of which the computer was 99% certain were correct. The overall accuracy increased from 48% with no decision aids to 69% with both decision aids and performance feedback; most of this was a result of NSAP being diagnosed in place of no diagnosis. Forty-three percent of the patients were admitted when diagnostic aids were not available vs. 34% when all aids were available. A decrease in operations resulted from decreased admission of patients with NSAP.

Conclusions.—The main benefit of diagnostic aids seems to be early and accurate diagnosis of NSAP, which in turn decreases admissions and the number of negative surgical explorations. Junior physicians should record clinical data about these patients on structured data forms and be encouraged to establish an early positive diagnosis before making decisions about patient management. Recent advances in computer hardware and software may soon provide further benefits of computer-aided diagnosis in the emergency department.

▶ What does an accurate diagnosis of NSAP mean? I think it means that there is a lack of a diagnosis. Can that term be accurate? It is good that the abdominal examination is being subjected to scrutiny and computerization, but I think this is a classic case of garbage in, garbage out.—E. Ruiz, M.D.

The Effect of the Treatment Setting on the Decision-Making Process: Acute Care Hospitals and Emergency Services

Weiss EC

Law Med Health Care 19:66–68, 1991 5–37

Background.—Acute-care hospitals and emergency services may have a twofold obligation to treat patients. First, they may be obligated to offer treatment and second, the health care professional may have an independent obligation to treat. These obligations, including the effects of the Cruzan decision, are examined.

Obligation to Treat and the Cruzan Decision.—Recently, the rights of private hospitals and physicians to refuse to treat patients have been limited. The multitude of complex payment systems also raises concerns about the appropriateness of care, and physicians may "overtreat" by way of protecting themselves from lawsuit. In the Cruzan decision, the U.S. Supreme Court found that an incompetent patient's refusal of treatment must be "clear and convincing."

Possible Outcomes.—The implications of this decision must be worked out on a case-by-case basis, but it could result in deterioration of the decision-making process. Generally, emergency treatment is not withheld until a surrogate consent or court order is obtained. On the other hand, if health care professionals believe that they are obligated to treat, they may refuse to discuss options with the patient or surrogate. If the surrogate has to go to court before treatment is withdrawn, the patient's interests are sacrificed for the protection of the hospital, and the court is forced to make a decision for which it is ill-equipped. Alternatively, health care professionals may decide not to begin treatment for fear that they will be unable to stop later. Thus, some patients would be denied potentially beneficial care. Likewise, patients and family may be resistant to hospitalization for fear that the physician or hospital will be unwilling to stop treatment later. All of these possible outcomes conflict with medical ethics and respect for patient autonomy.

Discussion.—The Cruzan decision should promote consideration of treatment preferences and encourage communication within the family and between the patient and physician. Individuals should consider these issues and communicate their wishes. Hospitals should understand the decisions that apply to them and form an institutional consensus on handling withdrawal of treatment.

► In the Cruzon decision, the U.S. Supreme Court upheld the Missouri Supreme Court's decision to deny the parents' request for termination of gastric tube feedings for a woman who had spent many years in a persistent vegitative state following traumatic cardiac arrest. The ruling held that "clear and convincing" evidence of the patient's own wishes was lacking. The court did not rule that withdrawal of feedings is *per se* not permissible.

The lesson from this tragic story is that *everyone* should have living wills or advance directives prepared to guide treatment if the person becomes unable to communicate following a medical catastrophe. This applies to healthy, young emergency physicians as well as "patients."

But in the absence of such directives, what do we do? The author expresses a number of concerns summarized in the abstract above. These include a reluctance of health care providers to discuss the issue with the patient's family, as well as a reluctance of providers or family members to initiate treatment that may be difficult to discontinue at a later time.

While one may debate whether these particular concerns influence initial resuscitative efforts in the emergency department, there can be no doubt that we are often placed in a difficult situation where we must make decisions regarding discontinuation or resuscitation despite having insufficient information about the patient's or family's wishes.

The author suggests that physicians, hospital personel, and families all be involved in such decisions, if possible, in an effort to apply the appropriate level of medical care. One can hardly disagree.—M.J. Bresler, M.D.

Rebound Tenderness Test

Liddington MI, Thomson WHF (Gloucestershire Royal Hosp, Gloucester, England)

Br J Surg 78:795–796, 1991 5–38

Background.—The rebound tenderness test (RTT) in the diagnosis of acute abdominal pain is performed by gradually increasing the pressure of the palpating hand over the tender spot and then suddenly removing it. A start of pain indicates a positive test and generally indicates a strong likelihood of peritonitis. Theoretically the test is of doubtful value because it may only indicate simple tenderness to abdominal palpation, which may have many causes. The usefulness of the RTT in indicating peritonitis was prospectively assessed.

Methods.—The RTT was performed on 142 unselected patients admitted on our emergency basis with abdominal pain and tenderness. The initial RTT result and the final diagnosis were recorded in each case.

Findings.—Eighty-eight patients had a positive RTT, and 43 of those had a final diagnosis of peritonitis. Forty-five patients had no peritonitis. Of the 54 patients with a negative RTT, 10 had peritonitis, and 44 did not.

Conclusions.—Teaching and practice of the RTT is not supported. The test has reasonably good sensitivity but low specificity. The positive predictive value was only 49%. In agreement with the findings of Prout and others, a demonstration of rebound tenderness has the disadvantage of being unpleasant to the patient and diagnostically useless.

▶ Rebound tenderness in the abdominal examination is a wonderful finding, if present. It is not a reliable test. Rebound should be tested for, but the absence of rebound does not exclude a serious problem. It is only one test in a battery of many that can aid in making a diagnosis.—S.B. Repasky, D.O.

Orthostatic Vital Signs: Variation With Age, Specificity, and Sensitivity in Detecting a 450-mL Blood Loss

Baraff LJ, Schriger DL (Univ of California, Los Angeles)

Am J Emerg Med 10:99–103, 1992 — 5–39

Introduction.—Although changes in orthostatic vital signs are used to assess syncope or possible hypovolemia, there have been no rigorous studies of normal values in elderly patients. The association between orthostatic vital sign changes and age in adults was studied.

Methods.—The sample consisted of 100 healthy blood donors and 100 ambulatory, self-sufficient individuals from a senior citizens' daytime activity center. The only exclusion criterion was a history of orthostatic hypotension. Each person underwent measurement of pulse and blood pressure after 1 minute in the recumbent position and again, in the same arm, 30 seconds after standing up. The same measurements were repeated after blood donation in the donors, who served as their own controls.

Findings.—The pulse increased by a mean of 2 beats per minute (bpm), systolic blood pressure decreased by 3 mm Hg, and diastolic blood pressure increased by 1 mm Hg. No clinically significant variations in orthostatic blood pressure change with age were noted. The most sensitive orthostatic vital sign used alone at a given specificity was an increase in pulse, a rise of more than 20 bpm having a sensitivity of 9% and a specificity of 98%. The sensitivity was improved with a minor loss in specificity by the addition of diastolic blood pressure change; the sensitivity was 17%, and the specificity was 98% with a pulse rise of more than 20 bpm or a diastolic blood pressure decrease of more than 10 mm Hg. No improvement in sensitivity was noted with the addition of systolic blood pressure change.

Conclusions.—Age does not appear to be related to any important difference in orthostatic changes in vital signs. At a specificity of 95% or higher, no combination of changes was sufficiently sensitive to detect a 450-ml blood loss. Individual clinicians should choose the definition of abnormal orthostatic signs that fulfills their desired level of sensitivity and specificity.

▶ This is really two different studies, one examining orthostatic vital signs before and after blood donation in adults of all ages and one examining orthostatic vital signs in the ambulatory elderly.

These data are helpful. They debunk a lot of the mythology surrounding orthostatic vital signs by showing that the "tilt test" is not nearly so useful in detecting blood loss as most of us were taught to believe during our residencies and that the average well elderly person is no more likely than his juniors to become orthostatic. We may conclude from this study that large changes in orthostatic vital signs in general are specific, but not sensitive for significant blood loss, i.e., a very positive tilt test is highly suggestive of blood loss, a negative one does not rule it out, and most patients with this degree of blood loss will fall into the gray zone in between.—J. Schoffstall, M.D.

Capillary Refill: Is It a Useful Predictor of Hypovolemic States?
Schriger DL, Baraff LJ (Univ of California, Los Angeles)
Ann Emerg Med 20:601–605, 1991 5–40

Introduction.—Capillary refill was introduced into clinical practice as part of the Trauma Score and life support courses before the test was subjected to experimental validation. Previous studies have shown that capillary refill varies with age, sex, and temperature. Capillary refill was measured to evaluate whether the test can correctly differentiate between hypovolemia and euvolemia in an emergency department (ED) setting.

Methods.—The first group included 47 volunteer blood donors aged 19 to 83 years. The second group included 32 ED patients who had a history consistent with hypovolemia and either a systolic blood pressure of less than 90 mm Hg (13 patients) or abnormal orthostatic vital signs (19 patients). Capillary refill was measured in donors before and after a 450-mL blood donation; the patients were tested before rehydration.

Results.—Blood donors had a mean capillary refill time of 1.4 seconds before donation and 1.1 seconds after donation. The mean capillary refill time was 2.8 seconds for the hypotensive group and 1.9 seconds for the orthostatic group. The sensitivity of the test in identifying hypovolemic patients, when scored with age- and sex-specific upper limits of normal, was 6% after donation, 46% for the hypotensive group, and 26% for the orthostatic group. Orthostatic vital signs were more sensitive and specific than capillary refill in detecting the 450-mL blood loss.

Conclusion.—Although capillary refill is not included in the Revised Trauma Score, the test continues to be taught in life support courses. The performance of capillary refill is inadequate to warrant its routine use in ED or pre-hospital settings as a method of detecting mild-to-moderate hypovolemia.

▶ It is always interesting to read an article that challenges a widely held belief and makes the reader think about and question something he has always taken for granted as being absolutely true. This article certainly accomplishes that very thing. But old habits are hard to break. We must emphasize that capillary refill by itself in adults is poorly reliable and that our time is better spent carefully determining blood pressures and pulse rates. However, capillary refill appears to be more useful in evaluating children.—E.J. Lucid, M.D.

Re-evaluation of the Tympanic Thermometer in the Emergency Department

Stewart JV, Webster D (Silver Cross Hosp, Joliet, Ill; Olympia Fields Osteopathic Med Ctr, Olympia Fields, Ill)

Ann Emerg Med 21:158–161, 1992 5–41

Introduction.—The accuracy of the infrared tympanic thermometer has been questioned recently. To investigate further, a study was designed to compare tympanic temperature with the conventional standard of rectal temperature.

Methods.—The study included 79 children, aged 3 weeks to 5 years who came to the emergency department. Rectal temperature was recorded with an electronic digital thermometer, followed by measurement of tympanic temperature with a commonly used portable infrared tympanic thermometer, First Temp. The latter was set to the core equivalency setting.

Results.—The mean tympanic temperature was 38.5°C, and the mean rectal temperature was 38.8°C. There was a highly significant correlation between tympanic and rectal temperatures. However, for patients younger than 3 months, the correlation coefficient was significantly weaker when compared with older patients. If fever is defined as a rectal temperature more than 38.0°C, the tympanic thermometer had a sensitivity of 96.6%, a specificity of 100%, a positive predictive value of 100%, and a negative predictive value of 90.1%. For patients older than 3 months, the values were 100% in all categories.

Conclusion.—The First Temp infrared tympanic thermometer accurately detects fever in pediatric patients older than 3 months, but results are inconclusive in children younger than 3 months.

▶ The use of tympanic thermometers in the emergency department has recently been challenged. Those studies that call the accuracy of tympanic thermometry into question have slight study flaws. This study is rather well designed and demonstrates both the accuracy and utility of infrared tympanic thermometry in patients older than 3 months of age.—E. J. Reisdorff, M.D.

6 Emergency Medical Education/Wellness

Emergency Medicine's Role in the Education of Medical Students: Directions for Change

Burdick WP (Med College of Pennsylvania, Philadelphia)

Ann Emerg Med 20:688–691, 1991 6–1

Introduction.—Because emergency medicine is a young field with an emphasis on basic clinical skills, educators in the field of emergency medicine are in a unique position to be in the forefront of the changes that are taking place in traditional undergraduate medical education. Teaching emergency medicine to undergraduate medical students should not concentrate only on those who choose to enter the field but should enable all graduating medical students to have the necessary clinical skills, including motor skills, to be able to provide immediate aid to prevent the loss of life. Fundamental goals in teaching emergency medicine to medical students were identified and recommendations made for change.

Goals.—The 6 fundamental goals in teaching emergency medicine to undergraduate medical students are the ability to provide immediate aid, identification of problems, the differential diagnosis and treatment of specific entities, understanding of societal issues as they relate to emergency care, and mastery of essential motor skills such as the control of bleeding, intravenous cannulation and infusion of saline and colloids, and needle or tube thoracostomy. In addition, the graduating student should be able to use data base resources, select appropriate specialties for consultation, work as a member of a health care team, and use time- and cost-efficient diagnostic modalities.

Recommendations.—The emergency medicine faculty must incorporate the goals of its institution into their courses by offering its services as preceptors, small group leaders, or lecturers. Educational techniques should be selected according to the subject at hand. For instance, prepackaged courses are most suitable for teaching the skills required for providing immediate aid, whereas problem-based learning may be a better approach to teaching how to work as a team or how to acquire the necessary information for solving a clinical problem at hand.

Conclusions.—Using educational methods creatively will improve undergraduate education in emergency medicine, as well as enhance emergency medicine's role in the overall undergraduate program.

▶ The author supports a problem-based approach to medical education. Conceptually, this provides the basis for curricular development based upon the actual clinical practice of medicine. When this occurs, emergency medicine is remarkably positioned to provide major input into such educational efforts. It is not an opportunity to be missed, and the author most appropriately indentifies the means by which emergency medicine can become a cornerstone of undergraduate medical education.—D.K. Wagner, M.D.

A Study of Occupational Stress and Depression Among Emergency Physicians

Gallery ME, Whitley TW, Klonis LK, Anzinger RK, Revicki DA (American College of Emergency Physicians, Dallas; Univ of Texas, Dallas; East Carolina Univ, Greenville, NC; Battelle Med Technology Assessment and Policy Research Ctr, Washington, DC)

Ann Emerg Med 21:58–64, 1992 6–2

Background.—In an early landmark study of residency-trained emergency physicians, Anwar attempted to measure "career commitment," but she did not specifically address attrition or "burnout." The levels of stress and depression among emergency physicians and whether these variables were related to the emergency physician's decision to leave the specialty were examined.

Methods.—The variable of fellowship in the American College of Emergency Physicians (ACEP) was used as a stratifying variable for a random sample of 1,350 emergency physicians. The questionnaire was based on locus of control, Work-Related Strain Inventory, Center for Epidemiologic Studies-Depression Scale, and other measures.

Findings.—In 763 usable surveys (56.5%), the mean scores for locus of control, Work-Related Strain Inventory, and Center for Epidemiologic Studies–Depression Scale were within normal ranges. However, a disproportionate number scored more than 2 SD from the mean vs. an expected distribution of 2.5% of the population. The scores of ACEP fellows and nonfellows differed on the work satisfaction scale but not on the locus of control, stress, or depression scales. The physicians most likely to leave the specialty over the next 10 years were older men, women, and those with high levels of stress and low job satisfaction.

Conclusions.—Although most emergency physicians reported normal levels of stress, a disproportionate number reported high levels of stress, tension, and depressive symptomatology and had plans to leave the specialty of emergency medicine. The number of physicians leaving appears to be greater than the number that will be replaced by residency training.

► This study addresses one of the sad truths of emergency medicine. More emergency physicians are leaving the specialty than are entering it despite the fact that more are needed every year. It would be nice to have a review of the factors that led to this trend. The major factors seem to be a lack of control over the practice, decreasing reimbursement, increasing liability risk, increasing legislation that restricts practice while increasing liability, and the dumping of noninsured patients on the emergency departments from all other specialties. Emergency physicians should be more aggressive in combating these problems. Unfortunately, at the present time, things are just getting worse. (See also Abstract 6–3.)—G.J. Ordog, M.D.

Work-Related Stress and Depression Among Physicians Pursuing Postgraduate Training in Emergency Medicine: An International Study

Whitley TW, Allison EJ Jr, Gallery ME, Heyworth J, Cockington RA, Gaudry P, Revicki DA (East Carolina Univ, Greenville, NC; American College of Emergency Physicians, Dallas, Tex; Queen Alexandra Hosp, Cosham, England; Australasian Society for Emergency Medicine, St Leonards, Australia; Battelle Human Affairs Research Ctrs, Washington, DC)

Ann Emerg Med 20:992–996, 1991 6–3

Background.—There is increasing interest in the work-related stresses perceived by physicians who pursue postgraduate training. Rotations in emergency departments reportedly are seen as stressful.

Objective.—Perceived levels of work-related stress and depression were examined in a cross-sectional mail survey of physicians in training in the United States, the United Kingdom, and Australasia. Respondents included 488 residents in the first 3 years of training in the United States, 365 senior house officers in the United Kingdom, and 82 basic and advanced trainees from Australasia.

Findings.—Respondents from the United Kingdom reported significantly more stress than those from the United States. Women reported significantly higher levels of stress than men. Trainees in the United States were more depressed than those from the United Kingdom or Australasia. Depression was more prominent in women than in men and in unmarried vs. married respondents.

Implication.—Women and all unmarried physicians pursuing postgraduate training in emergency medicine are especially at risk of experiencing high levels of work-related stress and symptoms of depression.

► This is an important study that specifically looks at emergency medicine house staff. The inclusion of data from the United Kingdom and Australia gives it an interesting twist. The conclusions emphasizing that female and unmarried physicians-in-training are more likely to experience higher levels of work-related stress and more frequent symptoms of depression are well stated, and this concept needs to be kept in mind for those who are faculty in residency programs or have contact with residents in the emergency department (ED).

Emergency physicians must be prepared to cope with the stress of day-to-day work in the ED; we all know what a strain it can be.—J.J. Kelly, D.O., F.A.C.E.P.

Autonomous Departments of Emergency Medicine in Contemporary Academic Medical Centers

Rusnak RA, Hamilton GC, Allison EJ Jr (Hennepin County Med Ctr, Minneapolis, Minn; Wright State Univ, Dayton, Ohio; East Carolina Univ, Greenville, NC)

Ann Emerg Med 20:680–687, 1991 6–4

Introduction.—With the approval of primary board certification for emergency medicine, the specialty has been recognized as an important area in modern medicine in the United States. The next step is a concentrated effort to establish autonomous academic departments of emergency medicine in U.S. medical schools. Issues related to seeking and achieving autonomous status for the emergency medicine department were examined.

Discussion.—Twenty autonomous emergency medicine departments currently exist in U.S. medical schools. Most of them achieved this status mainly through unplanned occurrences, for example, the salvage of a department with clinical service problems. More recently, it has been recognized that a more systematic approach is needed to establish the place of emergency medicine in academia. Two types of work are needed to accomplish the task: work within the residency program and work between the program and the medical school. Within the program, departments seeking autonomous status should devote faculty resources to worthwhile research projects, including protected time for these projects. These programs also need to develop their expertise in competing for extramural funding and to initiate intramural research programs to teach faculty members the basics of grantsmanship. Emergency medicine faculty members should also be involved in teaching health care issues in ambulatory medicine. Outside the department, faculty members must take part in interdisciplinary teaching programs and curriculum development. Preserving the commitment to 24-hour emergency department coverage demonstrates the program's commitment to excellence. Faculty should also work to create university-based programs that originate within the emergency department. It should be the program director's responsibility to acquaint the medical school dean with the advantages of an autonomous emergency medicine department. This person must seek other relationships as well to gauge support and opposition to autonomous status. By serving on committees, the program director can meet other faculty members, solve problems, and create trust, along with broad-based support for autonomous status both inside and outside the university.

Conclusions.—Emergency medicine must cultivate a more deliberate approach to achieving autonomous status in U.S. medical schools. This is the only way to ensure its continued growth in the years to come.

▶ This is a key article for those in academic emergency medicine, but also one with broader application to all emergency physicians. Ingredients to success are to deliver quality care and to demonstrate added value to your institution/hospital by stepping eagerly beyond the bounds of the emergency department. All emergency physicians, particularly academic faculty, can receive enormous return for teaching and committee activities outside their usual territory. The poor choice is to remain "those people down in the emergency *room*." (See also Abstract 6–5.)—R.M. McNamara, M.D.

Meeting the Goals of Academia: Characteristics of Emergency Medicine Faculty Academic Work Styles

Meislin HW, Spaite DW, Valenzuela TD (Univ of Arizona, Tucson)

Ann Emerg Med 21:298–302, 1992 6–5

Background.—Faculty members in emergency medicine training programs are responsible for 24-hour coverage of the emergency department in addition to their research, administrative, and teaching responsibilities. No studies have addressed how these faculty members fulfill their clinical responsibilities at the same time they pursue academic advancement. The ideal and actual work styles of emergency medicine faculty members were compared according to professorial rank, administrative title, and/or tenure vs. clinical track.

Methods.—A survey was sent to the 83 emergency medicine residency programs approved by the Accreditation Council for Graduate Medical Education. Program directors were asked to describe the actual and ideal

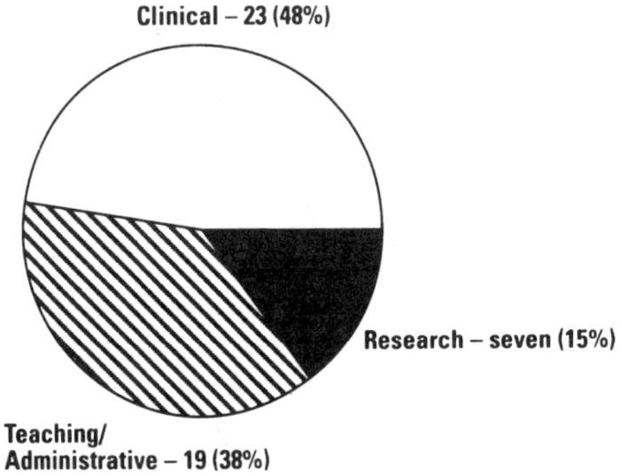

Fig 6–1.—Weekly mean hours (percent of total). (Courtesy of Meislin HW, Spaite DW, Valenzuela TD: *Ann Emerg Med* 21:298-302, 1992.)

academic work styles of their faculty, including the total number of weekly hours and how they broke down into clinical, research, and administrative or teaching time. Usable responses were submitted by 93% of the programs.

Findings.—The average program had 11 full-time and 4 part-time faculty members, who worked an average of 44 to 51 hr/wk. Clinical work accounted for a mean of 23 hr/wk and for 48% of the total work week. Administrative and teaching responsibilities accounted for a mean of 19 hr/wk and 38% of the total. Research time averaged 7 hr/wk, or 15% of the total (Fig 6–1). Clinical hours were fewer for physicians with greater administrative work loads and those with higher professorial ranks. The ideal work week was 40 to 42 hours but was quite similar to the actual work week, although with somewhat less administrative time.

Conclusions.—Emergency medicine programs appear to meet the demands placed on faculty members by increasing the number of faculty, varying responsibilities according to rank and title, and shortening the work week. These approaches appear to work quite well because the actual and ideal work situations are similar. Very little time appears to be available for research.

▶ Emergency physicians may work slightly fewer total hours than other academic physicians, but some of this time is spent on evening and night shifts, which require additional recovery time that goes uncounted. It appears from this study that senior faculty members trade less clinical time for more administrative teaching time but conserve research time. I wish we could all trade administrative for research time, which remains too low.—T. Stair, M.D.

Descriptive Analysis of Residency-Trained Emergency Medicine Physicians

Wakeman MA, Hall KN, Levy RC (Univ of Kansas Med Ctr, Kansas City; Univ of Cincinnati Med Ctr, Ohio)

J Emerg Med 9:379–384, 1991 6–6

Objective.—The emergency medicine residency program is relatively young, and there is little known about the career patterns of graduates in this specialty. Emergency medicine residency graduates between 1978 and 1982 were surveyed to analyze the demographics, practice characteristics, and job satisfaction in this specialty.

Subjects.—A questionnaire that covered personal and practice characteristics, training background, and career and training satisfaction was mailed to 858 physicians; 539 (62.8%) usable questionnaires were returned. The mean age of the respondents was 40.4 years, and 87.8% were men. Almost 94% achieved board certification in emergency medicine.

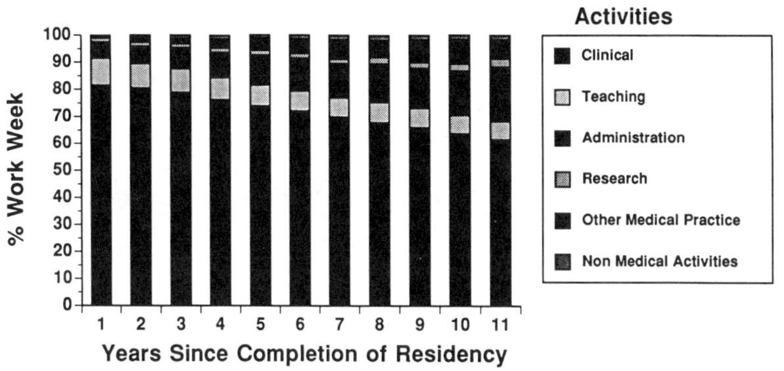

Fig 6–2.—Breakdown of work activities by years in practice. (Courtesy of Wakeman MA, Hall KN, Levy RC: *J Emerg Med* 9:379–384, 1991.)

Data Analysis.—The majority (87%) of respondents still practiced emergency medicine. The average number of hours worked per week was 49.8 hours, primarily in clinical practice. The percentage of time devoted to clinical work and teaching decreased each year after graduation, whereas the percentage of time spent in administrative duties increased steadily each year (Fig 6–2). The employment status varied widely, but the majority (62.5%) practiced in urban settings, particularly in states where emergency medicine residencies were located.

The majority of the respondents were satisfied or very satisfied with their choice of a career in emergency medicine and with the quality of their residency training. The most commonly cited strength of the training program was diversity of clinical experiences, while a significant weakness of the training program, according to 22.9% of respondents, was a lack of preparation for administrative duties.

Summary.—A majority of the emergency medicine residency graduates remain in clinical practice, although administrative tasks increased rapidly after graduation. When compared with graduates from 1972 to 1980, a lower percentage of graduates from 1978 to 1982 are involved in teaching and research. The increase in administrative functions and the lack of preparation for administrative responsibilities argue for greater emphasis in this area during residency training.

▶ There is considerable current talk and press regarding "burnout" in the specialty of emergency medicine. This study would tend to indicate that most (87.8%) of those physicians (n = 539) in this sample who completed training in 1978 through 1982 (5 years) were satisfied with practicing this chosen specialty. What is needed is a broad study across all specialties over a period of years to achieve a reliable comparison. The concern for the lack of administrative training in a residency of emergency medicine is understandable. How much of this can be taught? I would suspect that most of the founding fathers and leaders of emergency medicine like myself were trained on the job through the experience of learning from our mistakes.—G.V. Anderson, M.D.

Factors Associated With Career Longevity in Residency-Trained Emergency Physicians

Hall KN, Wakeman MA, Levy RC, Khoury J (Univ of Kansas, Kansas City; Univ of Cincinnati, Ohio)

Ann Emerg Med 21:291–297, 1992 6–7

Background.—The high level of stress associated with emergency medicine has led to speculation about physicians' ability to maintain a practice in this specialty over an entire career. The "survival rate" of residency-trained emergency physicians was studied, including a comparison of those who left the specialty with those who stayed.

Methods.—A questionnaire was sent to 858 physicians who had graduated from 46 accredited emergency medicine training programs from 1978 to 1982. Another survey was sent 6 weeks later to those who did not respond to the first mailing. A subgroup of nonrespondents was interviewed and compared with respondents on 5 variables. Physicians who did and did not leave the practice of emergency medicine were compared in terms of personal and professional demographics, career satisfaction, and satisfaction with training.

Results.—The response rate was 62.8%. The subgroup of nonrespondents studied showed no statistical differences from the respondents. The actuarial 10-year survival rate was 84.1%, with attrition continuing at a stable rate throughout the study period. A comparison showed that physicians who had left emergency medicine were less likely to have achieved board certification in emergency medicine and more likely to

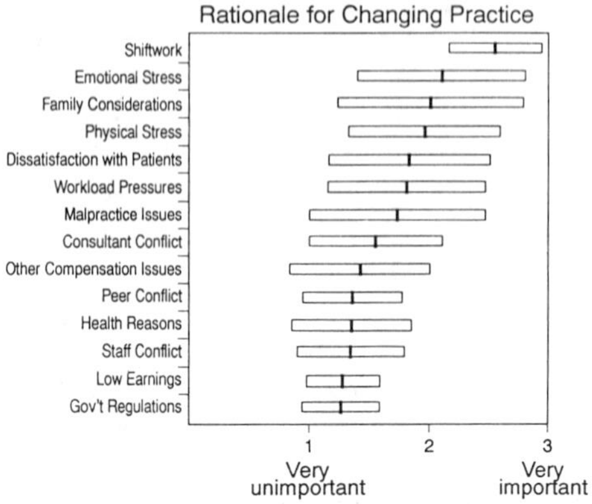

Fig 6–3.—Rating of reasons respondents left emergency medicine. These variables were rated on a 3-point scale. Hash marks indicate the mean of the answers, and length of the bars indicates ± SD. (Courtesy of Hall KN, Wakeman MA, Levy RC, et al: *Ann Emerg Med* 21:291–297, 1992.)

have achieved it in another field, less likely to work with emergency department residents in their practice, and more likely to have an annual gross income less than $100,000 per year. Those who left most often cited shift work, emotional and physical stress, and family considerations as the most important reasons (Fig 6–3). Those who left were less likely to report satisfaction with their initial choice of specialty, but the 2 groups were no different in their satisfaction with the quality of emergency medicine residency training.

Conclusions.—Residency-trained emergency physicians who work with residents, make more money, express satisfaction with their choice of specialty, and are board-certified in the field are less likely to leave this area of practice. The survival rate for these physicians appears to be higher than previously estimated.

▶ Emergency medicine residencies graduate just enough physicians to offset attrition, but not yet enough to make headway against the shortage of trained emergency physicians. Most leave the emergency department for jobs in primary-care clinics or urgent-care centers. Those who undertake additional specialty training gravitate to occupational medicine or the other hospital-based specialties of anesthesiology or radiology.—T. Stair, M.D.

Impact of an Emergency Medicine Residency Program on the Quality of Care in an Urban Community Hospital Emergency Department

McNamara RM, Kelly JJ (Medical College of Pennsylvania, Philadelphia)

Ann Emerg Med 21:528–533, 1992 6–8

Purpose.—Quality of care in the emergency department (ED) may be compromised by staff physicians who are not well trained in emergency care. No studies have addressed the effect of emergency medicine residency training on the quality of care. This issue was examined in an urban community hospital in which an emergency medicine residency program was introduced.

Methods.—The residency program took over ED coverage from non-residency-trained emergency physicians employed by a regional contract group. The retrospective analysis included ED encounters for a 3-month period 6 months before and for a 3-month period 6 months after institution of the residency program. The patients all had 1 of 5 common complaints: nontraumatic chest pain in a patient 30 years of age or older, lower abdominal pain in a 15- to 40-year-old woman, recent head trauma, headache of nontraumatic origin, and extremity laceration. Quality of care was measured by the frequency with which explicit criteria relating to these problems, including elements of the history and physical examination and diagnostic evaluations, were documented by the physician. Lists of criteria were assembled from the literature, including clinical policy guidelines.

Results.—For each problem, documentation in most areas was significantly better during the residency period. In no area did documentation decrease during the residency period. In the residency period, the emergency physicians were significantly more likely to order an ECG when indicated by the clinical policy guideline and not to order it when not indicated.

Conclusions.—Institution of an emergency medicine residency training program appears to improve the quality of care in the ED, as measured by documentation in the medical record. The number and geographic distribution of emergency medicine residency programs should be increased to encourage more widespread placement of residency-trained emergency physicians.

▶ This article examines only the process of care, not its outcome, and concludes that measurements of the quality of the process of evaluating 5 common and high-risk chief complaints show that better care is delivered when an academic emergency medicine program runs the show. Being part of such an academic program, I certainly welcome that finding! The best measure of the value of medical care, of course, is not the process that produced it but its outcome: did our treatment make the patient better?

Outcome is much more difficult to measure, however. In the meantime, this article should provide some ammunition to those who are trying to establish a new academic program.—J. Schoffstall, M.D.

Appropriate Management of Chemical Dependency in Emergency Medicine Residents

Steffen PD, Dailey RH (Univ of California, San Francisco; Samuel Merritt Hosp, Oakland, Calif)

Ann Emerg Med 21:559–564, 1992 6–9

Background.—When an emergency medicine resident physician is suspected of having a chemical dependency, prompt action must be taken to ensure the best possible outcome for all involved. One approach to intervening in such a situation was described.

Management.—When a staff member, family member, or another resident raises the suspicion of chemical dependency, the program director first seeks outside assistance from specialists in the treatment of chemical dependency. The director then confronts the resident under suspicion. If that suspicion is confirmed, the resident is admitted to a 28-day chemical dependency treatment center. Re-entry into residency after treatment is accompanied by ongoing monitoring. If relapse is suspected, further treatment or modification of monitoring is appropriate. If, at any stage, the resident is uncooperative, he is placed on probation with continued observation. Sometimes the initial suspicion of chemical dependency will prove ungrounded.

Conclusions.—Although residency program accreditation requires that program directors be able to manage a chemically dependent resident appropriately, most programs do not have a formal policy for such management. Chemical dependency in an emergency medicine resident must be dealt with immediately and appropriately. Early consultation with specialists in chemical dependency treatment should aid the director in giving the resident the best chance for a successful recovery.

▶ This article discusses, in a somewhat superficial manner, the problem of chemical dependency as it relates to emergency medicine residents and proposes an algorithm for dealing with the suspected drug-dependent physician. Most program and residency directors will have to deal with this problem sooner or later, and this article is a reasonable place to start their reading on the subject.

Unfortunately, it does not discuss in sufficient detail the nuts and bolts of managing such a case, and the reader must look elsewhere for this information. It also fails to discuss the difficult, but sometimes necessary decision to discharge a resident from the program if the drug dependency proves incorrigible or if a hazard to patients is suspected.—J. Schoffstall, M.D.

Emergency Physicians and the Biomedical Industry

Sanders AB, Keim SM, Sklar D, Adams J (Society for Academic Emergency Medicine, Lansing, Mich)

Ann Emerg Med 21:556–558, 1992 6–10

Background.—Ethical conflicts can arise when physicians have relationships with the biomedical industry. Three issues for emergency physicians to consider were discussed, and guidelines were offered.

Gift Giving.—Any gift given by a member of the biomedical industry to a physician should have an educational benefit to the physician or to his patients. These include textbooks of reasonable value, drug samples, and patient educational handouts. Physicians should not accept gifts that have no intrinsic educational value, such as tickets to sporting events and expensive dinners. Gifts offered because of prescribing patterns or other physician behaviors should not be accepted. Gifts of minimal value that relate to the physician's work, such as notepads, may be accepted.

Continuing Medical Education Activities.—Support from biomedical companies for educational activities should be in the form of educational grants payable to the continuing medical education (CME) sponsor. Although commercial support must be acknowledged in printed announcements, specific products should not be referred to. Only the sponsors determine the content, quality, and scientific integrity of CME activities. Presentations must provide a balanced view of all treatment options. Commercially supported social events should not compete with the educational events.

Academic Units.—Academicians have a special responsibility to articulate potential conflicts of interest when dealing with the biomedical industry and to resolve conflicts ethically. Academic training programs should provide educational sessions for residents and students about the ethical issues involved in having a relationship with a biomedical company.

Conclusions.—Gift giving, industry support for education and research, and industry promotional activities that reward physicians can cause a conflict of interest. Clinical, educational, and research decisions should be based on scientific evidence, not commercialism. Physicians may not be aware of the undue influence that promotional materials and gift giving have on their clinical decisions.

▶ In the last few years, there has been increasing scrutiny of the relationship between physicians and businesses that sell health care products or services, and we can expect this scrutiny to continue and intensify. Gifts from these companies, whether they take the form of expensive vacations, simple lunches, subsidized CME, speakers' honoraria, or ballpoint pens, are an example of such a relationship. This is a position paper from the Ethics Committee of the Society for Academic Emergency Medicine, emergency medicine's major academic organization. It takes a middle-of-the-road position regarding the ethical issues of physicians' relationships with biomedical companies. For a different, more puritanical point of view, see Waud's recent jeremiad in the *New England Journal of Medicine* (1).

I tend to side with Waud. I feel uncomfortable taking even so much as a pen from a drug representative. When I see my patient in a Guns 'n Roses T-shirt or a Hulk Hogan baseball cap, I know who his heros are. When he sees me with a Cipro pen in my pocket, and a Tylox notepad on my desk, who will he think mine are?—J. Schoffstall, M.D.

Reference

1. Waud DR: N *Engl J Med* 327:351, 1992.

SUBSPECIALTY EMERGENCY MEDICINE

7 Pediatric Emergency Medicine

Pediatric Emergency Medical Services

Pediatric EMS Transport: Are We Treating Children in a System Designed for Adults Only?

Sacchetti A, Carraccio C, Feder M (Our Lady of Lourdes Med Ctr, Camden, NJ; Univ of Maryland, Baltimore; Thomas Jefferson Univ, Philadelphia, Pa)

Pediatr Emerg Care 8:4–8, 1992 7–1

Background.—Unlike adults, small children and infants do not need stretchers or ambulances for transportation to the emergency department (ED). To determine the impact of this difference in transportation needs, a computer model was designed to compare pediatric treatment in a traditional adult transport system and a nonambulance transport system.

Methods and Findings.—A Macintosh Classic computer was programmed to simulate the treatment of a child with acute respiratory distress needing intubation. The time to intubation (TTI) of such a child treated in a standard ambulance transport system with paramedics was compared with that of such a child taken directly to an ED in a patrolling police car. In this computer model, police transport produces shorter TTIs for brief scene-to-ED travel times or limited paramedic success rates. Paramedic intubations produced shorter TTIs for long scene-to-ED transports.

Conclusions.—In cases of long transport times to the ED and high paramedic intubation success rates, field intervention and standard ambulance transport produce shorter TTIs. When travel times are short or paramedic success rates are low, police transport of children results in more expedient intubation.

▶ In developing emergency medical services for children, there is a need for this and other studies to help with the as yet unsettled questions of "scoop and run" vs. "stay and stabilize" (I never thought "play" was an appropriate term). This paper puts some logical dimensions on the issue and has us consider factors such as the length of transport time, paramedical skill level, types of alternative transports, and special needs of children. It is an excellent model. It would be a challenge to attempt a real-life application of the findings. (See also Abstracts 7–2 and 7–3.)—S. Ludwig, M.D.

Pediatric Interhospital Critical Care Transport: Consensus of a National Leadership Conference

Day S, McCloskey K, Orr R, Bolte R, Notterman D, Hackel A (Med College of Wisconsin, Milwaukee; Univ of Alabama, Birmingham; Univ of Pittsburgh, Pa; Univ of Utah, Salt Lake City; New York Hosp-Cornell Med Ctr, New York, NY; et al)

Pediatrics 88:696–704, 1991 7–2

Background.—Although pediatric interhospital critical care transport has evolved into a distinct discipline, guidelines for pediatric patient care have never been defined. The Pediatric Transport Leadership Conference was held in March 1990. The conference was attended by physician medical directors of pediatric transport programs and by representatives from the American Academy of Pediatrics and the Association of Air Medical Services.

Discussion.—At this conference, the following topics were discussed and consensus recommendations made for the major issues in each of the areas: existing guidelines for patient transport, team composition, and transport staffing; training requirements for pediatric and nonpediatric transport teams; goals and design of a transport data base; and medical-legal issues, including responsibilities of the referring and receiving institutions. By the end of the conference, many questions had been generated that may be answered by multi-institutional studies.

▶ Emergency departments and emergency physicians often play a role in pediatric critical care interhospital transport. As guidelines and standards are developed in this area, involvement of emergency physicians is necessary to ensure that both emergency departments and transport programs benefit.

Many important questions are raised in this paper, which emphasizes the need for more focused attention in this area. When is a physician needed on transport? What level of expertise in pediatric support should be required in rural areas where pediatric emergency or critical care specialists are not found? What are the medicolegal responsibilities of the referring and receiving hospitals at various points in time? The authors are very persuasive in arguing that developing a patient classification system, educational guidelines, and a standardized data base will help answer many of these questions. Listing the specific issues that need attention should help direct research efforts in the future.

The participants in the conference suggest that a separate transport team is preferable to one that extracts its personnel and equipment from existing units. There are specific needs in the areas of education, equipment, communication, and quality assurance that are better met by a separate team. Very few emergency departments are so well staffed that doctors and nurses can be sent out on transports without adversely affecting the care delivered in the emergency department. When the emergency physician is required to consult with and accompany the transport team, it comes at the expense of the primary responsibility. Hospital administrations must be made to understand that emergency departments that assume responsibilities for interhospital transport need to receive appropriate support for these activities.—M. Joffe, M.D.

Pediatric Prehospital Care in Urban and Rural Areas

Seidel JS, Henderson DP, Ward P, Wayland BW, Ness B (Univ of California, Los Angeles, Torrance; California EMSC Project)

Pediatrics 88:681–690, 1991 7–3

Background.—There are few studies of the management of children by emergency medical services (EMS), even though children account for 10% of EMS activity. An analysis was done to gather information about the pediatric population using prehospital care services.

Methods.—Data on pediatric prehospital runs were gathered from prehospital care reports of 4 EMS agencies. The services covered both rural and urban areas in 11 California counties. A total of 10,493 runs was analyzed, 88.2% of them in urban areas and 11.4% in rural areas.

Findings.—Urban vs. rural location made little difference in the parameters analyzed. The number of EMS calls involving children increased with age; however, 12.5% of all calls were for children younger than 2 years of age. Most calls were made in late spring and early fall and during nonschool hours. Most calls made after midnight were for adolescent motor vehicle accident or assault victims. For children younger than 5 years of age, medical problems were the most common reason for calls, especially respiratory distress and seizures. In rural areas, 64% of the calls were for trauma. Different regions assessed vital signs with varying frequency, and hospital contact varied as well. However, the services rarely performed a complete assessment, including full vital signs and neurologic assessment, in young children. Although the resources were available, advanced life support was infrequently used.

Conclusions.—The training of prehospital care providers must include special attention to pediatric medical problems and emergency care of younger children. Further study is needed of the optimum parameters and vital signs in the field assessment of children. Other topics for future research are suggested as well.

▶ This is a very detailed paper describing the scope of both urban and rural pediatric EMS in California. The authors emphasize the fact that nearly one third of calls for prehospital care in children occur in patients less than 5 years of age, the group that probably, with good reason, arouses the highest level of anxiety in prehospital providers. They are the group most likely to have critical illness as witnessed by the observation that the majority of cardiac arrests occurred in this group, and these are obviously the age and size of patients that differ most from the more commonly encountered adult patient and in whom the prehospital care providers have the least procedural and technical experience. It is also my anecdotal observation that prehospital providers often have a fair amount of anxiety and are less able to achieve an appropriate level of professional detachment when dealing with the occasional critically ill infant. For all these reasons, I think that Seidel and his coauthors have clearly provided the motivation for us to emphasize increased attention to pediatric education and experience for the hard-working members of our EMS corps.—F.M. Henretig, M.D.

Respiratory Effects of Spinal Immobilization in Children

Schafermeyer RW, Ribbeck BM, Gaskins J, Thomason S, Harlan M, Attkisson A (Carolinas Med Ctr; Mecklenburg County Ambulance Service, Charlotte, NC)

Ann Emerg Med 20:1017–1019, 1991 7–4

Objective.—A variety of methods, some of them untested, are used to stabilize the spine of injured persons. Two strapping techniques for spinal immobilization were compared to determine how they limit respiratory function.

Methods.—Fifty-one healthy children aged 6 to 15 years volunteered to be secured to a backboard by lateral or cross strapping (Fig 7–1). Forced vital capacity (FVC) was measured with the subjects upright, supine, and supine with the spine immobilized.

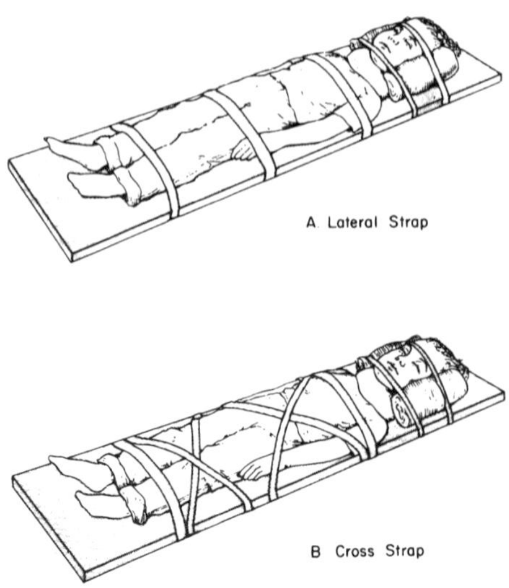

Fig 7–1.—Location of straps for immobilization with (**A**) lateral-strap technique and (**B**) cross-strap technique. (Courtesy of Schafermeyer RW, Ribbeck BM, Gaskins J, et al: *Ann Emerg Med* 20:1017–1019, 1991.)

Findings.—Values of FVC were consistently lower with the subjects supine than in the upright position. Most children aged 9 years and younger had a supine FVC less than calculated. Immobilization by either method further reduced the FVC. Neither of the techniques appeared to be advantageous. The mean FVC in the supine position without strapping was 2.45 L; with lateral strapping it was 1.98 L, and with cross strapping it was 1.97 L.

Implications.—There is no one best method of immobilizing the spine in an injured child. Pre-hospital personnel should determine whether the particular method used compromises ventilation.

▶ This interesting paper reminds us that spinal immobilization in the supine position significantly limits respiratory excursion in young children. The study utilized normal, healthy volunteers recruited from scouting camps between 6 and 15 years of age and found that strapping with both a lateral-strapping or cross-strapping technique in the supine position was associated with significantly lowered vital capacities when compared with that measured when the children were supine without strapping. Further, a number of children with multiple trauma who would likely be so immobilized may have concomitant pulmonary injuries. It is important to remind prehospital personnel to be especially aware of deterioration in respiratory status when a child is placed in the supine immobilization position.—F.M. Henretig, M.D.

Symptoms and Signs in Infants Younger Than 6 Months of Age Correlated With the Severity of Their Illness

Morley CJ, Thornton AJ, Cole TJ, Fowler MA, Hewson PH (Univ of Cambridge, England; MRC Dunn Nutrition Lab, Cambridge, England; Royal Children's Hosp, Melbourne, Australia)

Pediatrics 88:1119–1124, 1991 7–5

Background.—In a search for useful markers of serious illness in infants during the first 6 months of life, it is difficult to pinpoint which symptoms and signs are important and which are too common to be useful. The prevalence of individual symptoms and signs was examined in infants who were well, mildly ill, moderately ill, or seriously ill.

Methods.—Symptoms and signs were recorded for 1,007 infants younger than 6 months of age who were seen at home or in the hospital. The results were classified according to the 4 grades of illness severity.

Findings.—Most symptoms present in the preceding 3 days were associated with all grades of illness. Four symptoms that did not occur in well infants were a fluid intake of less than one third of normal in the last 24 hours, convulsions, frank blood in the stools, and bile-stained vomit. Signs that were sensitive indicators because they were only seen in moderately or seriously ill infants were obvious retraction of the lower ribs, a high-pitched or moaning cry, and an audible expiratory grunt. Seriously ill infants had signs that included no eye contact with the examiner, central cyanosis, a complete lack of awareness of surroundings, and an extended posture. The signs and symptoms of specific diseases and different grades of illness were not significantly different in the 2 centers where the study was conducted.

Conclusions.—Signs associated with moderate or serious illness were marked retraction of the lower ribs, high-pitched or moaning cry, expiratory grunt, loss of alertness, central cyanosis, and severe hypotonia. Both parents and health workers who look after infants should be taught to recognize these signs and symptoms of serious illness.

▶ This is another article in a series from this group on assessing the health of children by eliciting signs and symptoms as noted by mothers and child health personnel (1–3). The impetus for this study makes for an interesting contrast between child health care here and in Britain. In Britain, most, if not all early care is provided by child health providers and/or generalists. Each generalist has only 15 children less than 6 months of age on his patient panel at any one time. A study in the mid-1970s found that many infant deaths were associated with a delay in obtaining medical care and/or the failure of general practitioners to recognize serious illness (4, 5). In contrast, in the United States, most infants receive their care from pediatricians, and when they are ill, they can be taken to their physicians or to hospital emergency departments. In turn, the majority of pediatric patients are infants and young children.

The delineation of symptoms associated with serious illness noted here would not surprise any experienced pediatrician or emergency department physician: poor oral intake, bilious vomiting, blood in the stools, respiratory distress (retractions, grunting), and a high-pitched cry. The symptoms listed are useful in training physician assistants/extenders or providers not experienced in evaluating ill infants.

This study does not address the issue of predicting major illness in healthier-appearing children (for instance, the child with fever who is at risk for transient bacteremia). As many authors have noted, children with serious illness (meningitis, pneumonia) who are seen in our emergency departments can frequently be identified by physical examination, with attention to such details as interaction with the examiner and parents. There are, as yet, no clues on examination to predict the child at greatest risk for transient bacteremia. The search for that "holy grail" continues.—R.M. Rutstein, M.D.

References

1. Thornton AJ, et al: *Arch Dis Child* 65:280, 1990.
2. Morley CJ, et al: *Arch Dis Child* 65:834, 1990.
3. Morley CJ, et al: *Arch Dis Child* 66:100, 1991.
4. McWeeney PM, Emery JL: *Arch Dis Child* 50:191, 1975.
5. Stanton AN, et al: *BMJ* 2:1249, 1978.

Access to Care for Poor Children: Separate and Unequal?

St Peter RF, Newacheck PW, Halfon N (Univ of California, San Francisco; Univ of California, Los Angeles)

JAMA 267:2760–2764, 1992 7–6

Background.—The U.S. Congress has recently expanded the Medicaid program to include coverage for poor children by the year 2002. Currently, little information is available to assess whether these changes will improve access to basic preventive care for poor children or whether the care they receive will be comparable to what other children receive. A study was done to determine how Medicaid coverage affects the use of preventive care and how it affects the location and continuity of care for poor children.

Methods.—A nationally representative sample of 17,710 children younger than 18 years of age was selected in a stratified cluster sampling of U.S. households. The main outcome measures included the percentage of children with a usual source of routine care, the timeliness of routine care visits, the usual source where care is given, and the continuity between care sources.

Findings.—Ninety-one percent of poor children with Medicaid coverage had a usual source of routine care vs. 78% of those without Medicaid. Eighty-four percent of poor children with Medicaid received routine care within an appropriate time interval vs. 69% of poor children without Medicaid. Poor children with Medicaid coverage were less likely to receive routine care in physicians' offices than were children living above the poverty line. The former group was also more likely to lack continuity between usual sources of routine and sick care than the latter group was. Forty percent of children receiving routine care at community clinics received sick care elsewhere vs. 4% of those receiving care at physicians' offices. Children receiving routine care at community clinics were also more likely to use an emergency department as their usual source of sick care.

Conclusions.—Medicaid coverage does improve poor children's access to health care, but it does not ensure access to the continuity of care available to children living above the poverty line. Although recent changes in the Medicaid program may address some of these inequities, others are likely to persist.

▶ This is a distressing paper that, however, should come as no shock to anybody in the emergency medicine community. We all know that the United States has been unable to provide a top-notch quality of care to inner-city, poor children, as manifested in so many ways over recent years, including the increase in youthful victims of urban violence, the inability to decrease infant mortality rates, the widespread occurrence of measles outbreaks, and the depressingly low level of completion of primary immunization in the preschool years. We need a new system for guaranteeing access and availability of quality health care for our inner cities, and papers like this serve to remind us that this challenge is unmet.—F.M. Henretig, M.D.

Trauma Emergencies

Limitations of the Glasgow Coma Scale in Predicting Outcome in Children With Traumatic Brain Injury

Lieh-Lai MW, Theodorou AA, Sarnaik AP, Meert KL, Moylan PM, Canady AI (Children's Hosp of Michigan, Detroit)

J Pediatr 120:195–199, 1992 7–7

Background.—In patients with traumatic brain injury (TBI), the Glasgow Coma Scale (GCS) is the most commonly used prognostic scoring system. During the last decade, the authors' clinical experience suggested that many children with severe TBI and a relatively low GCS score recovered with a better-than-expected functional outcome. They evaluated the validity of the GCS score alone, with no assessment of the hypoxic-ischemic state, in predicting the outcome of severe TBI in children.

Patients.—The retrospective study included 79 children with TBI who were admitted to the intensive care unit during a 4-year period. The mean age was 6.6 years; 56% were boys, and most sustained their injury as pedestrians. The need for CPR and the presence of shock were among the data collected at the scene. Soon after admission and before the administration of sedatives or paralyzing agents, the GCS score was determined. In patients with GCS scores less than 8, intracranial pressure was continuously monitored; in all, it was maintained at less than 20 mm Hg. Cerebral perfusion pressure was maintained at more than 60 mm Hg. For survivors, the Glasgow Outcome Scale and a battery of neuropsychological tests were administered 2 to 12 months after the injury.

Results.—Eighty-nine percent of the children lived. Fourteen of 22 patients with a GCS score of 3 to 5 survived, a rate of 64%, vs. 58 of 59 with a GCS score of 6 or above. Shock and the need for CPR were significantly more common among those who died. The outcome was satisfactory—defined as a Glasgow Outcome Scale score of 4 or 5—in all children except for 2 who had prolonged periods of hypoxemia. The neuropsychological tests showed no significant differences between children with a GCS score of 3 to 5 and those with a GCS score of 6 or higher.

Conclusions.—In children who have sustained total TBI, a low GCS score is not the only predictor of a poor recovery. Many of those with a GCS score between 3 and 5 will return to independent function if they survive; thus aggressive neuroresuscitative measures should be taken. Hypoxic-ischemic insult must be considered independently when predicting outcome in these children.

▶ It is known that children seem to do better and recover faster than adults. It is also known that a GCS of less than 8 means a serious brain injury that requires aggressive airway management and shock therapy if the child is to have a chance at survival. The question was, what kind of survival. Part of the answer is related to the primary mechanism of injury and what effect hypoxia and ischemia have on the injured brain. Patients with rotational and shearing injury as well as those with subdural hematoma have poor outcomes. While the CT scan helps us initially, MRI will look at other aspects of the injured brain and allow the clinician to estimate the severity of injury and potential for neurologic recovery. The other part of the answer must lie in the recuperative processes of children that allow them to recover from injuries from which adults would not. The article brings us this good news.—R.W. Schafermeyer, M.D.

Predictors of Abdominal Injury in Children With Pelvic Fracture

Bond SJ, Gotschall CS, Eichelberger MR (Children's Natl Med Ctr, Washington DC)

J Trauma 31:1169–1173, 1991 7–8

Background.—Thoracic trauma seen on initial chest radiographs can identify severely injured children at increased risk of dying. A study was done to determine the best predictors of intra-abdominal injury in children with pelvic fractures.

Patients and Outcomes.—Of 2,248 children admitted to a pediatric trauma center with injuries from blunt trauma in a 48-month period, 54, or 2.4%, had radiographically diagnosed injury to the pelvic circle. Thirteen of the children had concomitant abdominal or genitourinary (GU) injury. Their mean age was 8.6 years. Eighty-nine percent of the injuries were sustained in motor vehicle accidents, with 59% of the children being pedestrians at the time. Six children died, a mortality rate of 11.1%. Pelvic fracture sites were the pubic rami in 59%, ilium or pelvic rim in 17%, and sacrum in 6%. Nineteen percent of the children had multiple pelvic fractures. Fracture location was highly associated with the probability of abdominal injury. In a backward-elimination, stepwise logistic model, the factors best predicting abdominal or GU injury were the presence of multiple pelvic fractures and the unweighted Revised Trauma Score. Factors not predictive were the patient's age, systolic blood pressure, respiration rate, Glasgow Coma Scale score, and mechanism of injury. In this model, the probability of abdominal injury, given physiologic stability, was less than 1% for isolated pubic fractures, 15% for iliac or sacral fractures, and 60% for multiple fractures of the pelvic ring.

Conclusions.—In this series, pelvic fracture occurred in 2.4% of children admitted with injury from blunt trauma. The death rate among these children was 11%, death usually resulting from an associated head injury. The unweighted Revised Trauma Score identifies children with the potential for abdominal or GU injury.

▶ Bond et al. provide useful information in this extensive retrospective review and analysis of associated abdominal injuries in children with pelvic fractures. The 2% mortality rate from pelvic fractures reported in this study (1/54, 95% confidence interval: 0% to 10%) is much lower than that reported in adult series. Children are more likely to die of associated head injury than hemorrhage from a pelvic fracture. The presence or absence of multiple pelvic fractures and the child's overall severity of illness will help guide us in selecting how best to assess injury to the abdomen.—K.N. Shaw, M.D.

Diaphragmatic Injury in Children

Brandt ML, Luks FI, Spigland NA, DiLorenzo M, Laberge J-M, Ouimet A (Hôpital Ste-Justine, Montreal; Montreal Children's Hosp, Canada)

J Trauma 32:298–300, 1992 7–9

Background.—Up to 5% of the patients with blunt abdominal trauma and up to 15% with penetrating lower chest wounds have diaphragmatic injury. However, such injuries may be overshadowed by the severity of associated wounds and easily missed. The treatment of diaphragmatic injury in 1 group of children was evaluated.

Patients and Methods.—Thirteen children were treated for diaphragmatic injury at Sainte Justine and Montreal Children's hospitals between 1972 and 1990. The patients were 6 girls and 7 boys aged 1½ to 15 years. Eight had penetrating trauma, and 5 had blunt trauma. Associated injuries, most commonly involving the liver, occurred in 9 patients. All 13 children had exploratory laparotomy with diaphragm repair.

Outcomes.—Two children died, both from causes unrelated to the diaphragmatic trauma. All survivors recovered without complications. One patient had cosmetic repair of a chest wall deformity 9 years after the trauma.

Conclusions.—Diaphragmatic injury in children is rare. It must be considered in any child sustaining blunt or penetrating thoracoabdominal trauma. Diaphragmatic rupture can occur without signs of external injury because of the increased compliance of the thoracic cage in children. Physicians can minimize morbidity and mortality by having a high index of suspicion, recognizing the injury promptly, and surgically repairing even the smallest diaphragmatic injury.

▶ This article is an excellent reminder to look for diaphragmatic injury in children with trauma. Cases of abdominal and chest trauma and blunt and penetrating injury are described. Like many of the injuries of childhood, there may be no external signs. Thus, one must maintain high surveillance and anticipation of potential injury. Although not part of the classic lap-belt complex, restraint device injuries to the abdomen may include diaphragmatic rupture. The authors also raise the problem of a lack of clear-cut physicial examination findings. The dyad of decreased breath sounds on the left along with Gibson's sign (scaphoid abdomen) may be a good indicator, but it is not constant. Most likely, the diagnosis will be made when difficulty is encountered in placing a nasogastric tube or when a chest radiograph is obtained. The authors also advise caution before placing a chest tube; however, such caution seems to be unwarranted with the relatively low incidence of diaphragmatic injury when compared with the rate of pneumothorax. I would hate to see a delay in the relief of a pneumothorax while a potential diaphragmatic rupture was being pondered.—S. Ludwig, M.D.

Management of Displaced Supracondylar Fractures of the Humerus in Children

Furrer M, Mark G, Rüedi T (Kantonsspital Chur, Chur, Switzerland)

Injury 22:259–262, 1991 7–10

Background.—Supracondylar fractures of the humerus (SFH) are very common in children. The great majority of them are extension fractures, with only about 5% being flexion-type fractures. The modified grading of Gartland and Wilkins is one of the best systems for classifying their degree of dislocation (Fig 7–2). Treatments for displaced SFH range from purely nonoperative treatment to open reduction, but nonoperative treatments can result in loss of motion and axial misalignment. The outcome of active treatment for displaced SFH was evaluated in 33 children averaging 6 years of age.

Methods.—The fractures were all Gartland and Wilkins grades IIB or III, and they included 32 closed and 1 open fracture. Primary neurovascular injury was found in 18% of the cases. Thirty-two patients had open reduction and internal fixation by Kirschner wires; only 1 patient was treated with closed reduction and percutaneous pinning. Nerves were visualized when preoperative neurologic deficits were found, but nerve suture was not required in those cases. In 1 case, intimal lesions totally occluded the brachial and radial arteries, which were therefore reconstructed. Follow-up averaged 29 months postinjury. Nine surgeons, including some in training, performed the operations.

Results.—No early complications occurred. The reconstructed arteries remained patent. The average hospital stay was 9 days. According to Innocenti's criteria, 27 of 30 patients had excellent results, and the remaining 3 had good results. Those 3 had a difference in carrying angle of <10 degrees as compared with the healthy side. Similarly, all deficits in range of motion were <10 degrees as compared with the healthy side. At follow-up, no neurologic deficits remained, no patient had pain, and all parents were satisfied with both the functional and cosmetic results despite the fact that most scars were 2 to 5 mm wide.

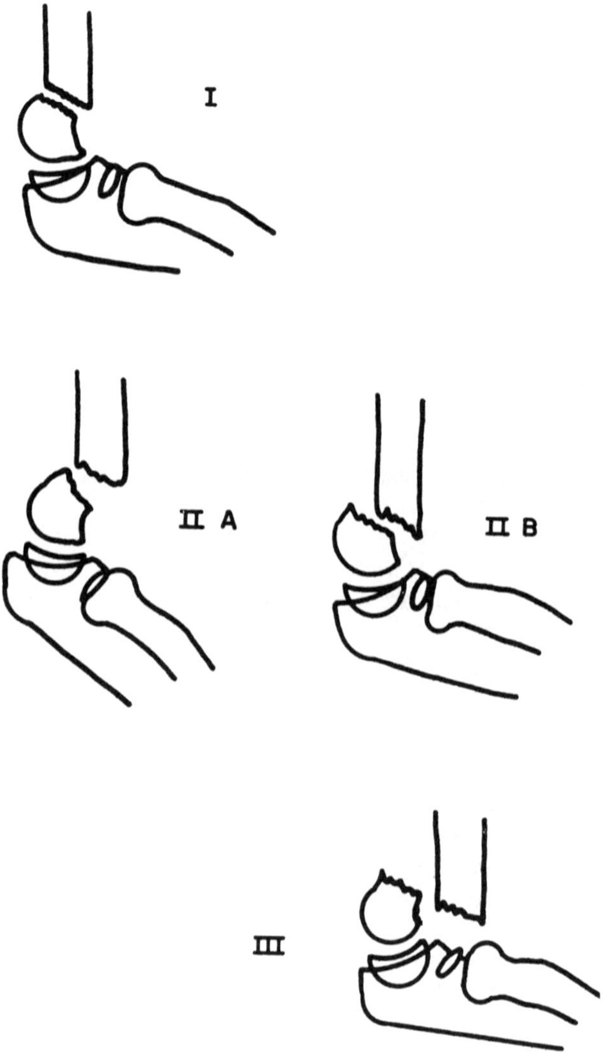

Fig 7–2.—Modified Gartland (1959) and Wilkins (1984) grading of SHF of children. (Courtesy of Furrer M, Mark G, Rüedi T: *Injury* 22:259–262, 1991.)

Conclusions.—Open reduction and internal K-wire fixation seem to give generally excellent results without complications or undue pain and with much shorter hospital stays than those required for treatment with traction. When closed reduction is successful at the first attempt, percutaneous pinning is a good alternative treatment.

▶ I become skeptical when surgeons recommend operative therapy without the benefit of a control group for statistical analysis. This is a descriptive series of children with displaced supracondylar fractures treated with open reduction and internal fixation (ORIF) and a discussion of the authors' opinions about optimal treatment.

Emergency physicians may be most interested in the 18% of patients with displaced supracondylar fractures with neurovascular injury and the 10% of children who had less-than-optimal long-term outcome despite aggressive therapy. Supracondylar fractures are a pediatric emergency that require careful assessment and prompt treatment.

The data show that 27 of 30 patients treated with ORIF had excellent results, as defined by previously published outcome criteria. There is no identified group treated nonoperatively to allow for valid statistical comparison. The authors mention historical controls from the literature, a method that does not control for differences in patient populations and changes in other aspects of therapy that occur over time. Furthermore, if they used the numbers from the studies they cite, a comparison of ORIF to nonoperative therapy would have demonstrated that there is no statistical difference in the likelihood of an excellent result ($P = .3$).

Children treated with ORIF remained hospitalized for an average of 9 days as compared with 17 days for those treated by closed reduction and traction. The negative impact that prolonged hospitalization has on children may justify operative therapy, even if the outcomes are similar. One study referenced in the paper shows percutaneous fixation yielding the best results. It appears that this approach can produce excellent results, minimal scarring, no operative risk, and shortened hospital stay. Larger studies assessing all methods of treatment and utilizing statistical methods are needed to determine the optimal approach for treating displaced supracondylar fractures in children.—M. Joffe, M.D.

Incidence, Mechanism of Injury, and Treatment of Fractures of the Patella in Children

Ray JM, Hendrix J (Univ of Kentucky, Lexington)

J Trauma 32:464–467, 1992 7–11

Background.—Fractures of the patella in children and adolescents are relatively rare. A retrospective review was done to determine the incidence, mechanism of injury, and most effective treatment for patellar fractures in this age group.

Methods and Findings.—The charts of 185 patients treated for fractures of the patella at 1 center between 1976 and 1988 were reviewed. Twelve patients were aged 8 to 16 years. Preoperative and postoperative radiographs were analyzed. Sleeve fractures were the most common type of patellar fracture and occurred in 5 patients. Transverse fractures were the next most common and occurred in 4. All of the children studied were boys with a mean age of 12.7 years. Ten boys needed surgery ranging from irrigation and debridement to open reduction and internal fixation. When indicated, partial patellectomy was done. Indications for surgery in these children were similar to the indications for surgery in adults. Also, as in the adult age group, the main mechanism of injury was motor vehicle and motorcycle accidents. One mechanism of injury not reported previously was noted: that of a flexed knee hitting the gym wall after a basketball lay-up shot because the basket was hung flush with the wall.

Conclusions.—In this series, 6.5% of all patellar fractures occurred in children aged 8 to 16 years. Seat belt laws requiring restraint of children should help reduce the incidence of patellar fractures from dashboard trauma. Placing basketball baskets away from gym walls should also reduce the danger of players striking their flexed knees on the walls. Young basketball players should be required to wear knee pads or protectors to prevent knee injuries.

▶ Not only are patellar fractures in children rare, but they can also be difficult to detect on roentgenograms. This case series of 12 patients alerts the emergency medicine physician to consider a patellar fracture when evaluating a child or adolescent with an acute blunt injury to the anterior aspect of a flexed knee as may occur during a motor vehicle accident (7/12) or when playing sports (4/12). The authors state that "a palpable defect located at the inferior pole of the patella is a clinical tip-off."—K.N. Shaw, M.D.

Tykes on Bikes: Injuries Associated With Bicycle-Mounted Child Seats

Tanz RR, Christoffel KK (Children's Mem Hosp; Northwestern Univ, Chicago, Ill)

Pediatr Emerg Care 7:297–301, 1991 7–12

Background.—Some common consumer products and recreational activities enjoyed by adults expose children to a risk of serious injury. Each year in the United States, bicycle-mounted child seats are associated with several hundred injuries to young children. The authors evaluate 2 such cases from their practice and examine data from the U.S. Consumer Product Safety Commission (CPSC).

Methods.—The CPS data covered the years 1978 to 1988. Injury estimates were calculated from reports received by the National Electronic Injury Surveillance System (NEISS), which codes information from emergency departments and distributes injury estimates for defined age groups. Injury severity was analyzed according to the CPSC 8-point scale.

Results.—There were 71 children with child-carried related injuries reported to NEISS. According to the NEISS weightings, an estimated 4,960 of such injuries occurred during the 11-year study period. The peak age of incidence for bicycle-mounted child seat injuries was 2 years.

Most (80%) of the estimated injuries resulted from falls; injuries to the head (51%) and face (21%) predominated. Severe injuries, accounting for 19% of the total, all involved the head or face. Less serious injuries involved the extremities. No deaths were reported. In the authors' experience, a 14-month-old girl injured her head when the seat fell off the bicycle. She has since had delayed development, left focal seizures, and residual left hemiparesis. A 4-year-old girl required skin grafting for a foot wound sustained because the bicycle lacked a spoke guard.

Conclusion.—A child's size and development and the bicycle's size, speed, and instability place children at risk for serious injury. Young children lack the ability to anticipate a crash and protect themselves. Recommendations include the use of helmets, improved seat design, and education of parents regarding the dangers of a seemingly pleasant activity.

▶ This study on childhood injuries associated with bicycle-mounted child seats demonstrates the value of a national data base. Unfortunately, many important questions are not answered about this particular childhood injury risk.

Epidemiologists love large data sets, but detailed information about a smaller number of injuries is often more useful. The data in this study are retrospective and based on emergency department charting. Are there certain errors in judgment by the adults that accounted for a large proportion of the injuries? How often were the seats used improperly, and are certain brands more frequently associated with injuries? Did helmets significantly reduce the severity of injury? Many important questions about the circumstances of injury cannot be answered. The authors compare the risk with other bicycle-related injuries, but how does the risk compare with other recreational activities? Is careful use of bicycle-mounted child seats reasonably safe, or should their use be discouraged?

New products create new injury risks. The CPSC collects data from a sample of emergency departments through the NEISS to identify injury risks that may be poorly recognized. The CPSC's role in identifying the risks from all-terrain vehicles, button batteries, microwave ovens, and many other products demonstrates that this is a worthwhile expenditure of public funds. The expanding role of information systems in health care delivery has great potential for improving public health. (See also Abstract 7–13.)—M. Joffe, M.D.

Bicycle-Associated Head Injuries and Deaths in the United States From 1984 Through 1988: How Many Are Preventable?

Sacks JJ, Holmgreen P, Smith SM, Sosin DM (Ctrs for Disease Control, Atlanta, Ga)

JAMA 266:3016–3018, 1991 — 7–13

Introduction.—Bicycle-related injuries are the cause of many fatalities and long-term disabilities in the United States. Safety helmets may reduce deaths and serious injuries, but fewer than 10% of all bicyclists use helmets. By reviewing death certificates and emergency department injury data for 1984 through 1988, the potential benefits from more widespread helmet use were estimated.

Methods.—Data were analyzed for bicycle-associated death and any injury occurring above the neck. Relative risks (RRs) of 3.85 and 6.67 were derived from a case-control study. By using these RR values and varying helmet usage from 10% to 100%, the population attributable risk was calculated to estimate the preventable deaths and injuries.

Results.—During the study period, 4,812 residents of the United States died of bicycle crashes. Head injury was involved in 62% of the deaths. Males (84.5%) and whites (84.2%) accounted for the majority of head injury bicycle-associated deaths (HIBADs). The peak age group for HIBADs was 15 to 19 years; the most common time of year for deaths was the summer (39.3%). Children younger than 15 years accounted for 76% of the head injuries and 41% of the head injury deaths. During the same 5-year period, an estimated 2,789,678 persons sustained bicycle-associated injuries.

Conclusion.—With a 6.67 increased RR of head injury from not wearing a helmet, 2,496 HIBADs and 757,341 bicycle-associated head injuries might have been prevented; with a 3.85 increased RR, 2,148 HIBADS and 651,684 bicycle-associated head injuries were potentially preventable. Physicians should strongly recommend helmets for their patients who bicycle, especially those younger than 15 years. Improvements in helmet design are needed to improve protection.

▶ This paper identified an area in which emergency physicians have an enormous impact. Our hospital and division of emergency medicine has conducted a helmet safety campaign that has reached over 6,000 school children since October 1991. We have been able to provide discount coupons for helmets by working with various bicycle shops and feel that we have had a significant impact on helmet usage. The attempt to legislate the use of helmets by motorcycle riders has met with significant opposition. However, bicycle injuries occur in a younger age group, and public safety campaigns can have an enormous impact on this age group. I encourage every emergency physician to become involved in your community's various public health and safety campaigns, and this is an excellent way to do it.—E.J. Lucid, M.D.

Fire Hydrant Play: Injuries and Their Prevention

Joffe M, Torrey SB, Baker MD (St Christopher's Hosp for Children, Philadelphia; Children's Hosp of Philadelphia, Pa)

Pediatrics 87:900–903, 1991 7–14

Background.—Poor urban children often injure themselves while playing in water from open fire hydrants during hot summer days. Information on the mechanisms, circumstances, and types of injury associated with this summer activity in poor urban areas was collected.

Patients.—During the summers of 1987 and 1988, 86 children in Philadelphia aged 25 to 206 months were treated for injuries that occurred while playing in water from open fire hydrants. Parents were interviewed either in the emergency department or by telephone within 2 days of the injury to collect data on the circumstances, mechanisms, and locations of the injury and on the patterns of play, the neighborbood, and the home environment. Data on weather conditions at the time of injury were obtained from the weather bureau. Injury severity was expressed as the Injury Severity Score.

Results.—Ninety-seven percent of the injured children were black or Hispanic. The mean maximum temperature on the days when the injuries occurred was 97.5°F. The children had few alternative means for keeping cool because only 22% of the injured children's homes had air conditioners. The mechanisms of injury were stepping on broken glass (40%), falling (24%), being hit by an oncoming car (22%), and other (14%). The types of injury were laceration (64%), abrasion/contusion (28%), fracture (4%), and concussion (4%). Broken glass in the street accounted for 55% of all injuries. Two thirds of the patients were barefoot when injured. Most injuries were minor, with motor vehicles causing all serious injuries. Water pressure that knocked children over or pushed them into traffic caused 11% of the injuries. Adults had opened fire hydrants in 90% of cases and were present when 68% of the injuries occurred, but their presence did not exert any beneficial effect.

Conclusions.—Public policy should be directed toward providing alternatives for cooling off on hot summer days. Public education should target adults to remove glass from the street and teach their children to wear shoes when playing outside. The placement of sprinklers on fire hydrants on hot summer days would reduce the water's force and make playing in it safer.

▶ The authors address an area of urban health concern in which the emergency physician can play an important part, both in the education of the public as well as the city agencies responsible for fire hydrant services. Emergency medicine is going to fulfill an expanded role in the health delivery system. Knowledge and concern involving traditional areas of preventive medicine must indeed become part of its purview. The authors point out that the utilization of inexpensive sprinkler devices saves money and minimizes injuries otherwise occurring with the uncontrolled exodus of water from fire hydrants, a useful example of the involvement of the emergency physician in urban preventive health activities.—D.K. Wagner, M.D.

Sweden's Experience in Reducing Childhood Injuries

Bergman AB, Rivara FP (Univ of Washington, Seattle)

Pediatrics 88:69–74, 1991 7–15

Introduction.—In 1957 to 1959, death rates from injuries in Sweden were greater than in the United States for children aged 1 to 4 years and similar for children aged 5 through 14 (Fig 7–3). Since 1959, Sweden has the lowest child injury death rate of any country in the world, primarily because of a systematic campaign undertaken by the Children's Accident Committee. Twenty-five individuals from 4 Swedish communities were interviewed to gain insight into this campaign.

Discussion.—The Swedish accomplishments in child injury prevention stem from a combination of factors, including special characteristics of the Swedish society and an energetic 35-year campaign spearheaded by the Joint Committee for the Prevention of Childhood Accidents. Sweden has had a stable government with a relatively homogenous population and little poverty. The Swedish population is small and consists of health-conscious law-abiding people who value children. The people believe that the government is an active instrument of bettering their lives.

The campaign to lower accident-related child mortality was spearheaded by the Children's Accident Committee, which is headed by a pediatrician, a pediatric surgeon, and a private individual, with strong support from the government and other private organizations. Key factors in the campaign have been support of trauma surveillance systems and injury prevention research, ensuring of safer environments and products through legislation and regulation, and a broad-based safety education campaign using a coalition of existing groups.

Implications.—The strategies used in the Swedish campaign can markedly reduce the number of children in the United States who are killed,

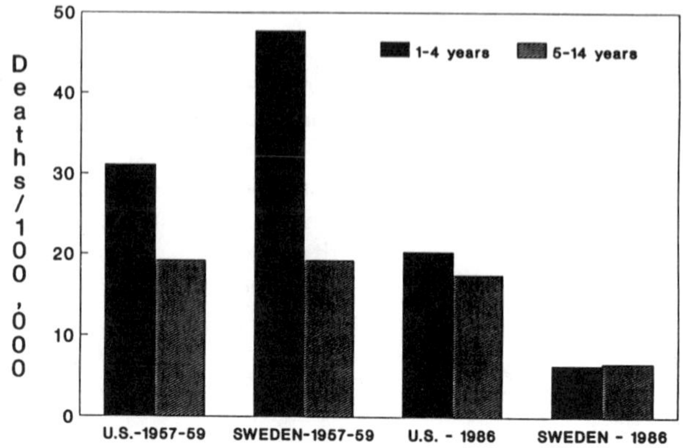

Fig 7–3.—Injury fatalities, Sweden and the United States, 1957 through 1959 and 1986. Data from World Health Organization. (Courtesy of Bergman AB, et al: *Pediatrics* 88:69–74, 1991.)

injured, and disabled from trauma. Despite the size and complexity of the U.S. society, these strategies are adaptable to this country, particularly in the presence of a serious national commitment to lower childhood injury mortality.

▶ It is refreshing to read about a comparison between the United States and a country other than Japan. Sweden is the world's leader in childhood safety, and we need to learn from the successes of others.

Sweden's very low child injury death rate is, in part, attributable to a 35-year campaign for childhood safety. United States initiatives in public health matters usually take the form of 1-year public awareness campaigns. The implication of having a "Year of the Child" is that other years are not. Short-term, intensive campaigns may suit the American attention span but do not provide a basis for long-term gains.

Sweden's Joint Committee for the Prevention of Childhood Accidents brought together a wide variety of existing public interest groups. This kind of cooperation is more difficult in an environment where groups and individuals need to take credit for successful programs in order to secure promotions and future funding. Sweden has been a leader in proving the effectiveness of their preventive efforts, but a 10-year interval between intervention and outcome requires patience and a long-term perspective. Direct government funding was not received for the program for 25 years, with reliance on insurance companies and automobile manufacturers for early support. The Swedes' prevailing belief in government as an active instrument led to secure funding once benefits of the childhood safety programs were apparent. Programs in the United States with long histories and impressive records of effectiveness, such as Regional Poison Control Centers, still suffer from insufficient and tenuous funding. Sweden's socialized health care delivery system made possible the comprehensive surveillance necessary to identify important childhood injury risks and to gain support from politicians, the media, and the public. In the United States, our fragmented health care system and emphasis on privacy and confidentiality make a comprehensive surveillance system difficult to realize.

Differences in size, homogeneity, and income distribution make comparisons between Swedish society and the United States problematic. The authors recognize these limitations. A less tangible, but perhaps more important factor in the success of Swedish programs relative to those in the United States is in the relationship between the individual and society. Swedes seem to feel more invested in the health and well-being of every Swedish child. The current state of economics, health care, and education for U.S. children does not reflect the same degree of shared responsibility.—M. Joffe, M.D.

Organ System Emergencies

A Treatment Protocol of the Acute Asthma Patient in a Pediatric Emergency Department

Press S, Lipkind RS (Univ of Miami; Jackson Mem Hosp, Miami, Fla)
Clin Pediatr 30:573–577, 1991 7–16

Background.—An estimated 5% to 12% of all children in Western countries have asthma and the prevalence appears to be increasing. Acute asthma is one of the most frequent reasons pediatric patients seek care in an emergency department. Increases in prevalence may be caused by a change in the epidemiology of asthma, increased exposure to environmental triggers, and inadequate or underutilized therapy. The adequacy of a treatment protocol used in an urban pediatric emergency department was evaluated.

Methods.—In a prospective 3-month study, 682 children aged 8 months to 15 years with acute asthma were treated. Patients with a first wheezing episode received a chest radiograph. Chest radiographs were also obtained when pneumonia or other pulmonary pathology was suspected. Patients were initially evaluated and treated by house staff physicians under the supervision of attending physicians.

Results.—During the study period 566 children were initially discharged, and 116 were admitted. There were no deaths in either group. All patients were treated with aerosol inhalation. Among the 247 patients who received both steroids and aminophylline, 15 had findings on chest radiographs consistent with pneumonia. Among the 566 discharged children, 131 had received intravenous aminophylline and steroids. Fourteen of the discharged patients were admitted during the subsequent 48 hours because of status asthmaticus. Approximately 1 in 6 asthma patients was admitted, thus making asthma the second most frequent reason for admission.

Conclusions.—This protocol for the treatment of acute asthma with mild to moderate respiratory distress in children was designed to standardize care and to define an end point in the decision-making process. The admission rate for asthma patients was 17%, or approximately 1 in 6 patients, as compared with rates of 9.9% to 26% in other studies. The admission of asthma patients was substantially reduced by administering intravenous aminophylline and steroids to patients who did not respond to aerosol treatment alone.

▶ Increased asthma prevalence, hospital emergency department visits, and mortality rates for asthma patients have provided the impetus to focus increased scrutiny of education and management on asthma for clinicians, researchers and agencies involved in quality assurance, and governmental agencies. A lot of questions are being asked about etiologies, therapeutic agents, and the overall management of asthma. In fact, there has been an explosion of articles over the past 2 years on these topics. Some are solid research papers with good design, whereas others are more of a view of how the authors treat asthma. In addition, this past year, the National Asthma Education Panel released its comprehensive report on the management of asthma (1).

With all of this activity, one would think that all the answers are in and there are 1 or 2 ways to treat asthma. Unfortunately, the debate will continue, with some advocates supporting the use of β-agonists and others supporting the use of aminophylline, and some believe that allergists should be the "primary-care physician" for children with moderate or severe asthma.

This prospective study uses a protocol to "simplify" the decision-making process for the management of asthma. I applaud the authors' use of chest radiographs in first wheezing episodes (2). Foreign bodies and other diseases are part of the differential diagnosis. Nowhere do I see that they used peak flow, pulsus paradoxus, or pulse oximetry to monitor and evaluate the patient objectively. Because blood gases and theophylline levels were utilized, the above parameters should be used to monitor patients and monitor progress.

Theophylline is a controversial agent these days. Its proponents say that it is safer than β-agonists and metered-dose inhalers and that drawing blood to monitor serum levels is not that difficult. The detractors believe that it is not indicated except for severe disease in children admitted to the hospital and that it can cause serious, life-threatening problems. Even the National Asthma Education Foundation booklet suggests the latter. There probably is a grain of truth to both sides of the issue. All parties seem to agree that steroids are underused and must be given to children with moderate to severe attacks.

Thus, the protocol is a start, but far from flawless. There needs to be more physical parameters monitored and additional patients studied to see whether the trends of low revisits for admission persists. (See also Abstract 7–17.)—R.W. Schafermeyer, M.D.

References

1. National Asthma Education Program: *Guidelines for the Diagnosis and Management of Asthma.* Bethesda, Md, National Heart, Lung and Blood Institute, 1991.
2. Muth D, Schafermeyer RW: *Pediatr Emerg Care* 6:110, 1990.

Randomized Trial of Salbutamol in Acute Bronchiolitis

Klassen TP, Rowe PC, Sutcliffe T, Ropp LJ, McDowell IW, Li MM (Univ of Ottawa, Canada)

J Pediatr 118:807–811, 1991 7–17

Introduction.—The treatment of infants with acute bronchiolitis has not been resolved, with recent studies demonstrating the limits of pulmonary function tests in these young patients. This randomized study assessed the safety and efficacy of nebulized salbutamol (albuterol) in the treatment of children younger than 2 years old with bronchiolitis.

Methods.—Young patients entering the emergency department were considered candidates for the trial if they were younger than 24 months of age, they had wheezing on auscultation, and they had a respiratory distress assessment instrument (RDAI) score of >3. After baseline assessments, the patients underwent random assignment to a nebulized salbutamol, .1 mg/kg, group or a .02 mL/kg, .9% saline group.

Results.—Of the 85 patients entered, 83 completed the study: the 2 exclusions included 1 patient with a respiration rate of 100 breaths per minute and 1 patient who had a previous chest tube insertion. Patients receiving salbutamol demonstrated significantly reduced RDAI results 30 minutes after initiation of the first treatment in comparison to controls. After 60 minutes, however, this difference did not reach significance. Of the 58% of patients with signs of infection, the patients receiving salbutamol had significantly better RDAI results than did the placebo patients. The drug therapy did not appear to affect oxygen saturation or the respiratory rate 30 or 60 minutes after drug administration. After 60 minutes, 50 patients did not experience a three-unit change in the RDAI scores, so 20 received salbutamol, and 30 were given placebo in an unblinded manner. Interestingly, the 30 patients who received placebo showed a larger improvement in RDAI scores 30 minutes after receiving salbutamol than the 20 patients in the treatment arm who had had 2 courses of salbutamol already.

Conclusions.—Nebulized salbutamol can significantly improve the clinical outcome of very young children with bronchiolitis. A longer study of salbutamol administration to this patient population would further elucidate the effects of the drug.

▶ The basis for this study was the development of a reliable scoring system for infants with bronchiolitis, which is similar to a scoring system that correlates well with pulmonary function measurements in older children with asthma. This scoring system has been called the "respiratory distress assessment instrument," or RDAI, and is based upon the severity of wheezing and retractions. The maximum score is 17 points or units. Inclusion criteria in this study included a RDAI score greater than 3. The baseline RDAI scores for both groups averaged approximately 8, with a wide range of values in both groups (4 to up to 14 points). Additional information might have been obtained if the patients had been grouped within RDAI score ranges (i.e., 4 to 7, 8 to 11) rather than assessed as a single group. To do so would have required a substantially greater number of patients. Patients with the higher RDAI scores may have been more likely to benefit from bronchodilator therapy. Nonetheless, this study does indicate that bronchodilator therapy in this patient population improves clinical variables measured 30 minutes after the first administration. A second treatment at 30 minutes does not appear to result in further improvement; however, this may well be due to sample size. It should be noted that the authors did not address the effect of bronchodilator therapy on disposition; admission or discharge was at the discretion of the treating physician.—J.T. Niemann, M.D.

Cardiotoxicity During Treatment of Severe Childhood Asthma

Maguire JF, O'Rourke PP, Colan SD, Geha RS, Crone R (Children's Hosp; Harvard Med School, Boston, Mass)

Pediatrics 88:1180–1186, 1991 7–18

Introduction.—Children with severe status asthmaticus have been treated successfully with intravenous isoproterenol infusion therapy. There is some concern, however, about the possible cardiotoxic effects of this treatment. The nature of cardiotoxicity associated with severe childhood asthma exacerbations was investigated to identify those at risk for cardiotoxicity during therapy.

Methods.—The 20 study participants had been admitted with severe bronchial obstruction resistant to initial therapy. The 6 patients in group 1 received intravenous isoproterenol infusion; the 14 patients in group 2 did not receive this treatment. The 12 patients in group 3, who served as a control group, each had a single measurement of serum creatine phosphokinase with isoenzyme fractionation (CPK-MB) during an outpatient visit while their asthma was stable. The 3 groups were similar in age and sex.

Results.—Group 1 had more severe illness than group 2. When compared with group 2, group 1 had a significantly higher mean peak heart rate (194 vs. 173 beats per minute), a significantly worse degree of hypercapnia, and a significantly more acidotic mean low arterial blood pH. Except for the intravenous isoproterenol infusion, the 2 groups were treated similarly. Group 1 showed markedly increased CPK-MB levels and ECG abnormalities consistent with transient myocardial ischemia. Tachycardia, hypercapnia, acidosis, and intravenous isoproterenol therapy were risk factors associated with cardiotoxicity.

Conclusion.—Cardiotoxicity is common in children undergoing treatment for severe status asthmaticus. In the absence of more serious and obvious complications, serum CPK-MB and ECG tests may be useful in detecting cardiotoxicity. There was no evidence of a dose relationship between the amount of isoproterenol received and the degree of CPK-MB increase. Calcium channel blockers may be useful in blocking some of the potential cardiotoxic effects of isoproterenol.

▶ Status asthmaticus, a common cause of emergency center visits and subsequent hospital admissions, can have serious, fatal complications. Mechanical ventilation, the treatment of last resort, carries a significant risk of complications in asthmatics, including pneumothorax or pneumopericardium. Fifteen years ago, the advent of intravenous isoproterenol was seen as a major advance in improving outcomes in patients with respiratory failure. Isoproterenol is not without problems, however, the most frequently encountered side effect being severe tachycardia. These authors now describe significant cardiotoxicity as measured by increased CPK levels. Practitioners need to be alert to the possible cardiac toxicity of isoproterenol and consider cardiac causes of sudden chest pain or respiratory decompensation in an ill asthmatic.

Based on recent reports, the use of continuous aerosol therapy with β-agonists may decrease the need for intravenous isoproterenol. In addition, the widespread adoption of recent national concensus statements on the treatment of chronic asthma, with an emphasis on chronic prevention therapy as well as early use of steroids for acute exacerbations, will, it is hoped, result in improved asthma control and fewer episodes of severe status asthmaticus.—R.M. Rutstein, M.D.

Relation Between Airway Responsiveness and Serum IgE in Children With Asthma and in Apparently Normal Children

Sears MR, Burrows B, Flannery EM, Herbison GP, Hewitt CJ, Holdaway MD (Univ of Otago, Dunedin, New Zealand; Univ of Arizona, Tucson)

N Engl J Med 325:1067–1071, 1991 7–19

Background.—There is a known association between diagnosed asthma and serum IgE levels. However, no conclusions can be drawn concerning the relationship between IgE level and hyperresponsiveness of the airway to a methacholine challenge. It is unknown what characteristics of asymptomatic individuals predispose them to airway hyperresponsiveness. The association between the total serum IgE level and airway hyperresponsiveness was evaluated in subjects with or without asthma or other atopic disease in a birth cohort of children.

Methods.—The subjects were 562 children 11 years of age who were participating in a longitudinal study of child health. All subjects included in the analysis responded to a questionnaire on respiratory symptoms, had measurements or total serum IgE levels, and were tested for airway responsiveness to inhaled methacholine. Children of non-European descent were excluded.

Results.—Thirteen percent of the boys and 6% of the girls had asthma diagnosed at the current examination. Symptoms of wheezing were noted in 22% of the boys and 15% of the girls, and airflow obstruction at baseline was 6% in the boys vs. 1% in the girls. The mean IgE levels were 120.8 IU/mL in the boys and 98.1 IU/mL in the girls; this difference was not significant, but the boys had a wider distribution.

There was a strong association between the prevalence of diagnosed asthma and the serum IgE level, with no asthma in children with levels below 32 IU/mL as compared with asthma present in 36% of children with levels of 1,000 IU/mL or higher. This correlation was not explained by concurrent diagnoses of allergic rhinitis or eczema. There was also a high correlation between airway hyperresponsiveness to methacholine and the serum IgE level, which remained significant even after exclusion of children with diagnosed asthma and those with a history of wheezing, allergic rhinitis, or eczema.

Conclusions.—There appears to be a close association between airway hyperresponsiveness and an allergic diathesis, as reflected by the total serum IgE level. This is the case even in children who have never had symptoms and have no history of atopy. Airway hyperresponsiveness may be either temporary or persistent.

▶ This study addresses the pathophysiology of airway hyperresponsiveness. The data support the close association between allergic diathesis, as measured by serum IgE levels, and positive methacholine challenge test results in children with and without histories of asthma. The study adds to our general knowledge but will have little impact on the practice of emergency medicine.

Children with chronic cough frequently present a diagnostic dilemma for emergency physicians. The usefulness of a previous history or family history of asthma or allergy in diagnosing "cough variant" asthma is well known, although the support of these data is welcome. Although the statistical relationship between airway hyperresponsiveness and IgE levels is strong, including a dose-response relationship, only 36% of those with the highest IgE levels have clinically significant asthma. The negative predictive value of IgE values less than 32 is good, but this occurred in only 22% of the patients. Serum IgE levels may occasionally be useful in selected patients, but it is unlikely that this would be measured in the emergency department setting. If a patient has a high IgE level and a positive methacholine challenge test but has never had a problem with bronchospasm, the clinician must ask a very pertient question: who cares?—M. Joffe, M.D.

Absence of Serum Chemistry Abnormalities in Pediatric Patients Presenting With Seizures

Kenney RD, Taylor JA (Carolinas Med Ctr, Charlotte, NC)

Pediatr Emerg Care 8:65–66, 1992 7–20

Background.—Traditionally, children with seizures have had evaluation of serum chemistry values. Although such studies may be helpful in certain cases, they may not be of use for most children with convulsions, febrile or nonfebrile, without clinical evidence of a metabolic or renal dysfunction. A retrospective study was done to determine the clinical value of routine serum chemistry tests in the initial management of children with seizures.

Methods and Outcomes.—The emergency department records of 241 seizure episodes in children were studied. Eighty-six febrile and 155 nonfebrile convulsive episodes were examined. Sixty-four percent of the patients had at least 1 serum chemistry value obtained. Clinically significant abnormalities were found in none of 149 serum sodium tests ordered, none of 148 glucose and blood urea nitrogen tests, none of 86 calcium tests, and none of 61 magnesium studies done. Clinical management was not changed in any case as the result of a laboratory value. The total cost of the laboratory tests was $8,200, which raised the emergency department cost by $31 to $80 for any patient having such a study.

Conclusions.—Routine serum chemistry studies in children with seizures treated in an emergency department are unnecessary unless specific clinical findings suggest otherwise. Such studies may be helpful in children with status epilepticus or a history of metabolic or gastrointestinal disease or in neonates or very young infants with convulsions.

▶ The article by Kenney and Taylor helps to slay another obsolete "sacred cow." We need to get rid of these beasts whenever possible. They need to be slain in order to promote thinking and to save money. Ordering laboratory tests in clusters or bundles may have led to completeness, but a lack of thought and excess expenses were the unfortunate by-products. We should order tests that will help establish a diagnosis or, more importantly, guide therapy. Emergency physicians and pediatricians are capable of deciding which tests these should be. Protocols are helpful guidelines to fall back upon in emergency situations. They should not be specific recipes to be followed from the cookbook of medical care. Rest in peace, seizure workup tests.—S. Ludwig, M.D.

Theophylline and Status Epilepticus in Children

Dunn DW, Parekh HU (Indiana Univ, Indianapolis)

Neuropediatrics 22:24–26, 1991 7–21

Background.—Theophylline is known to trigger seizures, but its effect on the outcome of seizures is unknown. The effect of theophylline on the occurrence and outcome of status epilepticus (SE) in children was evaluated.

Patients.—Of 114 episodes of SE occurring in 97 children during a 2-year period, 16 occurred in children receiving theophylline within the 24 hours before the seizure. In each case, serum theophylline levels were obtained within several hours. In 8 cases, the serum theophylline concentration appeared to be greater than 20 μg/mL at the onset of SE, and in 8 cases the theophylline level was either therapeutic or low.

Findings.—In the group with high theophylline levels, 5 of the children had possible precipitating factors. The mean duration of the episodes was 1.3 hours. One child died, and 3 sustained significant new neurologic damage. In the group with normal to low theophylline levels, all children were receiving long-term theophylline therapy, and 6 had possible precipitating factors. The mean duration of SE was 1.75 hours. There were no deaths in this group, and only 1 child had a transient neurologic deficit. In the overall group of 114 episodes of SE, the incidence of death or persistent neurologic deficit was 23%.

Conclusions.—At toxic levels, theophylline appears to be a significant factor in increased morbidity in children with SE. Failure to compensate for the increased cerebral metabolic rate seen in SE, resulting from hypoxia from the underlying respiratory disorder and the reduced cerebral blood flow that occurs with theophylline, increases the risk of a poor outcome. For asthmatic children who are at risk of seizures, theophylline is not the initial drug of choice.

▶ The conclusions these authors draw are not supported by their data and go beyond the scope of this case series. There is no significant statistical difference ($P > .05$) in morbidity and mortality between those patients with elevated theophylline levels and those without elevated theophylline levels in this study. Additionally, all children without epilepsy or a known CNS disorder who had status epilepticus and did not become hypoxic survived neurologically intact.

Of interest is that 75% of the patients with SF had a known seizure disorder or hydrocephalus. Certainly, one should try other bronchodilators in these children. In otherwise normal children, seizures occur at lower levels (42 vs. 100 μg/mL) in those taking theophylline for 72 hours or longer as compared with those with acute toxicity.—K.N. Shaw, M.D.

Oral Water Intoxication in Infants: An American Epidemic

Keating JP, Schears GJ, Dodge PR (Washington Univ, St Louis, Mo)

Am J Dis Child 145:985–990, 1991 7–22

Background.—Water intoxication has been considered a rare clinical event, but an increasing number of cases are being reported in infants. Thirty-four infants with water intoxication were seen in 1 institution over a 15-year period, 24 of them in the last 3 years. Most of the infants were living in poverty and had ingested excessive amounts of water offered at home by their caretakers when the supply of infant formula was exhausted.

Methods.—The 34 patients, 31 infants and 3 children, had an acute neurologic syndrome occurring in association with hyponatremia. The patients were treated with either a single infusion of hypertonic saline or a slow infusion of isotonic fluid. Data were gathered from the local offices of the Supplemental Food Program for Women, Infants, and Children (WIC) concerning the availability of food supplements and nutritional advice provided during the study period.

Findings.—The illness usually started suddenly with convulsions or apnea. Seizures occurred in all infants and usually consisted of generalized tonic-clonic activity. Respiratory failure occurred in 15 patients (48%). Despite some published suggestions that the rapid administration of hypertonic saline may cause central pontine myelinolysis, it was not observed as a complication. It is suggested that hunger overwhelms the infant's innate protective mechanisms and is the most important cause of infantile water intoxication. The unavailability of formula apparently plays a major causative role.

Conclusions.—Immediate consideration should be given to increasing the availability of formula through programs such as WIC to infants living in poverty, and there should be better education of mothers and medical personnel about the hazards of excessive water intake. With those measures, the life-threatening condition of water intoxication may be prevented.

▶ Hyponatremia is more common and probably more serious in infants, but it can be an unexpected finding in adult patients who arrive with some confusing scenarios such as seizures, altered mental status, generalized weakness, or leg cramps. In the case of infant hyponatremia, the history may be hard to ferret out because most parents think that water is harmless and even force it on a sick child. In the presence of symptomatic hyponatremia, the once-admonished rapid administration of hypertonic saline is now accepted therapy (1). This article emphasizes that too much of anything—even water—can be toxic. Many patients believe that vitamins, herbal preparations, or creams or ointments are likewise harmless, but the literature is replete with the toxicity from such "nonmedicines." Another unexpected problem for children given boiled tap water from old homes—even when it is properly mixed with formula—is lead poisoning (2).—J.R. Roberts, M.D.

References

1. *Crit Care Med* 19:758, 1991.
2. *Pediatrics* 89:87, 1992.

Severity of Childhood Bacterial Meningitis and Duration of Illness Before Diagnosis

Kilpi T, Anttila M, Kallio MJT, Peltola H (Univ of Helsinki, Finland)

Lancet 338:406–409, 1991 7–23

Background.—It is widely believed that rapid diagnosis is important in achieving good outcomes with childhood bacterial meningitis (BM), but some evidence suggests that poor outcomes can sometimes occur with illnesses of short rather than long duration. The relationship of the severity of illness to the duration of illness before admission was studied prospectively.

Methods.—Two hundred eighty-six children with culture-positive CSF from 18 hospitals in Finland were studied from 1984 to 1989. They included 141 who had been ill less than 24 hours before diagnosis, 75 with illness between 24 and 48 hours before diagnosis, and 70 who had been

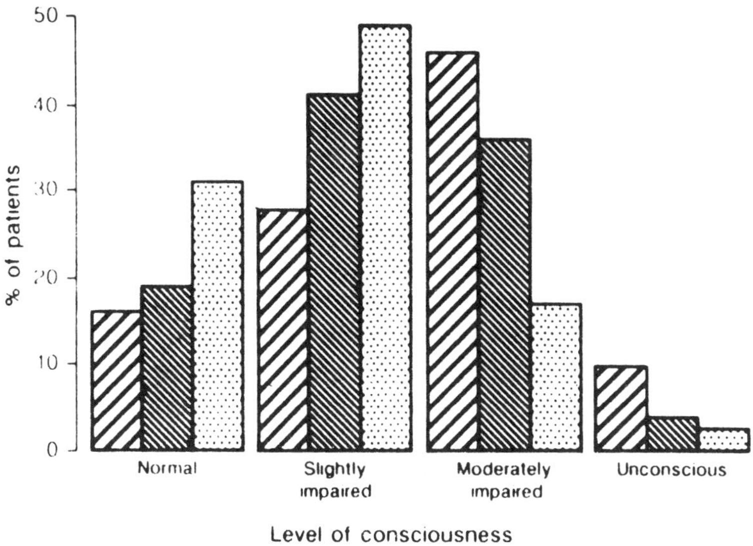

Fig 7–4.—Relation of level of consciousness on admission to duration of illness in bacterial meningitis. *Note: Hatched bars,* ≤ 24 hours; *filled bars,* > 24–48 hours; *shaded bars,* > 48 hours. $P < .001$ (≤ 24 hours vs. > 48 hours). (Courtesy of Kilpi T, Anttila M, Kallio MJT, et al: *Lancet* 338:406–409, 1991.)

ill for more than 48 hours before diagnosis. The relationships between the length of history and various clinical and laboratory parameters were determined.

Results.—Children with short histories of illness had greater impairments of consciousness than did those with longer histories (Fig 7–4). Seizures before or at admission occurred in 24% of patients with short histories, significantly more than the 9% of those with long durations of illness. Other variables that were significantly worse in children with symptoms or signs of BM for 48 hours or less included CSF protein concentrations, a positive CSF Gram stain, positive blood cultures, serum C-reactive protein (CRP), and the urinary sodium concentration. Neither causative organism, sex, age, nor preadmission antimicrobial treatment accounted for the differences. A multiple regression analysis showed that significant differences existed between the groups with histories of different duration for levels of consciousness, seizures, otitis media, systolic blood pressure, CSF protein, serum CRP, blood hemoglobin concentration, and urine electrolyte concentrations.

Conclusions.—Children with symptoms of BM for more than 48 hours before diagnosis appear to do significantly better than those with a shorter history of illness. On the basis of the level of consciousness and seizures, those with symptoms for less than 24 hours were in the worst clinical condition and experienced higher mortality rates. When BM occurs in its acute form, sepsis and meningitis may develop in a few hours. In these cases, diagnostic delay may be unavoidable.

▶ Studies that turn conventional wisdom on its head are always interesting. The implications of these data are important for our understanding of BM but also extend to the medicolegal arena (see also Abstract 7–24).

The organization of Finland's health care system allowed the authors to collect a larger series of patients than previous prospective studies of BM. When divided by duration of illness or other variables, the groups remain large enough for statistical analysis. The strength of the study is in the statistical significance of many clinical and laboratory parameters showing a greater severity of illness in patients with a shorter duration of symptoms. The surprising results need replication to reconcile the authors' conclusions with other studies, both laboratory and clinical, that show progression of the severity of illness and laboratory abnormalities over time.

Differences in virulence factors of the organisms or host factors need to be better understood to explain the variability in clinical presentation. The authors should look at outcome as related to the duration of symptoms prior to diagnosis. The development of *Haemophilus influenzae* vaccine and steroid therapy was necessitated by the observation that even with early diagnosis and prompt treatment, some children had neurologic sequelae.

Allegations of a failure to diagnose BM are the most costly and painful type of litigation for pediatric emergency physicians. The understanding that some children with BM become very ill very fast and that others have a more insidious course demonstrates that sequelae and delays in diagnosis may indeed be unavoidable.—M. Joffe, M.D.

Pediatric Bacterial Meningitis: Is Prior Antibiotic Therapy Associated With an Altered Clinical Presentation?

Rothrock SG, Green SM, Wren J, Letai D, Daniel-Underwood L, Pillar E (Loma Linda Univ; Riverside Gen Hosp, Calif; California Emergency Physicians' Med Group, Oakland)

Ann Emerg Med 21:146–152, 1992 7–24

Introduction.—The initiation of antibiotic therapy before hospital admission may mask the diagnosis of meningitis. The clinical features of children treated orally with antibiotics were retrospectively compared with those who were not treated before bacterial meningitis was diagnosed.

Methods.—Between 1979 and 1990, 258 children 24 months old or younger were hospitalized for bacterial meningitis proven by culture, antigen study, or Gram's stain. In the 24 hours before the detection of meningitis, 83 children were treated with antibiotics, and 175 were not. Their records were reviewed for demographic, historic, physical examination, and laboratory features.

Results.—Although the duration of symptoms before diagnosis was longer in pretreated patients, they exhibited significantly lower rates of altered mental status and temperatures of 38.3°C or higher. Pretreated children had more frequent vomiting, ear, nose, and throat infections, and physician visits before detection of meinigitis than did untreated children. There were no significant differences between groups in the incidence of upper respiratory symptoms, seizures, nuchal rigidity, Kernig's and Brudzinki's signs, focal neurologic signs, mortality, or the length of hospitalization.

Conclusions.—Children 24 months old or younger who receive antibiotics before the detection of meningitis have a more subtle presentation than untreated children do. A high index of suspicion should be maintained when evaluating children who were given antibiotics for a seemingly minor illness.

▶ The standard teaching was that children with partially treated meningitis had a modified set of signs and symptoms on the assumption that antibiotic therapy suppressed the manifestations of the illness at first. Once several days passed, the illness would re-emerge more fulminantly. While this is a retrospective review, it still confirms that we must be especially careful in evaluating children who are currently taking antibiotics. This paper points out that these children have not only a lower rate of altered mental status but also concurrent illnesses that could lead one astray.

Antibiotics also affect CSF studies and, in the case of ceftriaxone, may make the diagnosis difficult and easily missed. Additional CSF studies are warranted in children pretreated with antibiotics. If the suspicion is high enough, then hospital admission is warranted until cultures are negative or the child recovers. This article reminds us of the dangers inherent in return visits to the emergency department.—R.W. Schafermeyer, M.D.

The Changing Spectrum of Neonatal Meningitis Over a Fifteen-Year Period

Shattuck KE, Chonmaitree T (Univ of Texas, Galveston)

Clin Pediatr 31:130–136, 1992 7–25

Background.—Meningitis remains a significant cause of mortality and morbidity in neonates. A study was done to determine whether the etiology of neonatal meningitis is changing over time, to characterize the presentation of different types of meningitis in 1 neonatal population, and to assess the necessity of lumbar puncture in the routine sepsis workup.

Methods.—One hundred seventy-seven cases of neonatal meningitis treated at the University of Texas Medical Branch at Galveston between 1974 and 1988 were studied. Medical records were examined for age, gestational age, birth history, gender, race, interval between illness onset and diagnostic lumbar puncture, clinical presentation, laboratory findings, culture results, treatment, and follow-up.

Findings.—During the 15-year period of the study, the incidence of bacterial meningitis declined. The incidence of aseptic meningitis remained the same, and the diagnosis of enteroviral meningitis was made more frequently. Between 1984 and 1988, the most common cause of meningitis in neonates older than 7 days was enterovirus, which accounted for one third of all cases of neonatal meningitis. Half of all the infants with bacterial meningitis had negative results on their blood cultures.

Conclusions.—Diagnostic lumbar puncture should remain part of the routine assessment of neonates with suspected sepsis. Cerebrospinal fluid should be cultured for enterovirus and for bacteria when an infant older than 7 days is seen with suspected sepsis.

▶ The incidence of neonatal meningitis has gone down, but no one is sure of the reasons for the decline. Certainly, this good fortune should have no impact on the way we manage individual neonates with fever. They all must receive a complete septic workup. It is hoped that neonatal meningitis will continue to have a declining incidence, but I believe in the jinx factor, so such blessings are better left unmentioned.—S. Ludwig, M.D.

Seizures Associated With Meningitis

Rosenberg NM, Meert K, Marino D, De Baker K (Children's Hosp of Michigan, Detroit)

Pediatr Emerg Care 8:67–69, 1992 7–26

Introduction.—Seizures have been described in 11% to 53% of children with bacterial meningitis. The records of 187 such patients who were admitted in 1981 through 1987 to an urban children's hospital were reviewed. Two thirds of the children were admitted through the emergency department.

Findings.—Twenty-five patients (13%) were admitted with seizures. Seven of the 25 patients with seizures had received antibiotics before the diagnosis was made. Four of those patients but none of those not given antibiotics lacked other initial signs and symptoms. One fourth of all patients had received oral antibiotics. All pretreated patients survived intact, but 13 who were not pretreated died or remained in a vegetative state. The 33 patients who had seizures after admission had a poorer outcome than the others; their CSF protein levels were significantly higher.

Recommendations.—Children who have seizures before arrival at the emergency department but who have no other signs or symptoms of meningitis do not require lumbar puncture. Those having a seizure after receiving antibiotics are an exception.

▶ The average age of the 25 babies who had seizures as their initial symptom of meningitis was 14 ± 17 months in this study. Their average temperature was 37.4 ± 1.6°C. The signs and symptoms of meningitis are often nonspecific in young babies. Lethargy, irritability, and vomiting are more common than fever, nuchal rigidity, and bulging fontanelles. One could argue that any child with seizures who is less than 18 months of age and does not have a clear traumatic or metabolic etiology needs to be evaluated for meningitis. Clearly, babies pretreated with antibiotics that may mask symptoms deserve a lumbar puncture. (See also Abstract 9–4.) —K.N. Shaw, M.D.

Management of the Febrile Child: A Survey of Pediatric and Emergency Medicine Residency Directors

Baraff LJ (Univ of California, Los Angeles)

Pediatr Infect Dis J 10:795–800, 1991 7–27

Objective.—There is not yet any standard of care for the management of febrile children. A survey of all residency directors of post graduate training programs in pediatrics and emergency medicine was conducted to determine whether there is uniformity in the training of residents regarding this issue.

Methods.—A survey instrument was sent to the directors of 231 pediatric and 76 emergency medicine residency programs. Ten specific questions regarding the definition, evaluation, and treatment of febrile children were included.

Findings.—Response rates were 62% among pediatric and 53% among emergency medicine residency directors. There was no uniformity in the definition of fever; suggested temperatures ranged from 37.4° C to 38.6°C, and no temperature was used by more than 40% of the teaching programs. Likewise, there was no consensus about what age febrile children should be admitted to the hospital, although significantly more pediatric (99%) than emergency medicine (82%) respondents indicated that all febrile infants younger than 4 weeks should be admitted. Forty-eight percent of pediatric respondents and 42% of emergency medicine respondents taught that lumbar puncture should be performed for all children younger than 12 months when they have their first febrile convulsion. Thirty percent and 61%, respectively, taught that blood cultures should be obtained for children with fever without a source who are younger than 24 months. The teachings regarding the use of nonspecific and specific tests also varied. Interestingly, almost no program taught that the Yale observation scale should be used in the evaluation of febrile children. Although the majority of directors taught that antibotics should not be prescribed for children with fever of unknown source, approximately 45% allowed this practice for children younger than 2 months.

Conclusions.—The survey quantified substantial variation in the approach to febrile children and there were significant differences in training by specialty. There is a need to develop objective criteria that will facilitate a more uniform approach to the febrile child.

▶ Dr. Baraff is right. There is no standard of care for the management of the febrile child. Everyone does it differently. Each academician has a study supporting his view, and each practitioner has his favorite test and antibiotics to combat fever. Many studies, almost too numerous to count, have tried to shed light on this issue, yet it is still confusing, and emergency department management is hampered by noncompliant parents and the uncertainty of follow-up. At times, the stakes are high, as in the febrile patient less than 1 month of age. I am surprised that emergency medicine respondents did not think that more of these children should be admitted because they are the highest-risk group with poorly localizing symptoms when infected with a serious bacterial infection. At the least, they should consider hospitalizing children for inpatient observation. The same caution is true for patients with sickle cell anemia and other children with immunocompromising illnesses.

On the other hand, many viral illnesses cause children to undergo additional testing and possibly antibiotic therapy because the child's parent chose to bring the child to the doctor or emergency department. It is not surprising to see blood cultures obtained more frequently in the emergency department than in the clinic setting. Urinalysis is probably obtained less often than it should be.

While the Yale observation scale continues to get press coverage, it has never been validated as the magic bullet that has the sensitivity, specificity, and predictive values to make it a gold standard. A different scale could be developed and validated, but until then, every physician needs to evaluate the child's behavior and mental status, document that status, and treat according to what the history and physical examination suggest as the most prudent management.—R.W. Schafermeyer, M.D.

Diagnosis of Urinary Tract Infection in Children: Fresh Urine Microscopy or Culture?

Vickers D, Ahmad T, Coulthard MG (Royal Victoria Infirmary, Newcastle upon Tyne, England)

Lancet 338:767–770, 1991 7–28

Background.—Urinary-tract infection in children requires prompt treatment to avoid serious, debilitating illness, but diagnosis by culture requires some time. Clinicians occasionally do not receive confirmation for 3 days or longer after urine collection.

Methods.—The value of microscopy was examined in 342 children who either had a history of urinary tract infection or had symptoms consistent with infection. Fresh unspun, unstained specimens were examined at × 400 in a mirrored counting chamber and were also sent to a microbiology laboratory for culture. Many samples were also plated onto dip slides.

Findings.—The initial microscopic study identified all but 1 of 24 urinary tract infections, with 1 false positive report due to vaginal contamination by lactobacilli. Nine percent of the specimens were equivocal. More than 6% of the urine cultures yielded false positive results, with growth of more than 10^5 colony-forming units per milliliter on a single organism. True infections were associated with counts higher than 10^7/mL.

Conclusions.—Microscopic examination of urine by a clinician is a more reliable screening test for urinary tract infection in children than is routine culture in a microbiology laboratory. It also is less expensive and more expeditious.

▶ Emergency physicians frequently decide on presumptive therapy for urinary tract infections (UTIs) on the basis of clinical information and screening laboratory tests. The optimal screening test is accurate, rapid, easy to perform, and inexpensive. This study comparing fresh urine microscopy with culture is well designed and interesting but does not address significant recent developments in this area.

The study was performed by physicians in a pediatric renal unit, who presumably have considerable expertise in urine microscopy. The sample included only patients referred to the specialty clinic or inpatient unit. One should not assume that an emergency physician using a microscope available in the emergency department in a different population would achieve the same accuracy.

Urine dipsticks for leukocyte esterase and nitrite are more rapid, easier, and probably less expensive, considering time and equipment, than fresh urine microscopy. Studies in children have shown sensitivities and specificities that approach laboratory urinalysis. The study should have compared fresh urine microscopy with dipsticks as well as culture. There are data to suggest that young infants, who are at greater risk of urosepsis, are more likely to have a positive urine culture with an unremarkable urinalysis. The authors should have called attention to these important differences with young infants.

Sensitivity is the more important parameter when developing a screening test. False positives may result in some unnecessary testing and treatment, but this is of less importance than the serious consequences that can occur from a false negative. Fresh urine microscopy missed a UTI that was subsequently proved by culture. The better performance of microscopy was primarily related to its better specificity.

Recent CLIA regulations limit the ability of physicians to perform laboratory tests on their own. Trends in the United States have been to send more specimens to certified laboratories, where quality control can be more carefully monitored. The recommendation for fresh urine microscopy over culture may be reasonable in Great Britain, but in 1992 it is not a realistic possibility in many emergency departments in the United States.—M. Joffe, M.D.

Sleep Apnea in Infants Who Succumb to the Sudden Infant Death Syndrome

Schechtman VL, Harper RM, Wilson AJ, Southall DP (Univ of California, Los Angeles; Royal Hallamshire Hosp, Sheffield, England; Natl Heart and Lung Inst, London, England)

Pediatrics 87:841–846, 1991 7–29

Background.—Studies of apnea in infants at risk of sudden infant death syndrome (SIDS) have given inconsistent results. Siblings of SIDS victims have been noted to have increased brief apneic pauses and more frequent periodic breathing during quiet sleep than did control infants in some studies but not in others. Infants who have had an apparent life-threatening event are also found to breath periodically more often than expected.

Study Design.—Sleep recordings were available for 22 healthy infants aged 2 to 65 days who later died of SIDS and for 66 matched control infants. The number of apneic pauses and the total duration of apnea during quiet sleep and rapid eye movement (REM) sleep were compared in those groups in the first month of life and at the age of 40 to 65 days.

Findings.—Victims of SIDS had fewer apenic pauses than did control infants after the age of 1 month but not before. The total duration of apneic pauses tended to be shorter in older SIDS victims than in controls. Brief apneic pauses were less frequent in SIDS victims during both quiet sleep and REM sleep.

Interpretation.—A reduced number of apneic pauses is the first finding of a difference in victims of SIDS in the second month of life that is not apparent in the early postnatal period. Few SIDS-related deaths occur before the age of 1 month; the great majority take place at 2 to 6 months of age, thus indicating some vulnerability in older SIDS victims.

► The evaluation of infants at risk for SIDS is widely discussed in pediatric emergency medicine literature. There have been innumerable studies testing infants who are near-miss SIDS survivors, siblings of SIDS patients, and other assorted groups of babies who are felt to be at high risk. The results of apnea studies on these infants during different periods of sleep and under different conditions have had widely varying results as reviewed in this paper from UCLA. This group finds that when compared with controls, there are actually fewer respiratory pauses during both quiet sleep and REM sleep in those babies studied during the second month of life who went on to die of SIDS later in infancy. This finding may have important implications for the etiology of SIDS, although the relationship would seem intuitively to be the inverse of what one might expect. I think the bottom line is that we still have very little actual insight into the ultimate causes of SIDS, but it is probably a multifactorial problem that involves alterations in central control of respiration during sleep in some groups of babies, as well as obstructive airway problems in other babies, and perhaps primary cardiovascular dysfunction in yet another group.—F.M. Henretig, M.D.

Blood Lead Levels in Children With Foreign Bodies

Wiley JF II, Henretig FM, Selbst SM (The Children's Hosp of Philadelphia, Pa)

Pediatrics 89:593–596, 1992 7–30

Background.—Inner-city children remain at high risk for lead poisoning. Previous studies have reported an association between increased lead absorption and increases in certain behaviors such as pica, finger sucking, mouthing of nonfood items, and accidental poison ingestion. Whether children with aural, nasal, or gastrointestinal (GI) foreign bodies also have increased blood lead levels and whether such behavior could be considered an additional marker for lead poisoning was investigated.

Patients.—The study population consisted of 40 children with a mean age of 39 months who were brought to an urban pediatric emergency department (ED) with aural, nasal, or GI foreign bodies; 40 children with a mean age of 44 months who were seen in the same ED for other reasons, and 65 children with a mean age of 35 months who were attending a pediatric clinic in the same hospital. All children were younger than 6 years of age, and none had a previous diagnosis of lead poisoning. Venous blood samples were obtained for lead and erythrocyte protoporphyrin (EP) determinations. All parents were interviewed to obtain data on environmental and behavioral risk factors for lead poisoning.

Results.—Children with foreign bodies had a higher mean venous blood lead level and were more likely to have an elevated blood lead value than did patients in either control group. Emergency department clinic controls had the same incidence of elevated blood lead values. Among all children with elevated blood lead levels, those with foreign bodies had a greater degree of blood lead elevation than did those in either control group. Children with foreign bodies also had a higher incidence of prior pica or prior poison ingestion than did controls attending the pediatric medical clinic. There was no significant difference in environmental risk factors among the 3 groups.

Conclusions.—Inner-city children living in areas with a high prevalence of lead poisoning when seen in the ED with foreign bodies should be screened for lead poisoning while in the ED.

▶ The authors call attention to the fact that asymptomatic early lead poisoning remains a public health problem, particularly for inner-city children. While previous authors have identified other behavioral characteristics, notably pica, as associated with increased lead absorbtion, the association of such findings with the presence of foreign bodies has not previously been reported. While the authors address the problem predominantly in infants and children with acutely placed foreign bodies, other investigators at our institution are currently looking at the risk of elevated blood lead levels in adolescents with persistent retained foreign bodies. As the authors note, it may be necessary to exclude primary behavioral characteristics. Additionally, the authors call attention to the case for utilizing the emergency center as a vehicle to develop appropriate public health screening programs, a substantial area for growth of the specialty in an ever-increasing cost-conscious and preventive health environment.—D.K. Wagner, M.D.

The Clinical Features of Children With Malrotation of the Intestine

Bonadio WA, Clarkson T, Naus J (Med College of Wisconsin, Milwaukee)

Pediatr Emerg Care 7:348–349, 1991 7–31

Introduction.—Malrotation of the intestine is a relatively uncommon condition that usually occurs in young infants and can be serious or even fatal when accompanied by volvulus of the midgut. Early diagnosis and prompt surgical intervention are required for a favorable outcome. Data on 37 patients with malrotation of the intestine were reviewed.

Methods.—The children were initially seen in 1977 to 1988. All were previously healthy when they came to the emergency department with bilious vomiting (97%) or constipation (89%). The group included 20 boys and 17 girls aged younger than 1 week to older than 10 years. Most (33) were aged 8 weeks or younger. A barium contrast study of the upper gastrointestinal tract was performed in 36 patients and revealed an obstructive process of the duodenum. Laparotomy was performed in all 37 patients.

Results.—In 25 children there was volvulus of the midgut, although 23 appeared well and 15 had no abnormal findings at the initial abdominal examination. The 2 infants younger than 10 days who died were in shock with extensive gangrene of the bowel.

Conclusion.—Infants and children with malrotation of the bowel may not appear ill at presentation. All young infants with bilious vomiting should undergo a radiographic study of the upper gastrointestinal tract.

▶ An imminently treatable, yet frequently overlooked condition, malrotation should rarely be missed. The majority of infants with malrotation will be seen in the first 8 weeks of age. Any infant with bilious vomiting deserves a radiographic evaluation, even if healthy appearing.

Occasionally, patients with malrotation may have a benign, relatively symptom-free course, with the malrotation being discovered serendipitously. Alternatively, older children may have a long history of chronic gastrointestinal complaints such as chronic abdominal pain with intermittent vomiting. Several children have had alternating bouts of diarrhea, bulky stools, and evidence of malabsorption. Children with a history of long-standing chronic vomiting, abdominal pain, and/or episodes of abdominal distension deserve consideration of malrotation as the cause, with appropriate diagnostic studies.—R.M. Rutstein, M.D.

Aicardi Syndrome: A Clinicopathologic Case Report Including Electron Microscopic Observations

Font RL, Marines HM, Cartwright J Jr., Bauserman SC (Cullen Eye Institute; The Methodist Hosp, Houston, Tex; Texas A&M Univ, Temple)

Ophthalmology 98:1727–1731, 1991 7–32

Background.—Aicardi syndrome, characterized by infantile spasms, agenesis of the corpus callosum, severe mental retardation, and chorioreti-nopathy with lacunar defects, is thought to be an X-linked dominant disorder. It is found mostly in girls. A patient with Aicardi syndrome was studied.

Case Report.—A 2-year-old girl was found unresponsive by her babysitter and taken to the hospital emergency room. The girl died about 1 hour later despite extensive attempts to resuscitate her. Histopathologic findings at autopsy, confined to the brain and eyes, were highly characteristic of Aicardi syndrome. The primary abnormalities were agenesis of the corpus callosum, micro-polygyria, bilateral papillomas of the choroid plexi, and bilateral microph-thalmos. Bilateral hypoplasia of the optic nerves, bilateral colobomas of the juxtapapillaris choroid and optic disk, bilateral total retinal detachment with dysplastic rosettes and chorioretinal lacunae with focal thinning, and atrophy of the retinal pigment epithelium and choroid were also seen. Scanning electron microscopy of the chorioretinal lacunae showed peculiar papillary proliferations of the retinal pigment epithelium in both eyes.

Conclusions.—The histopathologic abnormalities in this case were consistent with Aicardi syndrome. Chorioretinal lacunae, believed to be pathognomonic, were found in both eyes. The cause of this syndrome is not known. More than 100 cases of it have been reported.

▶ This article contains some interesting information about the unfortunate genetic defect called Aicardi syndrome. This is a rare condition that should be confirmed and reported to the parents prior to a child's arrival at the emergency center. For me, this article raises a more generic issue—how do we identify children on an outpatient basis who fall into a "do not resuscitate" (DNR) category? How can we develop mechanisms that are safe, caring, and legally responsible so that an infant need not endure an hour of resuscitative effort that is not necessary? We seem to have come to some peace with DNRs on the inpatient side. How do we conduct the same type of ethical discussion and put outpatient DNRs into practice when appropriate?—S. Ludwig, M.D.

Sudden Cardiac Death in the Pediatric Population

Gillette PC, Garson A Jr (Med Univ of South Carolina, Charleston; Baylor College of Medicine, Houston, Tex)

Circulation 85:(suppl 1):64–69, 1992 7–33

Introduction.—Although sudden deaths are less frequent in children than in adults, many are preventable, and others are potentially preventable. Sudden nontraumatic death accounts for as many as 20% of deaths in the age range 1 to 20 years.

Apparently Normal Children.—There are 6,000 to 7,000 cases of sudden infant death syndrome each year in the United States. The cause remains unknown, but one suggestion is that a sudden increase in sympathetic activity, as may result from emotion or physical stress, initiates sudden arrhythmic death associated with a long QT interval. Sudden deaths also occasionally occur in older children. Patients with idiopathic hypertrophic subaortic stenosis may die during exercise.

Cardiac Patients.—Sudden death may occur in 1% of children with aortic stenosis each year. In some series, mitral valve prolapse is the most common cardiac diagnosis associated with sudden death. Cardiac surgery has not eliminated the risk of sudden death for children who have congenital cardiac defects. Sudden deaths of patients with Fallot's tetralogy may represent conduction disorder with a complete atrioventricular or ventricular arrhythmia. Arrhythmias are not infrequent after the Mustard or Senning operation for transposition of the great arteries.

Specific Arrhythmias.—Patients with Wolff-Parkinson-White syndrome who have a short antegrade refractory period of the accessory pathway or who receive digoxin are at risk of dying suddenly. Sick sinus syndrome is a risk factor when it follows cardiac surgery. Complete atrioventricular block is a potential cause of sudden death in children. Ventricular arrhythmias are a particular risk in those having repair of congential heart defects.

▶ The authors review the current literature on sudden death in children. For the emergency physician, it is stressed that a cardiac evaluation including a good physical examination, chest radiograph, ECG, and referral or consultation with cardiology for echocardiography, exercise testing, and halter monitoring be done for all children with syncope. Acute myocarditis and previously undetected abnormalities such as QT prolongation, hypertrophic cardiomyopathy, aortic stenosis, mitral valve prolapse, coronary artery abnormalities, and Marfan's syndrome are reasons for sudden death in children without known cardiac disease. However, all syncope is not cardiac in origin. Seizures should also be considered. Additionally, make sure that it was not a simple vasovagal episode prior to this workup. (See Abstract 3–21.)—K.N. Shaw, M.D.

Sickle Cell Screening Practice in Pediatric Emergency Departments
Losek JD (Med College of Wisconsin, Milwaukee)
Pediatr Emerg Care 7:278–280, 1991 7–34

Background.—Sepsis is the leading cause of death in children with sickle cell disease, and most of these children are younger than 3 years of age. The impact of sickle cell disease status on the management of black children with unknown status who come to an emergency department (ED) is unknown. The need and method of screening for sickle cell disease in black children who come to a pediatric ED was determined.

Method.—A mail survey of 32 pediatric ED directors was conducted by a brief written case presentation and questions. In a prospective review parents of black children younger than 2 years of age who were seen in the ED were questioned about their child's sickle cell disease status.

Findings.—Twenty-two of 28 EDs surveyed included sickle cell screening by the differential solubility test for hemoglobin S in the management of the hypothetical case of a febrile black infant aged 6 months. The parents of only 9 of 51 patients whose condition warranted knowledge of their sickle cell status knew their child's status. Thirty-five of the patients (69%) had a presumptive newborn screening test for sickle cell disease, but only 15 were present when the test results were readily available from the laboratory. Thirteen of these 15 patients had private physicians, but only 3 physicians had the results of newborn sickle cell screening tests. A review of the patients' hospital records revealed that 9 patients had prior screening tests and 30 required a sickle cell screening test in the ED. The ED screening detected 3 patients with newly diagnosed sickle cell trait.

Conclusions.—Newborn sickle cell screening data are a dependable source of determining disease status, but in this study, parental knowledge and hospital and physician medical records were not good sources of the data. Unless the data are available from records, personal knowledge, or the laboratory at all times, double screening may be necessary for ED management of young black children. A sickle cell screening test is recommended for a young black child in the ED if newborn screening results are not available.

▶ Previous studies have noted improved survival in children with sickle cell disease diagnosed early in infancy. The benefits of early diagnosis are dependent on contacting identified families, and providing extensive parental education, expectant therapy for febrile illnesses and sequestration, and penicillin prophylaxis. On the basis of these studies, many states now routinely test for hemoglobinopathies at birth. In all states now performing newborn screening, only children with abnormal results are notified (much as with phenylketonuria and thyroid testing). The majority of parents, therefore, will not be informed of their newborns' hemoglobin test results.

In our city, over the last 2 years some 50,000 newborns have been screened. The screening center has been able to contact 60 of the 65 families of newborns identified with either homozygous hemoglobin sickle cell disease or thalassemia. When a child comes to the emergency center or physician's office and the family is unaware of the sickle cell status, only very rarely will the child have an undiagnosed hemoglobinopathy (approximately 1 in 10,000 infants in our area).

It would certainly improve medical care if the parents were notified of all results or, alternatively, if there were a 24-hour hotline to call for newborn screening results. Several jurisdictions are experimenting with such a system where physicians can access computerized results from office phones.

The cost of rescreening all febrile African-American infants seen in the emergency center and then admitting the 8% with abnormal screening test results (>90% of the time from the presence of sickle trait, not disease) is quite high; we can deliver lower-cost, better-quality care by providing newborn screening results to parents and health care providers.—R.M. Rutstein, M.D.

Pain in Sickle Cell Disease: Rates and Risk Factors

Platt OS, Thorington BD, Brambilla DJ, Milner PF, Rosse WF, Vichinsky E, Kinney TR (Children's Hosp, Boston; New England Research Inst, Watertown, Mass; Med College of Georgia, Augusta; Duke Univ, Durham, NC; Oakland Children's Hosp, Calif)

N Engl J Med 325:11–16, 1991 7–35

Introduction.—Patients with sickle cell disease experience periodic episodes of acute muscoloskeletal pain known as "crises." Little is known about the epidemiologic characteristics of this clinical syndrome.

Methods.—The 3,578 study participants were enrolled at 23 clinical centers. Patients ranged in age from newborn to 66 years and were followed between 1979 and 1988. A pain rate was calculated by dividing the number of episodes by the number of patient-years. Findings were categorized according to the 4 hemoglobinopathy groups: sickle cell anemia, sickle β^0-thalassemia, hemoglobin SC disease, and sickle β^+-thalassemia.

Results.—There were 12,290 episodes of pain with a wide variation within each of the 4 hemoglobinopathy groups. Patients with sickle cell anemia who averaged 3 to 10 episodes a year represented only 5.2% of that group but accounted for 32.9% of the pain episodes. Patients with sickle cell anemia who were over the age of 20 years and had a high rate of pain episodes tended to die earlier than those with low rates. Of all the laboratory values tested, only hematocrit and fetal hemoglobin level appeared to be important risk factors for pain. Few patients entering the study between 10 and 19 years of age died, but there appeared to be no relation between mortality and pain rates in this age group. Apart from its association with an increased hematocrit, α-thalassemia had no effect on pain.

Conclusion.—In patients with sickle cell anemia over the age of 20 years, the number of pain episodes a year is a measure of clinical severity and is correlated with early death. The relationship between low fetal hemoglobin levels and high rates of pain suggest that treatments designed to increase these levels may also improve survival.

▶ Emergency physicians care about sickle cell disease because they must provide early care to many patients in crisis. Factors affecting the severity of the disease and survival of the patients are of interest.

Patients with frequent crises have a poorer prognosis. An elevation of fetal hemoglobin levels will improve prognoses. Identification of patients in recurrent crisis may be an important role for emergency medicine.

Specific therapy to limit recurrences will be a welcome advance in this chronic condition.—J.E. Clinton, M.D.

Procedures and Techniques

Retrograde-Assisted Fiberoptic Tracheal Intubation in Children With Difficult Airways

Audenaert SM, Montgomery CL, Stone B, Akins RE, Lock RL (Univ of Kentucky; Shriners Hosp for Crippled Children, Lexington, Ky)
Anesth Analg 73:660–664, 1991 7–36

Background.—Retrograde and flexible fiber-optic techniques can be used for clinical management of difficult pediatric airways. Retrograde-assisted fiber-optic intubation in 20 pediatric patients, 7 of whom were less than 16 months of age, is reported.

Case Report.—An 11-month-old, 7.8-kg boy with mandibular hypoplasia and Klippel-Feil anomaly was admitted for elective surgery. He received methohexital administered rectally for general anesthesia, 0.16 mg of glycopyrrolate through intravenous access, and incremental halothane in oxygen via a Patil-Syracuse mask to deepen anesthesia. Spontaneous ventilation was maintained. The airway was secured by the following method: needle cricothyrotomy was performed by using a 22-guage Teflon catheter over a needle. The needle and catheter were advanced until there was free aspiration of air. The needle was withdrawn, and a guidewire was passed through the catheter and cephalad to exit through the left nostril. The cephalad end of the wire was fed through the suction port of an intubating bronchoscope loaded with a softened, lubricated endotracheal tube. Phenylephrine was applied to the nasal mucosa, and the bronchoscope was fed along the wire past the vocal cords. The wire was withdrawn. The bronchoscope was then further advanced, and the endotracheal tube was inserted to an appropriate depth.

Discussion.—Use of the pediatric bronchoscope makes “intubation over the scope” possible with endotracheal tubes as small as 3 mm internal diameter. The use of the retrograde wire allows even an inexperienced bronchoscopist to quickly follow the wire to the glottic opening. These combined techniques permit one to bypass abnormal landmarks, edema, and small amounts of blood. The bronchoscopist can also perform oxygen insufflation throughout bronchoscopy and intubation. Retrograde-assisted fiber-optic intubation, while not frequently used, is a useful method of securing a difficult pediatric airway.

▶ This is an interesting description of the use of retrograde-wire assisted, fiber-optic guided bronchoscopic intubation of the trachea in children with complicated airway management problems primarily resulting from congenital anomalies of the head, neck, and face. These patients were all intubated in the operating room for elective surgical procedures, and although the authors describe the technique as being relatively easy and straightforward, there are few details given as to the typical length of time to perform the procedure. We presume that the authors are all members of the department of anesthesia at their institution. Whether this technique would be immediately adaptable to the emergency department setting, particularly for practitioners who are relatively inexperienced with pediatric airway management, remains to be seen. To my knowledge, there have been no formal studies of retrograde-wire assisted tracheal intubation in children under any circumstances as yet, although I think that there might be a role for the use of such a techninque in a severely facially injured young infant or child, as has been described in the adult population.—F.M. Henretig, M.D.

Subclavian Vein Catheterization in Critically Ill Children: Analysis of 322 Cannulations

Casado-Flores J, Valdivielso-Serna A, Pérez-Jurado L, Pozo-Román J, Monleón-Luque M, García-Pérez J, Ruiz-Beltran A, García-Teresa MA (Niño Jesús Hosp, Madrid)

Intensive Care Med 17:350–354, 1991 7–37

Background.—Percutaneous subclavian vein catheterization (SCVC) has become a vital technique for proper emergency treatment in adults. However, there is still concern about the potential complications of this technique in children. This prospective study assessed the technical difficulties and complications of SCVC in children.

Methods.—During an 8.5-year period, 322 SCVCs were done in 272 children with a mean age of 2.6 years. The most common reason for intensive care unit admission was sepsis. Catheters were placed at the bedside by critical-care pediatricians via the infraclavicular route; reasons for placement were hemodynamic monitoring in 48%, lack of peripheral venous access in 22%, parenteral nutrition in 13%, CPR in 13%, or other emergency situations. Catheters were cultured on removal in most cases.

Results.—The success rate of SCVC was 93%; 70% of insertions were done under routine conditions, and 30% were performed in emergencies. There was a 13% occurrence of incidents during the cannulation procedure. Nine of these 41 incidents required emergency therapy, including 6 cases of pneumothorax, 2 of hemothorax, and 1 of hydrothorax. Misplacement of the catheter tip was more common when inserted on the right side. While the catheter was in place, there was a 6.5% incidence of complications, including 7 cases in which the catheter migrated out of position, 3 venous thromboses, and 3 catheter obstructions. Of 190 catheters cultured, there was a 17% incidence of positive cultures, most through colonization. The most common organism isolated was *Staphylococcus epidermidis*. Significant associations were seen between catheterization for more than 5 days and catheter-related sepsis and between isolation of *S. epidermidis* and the duration of cannula use. No deaths were ascribed to use of the catheter.

Conclusions.—As in adults, percutaneous SCVC is a nearly essential technique in the treatment of critically ill children. Regardless of the routine or emergency nature of the insertion, it is relatively easy and safe when performed by trained, nonsurgical pediatricians. There appear to be fewer complications when the left subclavian vein is used, so it should perhaps be used first. Complications can be prevented by having a complete and rigorously defined procedure for insertion and removal.

▶ Cannulation of the subclavian vein is a technical procedure that should be familiar to every pediatric emergency medicine specialist. Nonetheless, this report confirms the existing body of thought, i.e., that the subclavian route should not be the technique of first choice. The authors demonstrate that there are a number of significant, serious complications even when the procedure is performed in the relative "calm" of the intensive care unit. A similar study done in the emergency center would no doubt result in more untoward results. It is also important to note that many of the complications required additional emergency treatment. I disagree with the conclusion drawn by the authors who write, "Subclavian vein catheterization is a procedure that has become almost essential for the beneficial handling of critically ill children. It can be performed easily and with relatively few serious complications. . . ." Knowing that there is greater than a 1 in 10 chance of being unsuccessful or harmful to the patient does not qualify as easy or simple. Other intravenous routes work as well and are safer, particularly in the emergency center.—S. Ludwig, M.D.

Complications of Endotracheal Intubation and Mechanical Ventilation in Infants and Children

Rivera R, Tibballs J (Royal Children's Hosp, Parkville, Victoria, Australia)
Crit Care Med 20:193–199, 1992 7–38

Background.—Endotracheal intubation and mechanical ventilation can be lifesaving in patients with airway obstruction and respiratory failure. In children, however, these procedures can have complications. The frequency of complications of endotracheal intubation and mechanical ventilation in infants and children was investigated.

Methods.—Eight hundred sixty-nine patients were assessed in this prospective cohort study. All were in a pediatric tertiary multidisciplinary intensive care unit. Five hundred patients were endotracheally intubated, and 431 were ventilated mechanically. The median patient age was 10 months. The median duration of endotracheal intubation was 4 days, and the median duration of mechanical ventilation was 2 days.

Findings.—One hundred eighty-six complications occurred in 119 patients for an incidence of 24%. No person died from intubation- or ventilation-related causes. The overall frequency of accidental extubation was 3.2%, which occurred at a rate of 1.26 extubations per 100 intubation days. The frequency of accidental extubation was higher in nonventilated, unsedated patients with croup or epiglottiditis, being 23% at a rate of 11.83 extubations per 100 intubation days. Lung atelectasis was seen in 7.8% of the patients. Air leaks occurred in 6.8%, and infection occurred in 2.3%. Other complications were tissue damage in 3.4%, endobronchial intubation in 2.4%, postintubation stridor in 2.4%, bronchopulmonary dysplasia in 2.3%, and endobronchial tube blockage in .8%.

Conclusions.—In this cohort, 24% of the infants and children had complications related to endotracheal intubation or mechanical ventilation. Complications were related to the duration of these interventions.

▶ It seems to me that more children and adolescents are intubated and ventilated in our emergency department (ED) than in previous years. Part of the cause is the increased acuity of illness and injury and increased regionalization of resources. Another reason is our improved understanding of the management of severe head trauma. We usually do not see the complications listed in this article. However, if overcrowding forces you to keep patients in the ED, it behooves you and your colleagues to understand the complications of mechanical ventilation.

The most common ED problems with intubation include right main stem intubation, esophageal placement, dislodgment of the tube, and air leak due to a damaged cuff. With mechanical ventilation, high- and low-pressure monitors must be on, and any patient who deteriorates while being mechanically ventilated must be taken off the ventilator and bag-ventilated while someone checks out the ventilator. If the patient does not improve, you must check tube placement and check for a pneumothorax or tension pneumothorax. (See also Abstract 7–39.)—R.W. Schafermeyer, M.D.

Validity of a Disposable End-Tidal CO_2 Detector in Verifying Endotracheal Tube Placement in Infants and Children

Bhende MS, Thompson AE, Cook DR, Saville AL (Children's Hosp of Pittsburgh, Pa)

Ann Emerg Med 21:142–145, 1992 7–39

Objective.—A disposable, colorimetric end-tidal CO^2 ($PETCO^2$) detector is available for identifying endotracheal tube (ETT) position in adults. Its validity in identifying ETT position in infants and children was evaluated in a prospective study.

Study Design.—A total of 151 intubations in 137 infants and children aged 1 day to 17 years and weighing 1.1 to 70 kg were studied. Endotracheal intubation was performed in the operating room, intensive care unit, or emergency department, both in cardiac and non-cardiac arrest settings. The tube position was verified, the $PETCO^2$ detector was attached, and the test was read as positive if there was any change to yellow and negative if it remained purple.

Findings.—In all 120 patients with spontaneous circulation, the $PETCO^2$ detector correctly identified ETT position, including 124 tracheal and 4 esophageal positions. In 17 patients in cardiopulmonary arrest, the $PETCO^2$ detector identified all 6 esophageal tube positions but incorrectly interpreted 2 of 17 endotracheal positions as esophageal intubations.

Conclusion.—The $PETCO^2$ detector is accurate in confirming ETT position in infants and children with spontaneous circulation who weigh more than 2 kg. During resuscitation a positive result confirms the tracheal position, but a negative result requires an alternative method of confirming ETT position. It is recommended that the $PETCO^2$ detector be incorporated in routine care, in the absence of other means of detecting expired CO^2, as a vital step in avoiding catastrophic esophageal intubation.

▶ How many times have you asked yourself, "Am I in the trachea?" or been asked this question by the intubationist—probably more times than you can remember. You sweat, work hard, see the cords, and then hope that the tube really did go into the trachea. You listen over the lung fields, axilla, and stomach. In this day and age, you probably look at chest rise with bag ventilation and the oxygen saturation on your pulse oximeter. Yes, it's in and you get a chest radiograph.

The $PETCO^2$ detector is a quick and easy method to verify ETT placement in adults with spontaneous circulation. Would it work in children, especially small children? It is not always safe to assume that technology that is safe in adults is safe in children. This prospective study demonstrates its usefulness in children with spontaneous circulation regardless of age or size. This technology may be especially useful for those of you who are doing rapid-sequence induction and intubation more frequently.—R.W. Schafermeyer, M.D.

The Influence of Diazepam or Lorazepam on the Frequency of Endotracheal Intubation in Childhood Status Epilepticus
Chiulli DA, Terndrup TE, Kanter RK (State Univ of New York, Syracuse)
J Emerg Med 9:13–17, 1991 7–40

Objective.—In patients with status epilepticus (SE), the use of anticonvulsant drugs can result in respiratory depression, sometimes necessitating endotracheal intubation (ETI). Diazepam has recognized respiratory depressant effects at dosages used to treat SE, whereas those of lorazepam at comparable dosages are minimal. This retrospective study compared the frequency of ETI in children with SE treated with intravenously administered diazepam or lorazepam.

Patients.—One hundred forty-two consecutive children were admitted with a diagnosis of seizure disorder or SE during a 28-month period. Of these, 38 had SE for an incidence of 27%. Twelve patients were excluded from the analysis, 10 of them because they were receiving concomitant phenobarbital. Fifteen children were treated with lorazepam, and 11 were treated with diazepam, alone or with phenytoin. These 2 groups were evaluated for demographic, seizure severity, and management variables.

Findings.—The rate of ETI was 27% in the lorazepam group vs. 73% in the diazepam group. Preintubation drug dosages—.14 mg/kg for lorazepam and .26 mg/kg for diazepam—were well within recommended limits, and their efficacy was more than 91% in both groups. There were no differences in age, weight, sex, seizure type or duration, and appropriate anticonvulsant dosage.

Conclusions.—In children with SE, lorazepam appears to reduce the incidence of ETI when compared with diazepam, regardless of whether concomitant phenytoin is given. Lorazepam may thus be preferred as the initial anticonvulsant drug. Prospective, randomized trials are needed for confirmation.

▶ This is a retrospective chart review study of the incidence of respiratory depression necessitating ETI in children being treated with diazepam vs. lorazepam for status epilepticus. The major finding, in a relatively small number of children, is a significantly higher rate of ETI in the diazepam group (73% as compared with 27% in the lorazepam group). There were actually only 26 patients, 15 treated with lorazepam and 11 treated with diazepam. The authors comment that the retrospective design of their study did not allow them to make detailed analyses of the factors that entered into the decision for ETI or to compare the precise details of drug administration in either group. It has been my own experience that while lorazepam is touted as having less respiratory depression for a given degree of anticonvulsant effect and has, in fact, become the status epilepticus anticonvulsant of choice for most pediatric emergency departments, there is one scenario that I have observed and that needs to be cautioned against. Lorazepam has a perceptible delay in onset of action on the order of 1 to 2 minutes; diazepam usually has its onset of action within seconds of the time the drug is administered. If clinicians are expecting an instantaneous cessation of seizures with the administration of their anticonvulsant and start out with a single dose of lorazepam and decide after 30 sections that they are not getting the desired effect and give a second and then possibly a third dose, they may well find that they have an apneic patient 5 minutes later, and in that context, the apnea will last for several hours, as opposed to the much shorter duration of effect that we used to observe with diazepam. This is not to be construed as a vote in favor of the routine use of diazepam over lorazepam, but rather I am counseling a little bit of patience in awaiting the onset of action of lorazepam, particularly for those of you who are more used to the nearly instantaneous effects of diazepam. As the authors point out, it is hard to compare the likelihood of the current generation of benzodiazepines to cause respiratory depression with the classic anticonvulsant regimens including phenobarbital and phenytoin from years gone by. Prior to about the past decade, it was generally considered that seizures lasting anywhere from 20 to 30 minutes were of no clinical significance to patients, and emergency medicine practitioners and pediatricians had a higher tolerance for watching and waiting as their pediatric patients continued to convulse. We now believe, based on a variety of animal studies, primarily, and more intensive investigations into the metabolic consequences of prolonged seizure activity, that status epilepticus may indeed be harmful to the cerebral metabolic state and may result in at least subtle neurologic sequelae. Thus, a more aggressive approach to stopping seizures in a timely manner is more recently advocated and, with that, undoubtedly the consequence of more frequent observation of respiratory depression and the need to provide at least temporary airway support than was previously encountered.—F.M. Henretig, M.D.

Chloral Hydrate for Emergent Pediatric Procedural Sedation: A New Look at an Old Drug

Binder LS, Leake LA (Texas Tech Univ, El Paso)
Am J Emerg Med 9:530–534, 1991 7–41

Background.—Procedural sedation is difficult to administer to children admitted to the emergency department (ED). The child is usually quite anxious, may recently have eaten, and needs immediate attention in the hurried setting of the ED. Thus, established guidelines and monitoring protocols are not always followed. Whether chloral hydrate might be safe and suitable for children in an ED setting was determined.

Methods.—The 95 children (aged 1 to 10 years) enrolled in the study were seen in an ED during a 10-month period. They received either chloral hydrate (25 to 50 mg/kg orally) or no medication before procedural intervention. The 42 given chloral hydrate were selected at physician discretion. All children were monitored by the ED staff and continuously observed by their parents.

Results.—The chloral hydrate group was significantly younger (3 vs. 4.7 years) than the control group and had significantly fewer cases of wound repair only (67% vs. 96%). The time to sedation was 42.7 minutes with chloral hydrate; the time to recovery was 42 minutes. There was no vomiting or problems with oral administration of the sedative. In 2 sub-groups examined (children younger than 6 years of age and younger than 4 years of age), sedation scores were significantly higher in the chloral hydrate group.

Conclusion.—Oral administration of chloral hydrate offers a wide margin of clinical safety well suited to ED requirements. Some children had a minimal response, perhaps because of their gastric contents. Rectal administration might improve absorption in some cases. Overall, chloral hydrate appears to fulfill many characteristics of an ideal ED pediatric sedative.

▶ These authors report a prospective study on the use of chloral hydrate for procedural sedation in children in the ED setting. Although this drug has been around for years and enjoys wide popularity in the radiologic community for pediatric sedation during CT and MRI scans, it has not been particularly popular as a procedural sedative in pediatric emergency medicine (PEM) circles due to the perception that it is relatively delayed in onset and provides a longer-than-desirable duration of action. Indeed, this study found a mean time to sedation of 42 minutes and a time to recovery of 42 minutes; the former, in particular, is considerably longer than that typically experienced with the use of the more modern parenteral agents such as midazolam. However, as the authors comment, the drug has an exceedingly high margin of safety, is easily administered orally, and may be particularly suited to procedures that are high on the anxiety scale but in which analgesia is relatively easily provided, e.g., drainage of an abscess with concurrent, local anesthesia. Most PEM practitioners are currently relying on oral or intranasal midazolam in these kinds of situations. However, I am not aware of a carefully controlled study comparing midazolam by those routes and oral chloral hydrate. In my own practice, I still prefer to establish intravenous access and use intravenous morphine or fentanyl in addition to midazolam for procedures that are likely to be significantly painful or more prolonged than those described in this paper.—F.M. Henretig, M.D.

Steroid Use Is Associated With Pneumonia in Pediatric Chest Trauma

Williams MD, Reckard PE, Knox R, Petersen SR, Schiller WR (Saint Joseph Hosp and Med Ctr, Phoenix, Ariz)

J Trauma 32:520–525, 1992 7–42

Background.—Corticosteroids are commonly used in severe closed head injuries, although their effectiveness is unproved. Endogenous, global, nonspecific immunosuppression results from major trauma, and steroid immunosuppression may have additional deleterious effects. A series of pediatric chest trauma patients were studied to identify risk factors associated with pulmonary infection.

Patients.—During a 5-year period, 342 children with traumatic injury were admitted to a trauma center specializing in neurologic trauma. Eighty of these patients had chest trauma, a rate of 23%. There were 45 boys and 33 girls ranging in age from 6 weeks to 15 years. Thirty-four children were aged 10 to 15 years. The mean Injury Severity Score was 32, and the mean Glasgow Coma Score was 9.1. Ninety percent of the patients had blunt injury, with nearly half being hit by motor vehicles. Records of 78 children were available for evaluation.

Findings.—Pulmonary infections developed in 16 children, a rate of 20%. The children with pneumonia were in the hospital for a mean of 43 days vs. 12.7 for noninfected children. They were intubated for 8.4 vs. 1.5 days and had chest tubes in place for 2.2 vs. 1.4 days. Pneumonia was significantly associated with a longer mean duration of steroid usage, 6.4 days in the infected patients vs. .8 days for noninfected patients. The duration of steroid treatment for the treatment of concomitant brain injury was a significant independent risk factor for pneumonia.

Conclusions.—In children with chest injuries, steroid treatment for concomitant brain injuries is an independent risk factor for pulmonary infection. More sparing use of steroids might help to decrease pneumonia in these patients; the indication for such treatment should be carefully evaluated. Not surprisingly, the duration of endotracheal intubation and chest tube placement are also independent risk factors for pulmonary infection.

▶ It is probably not surprising that corticosteroids increase the incidence of pneumonia in children admitted to critical care units for multiple trauma. They have never been proved to have a significant, beneficial effect in pediatric head trauma and are probably relatively unimportant in the overall scheme of things. We can probably put steroids in the same category as hypothermia vis-à-vis adjuncts to the pediatric critical care of serious trauma victims, with relatively few indications for the use of either modality in this context. I personally agree with the authors' conclusion that a careful assessment of the importance of steroid treatment, particularly the duration of treatment, for pediatric head trauma ought to be considered.—F.M. Henretig, M.D.

8 Emergency Medical Service Systems

Prehospital Care ACLS/ATLS

The Impact of Injury Severity and Prehospital Procedures on Scene Time in Victims of Major Trauma

Spaite DW, Tse DJ, Valenzuela TD, Criss EA, Meislin HW, Mahoney M, Ross J (Univ of Arizona; Tucson Fire Dept)

Ann Emerg Med 20:1299–1305, 1991 8–1

Background.—In advanced life support for victims of major trauma, it is assumed that the benefits of various procedures must be weighed against the potential negative effects of delaying definitive care. A retrospective study of severely injured patients was performed to assess the relationship among injury severity, prehospital procedures, and time spent at the scene.

Methods.—The analysis included 98 consecutive trauma patients with an Injury Severity Score greater than 15 who were brought to a level 1 trauma center. Prehospital and hospital records were evaluated for each patient. The analysis considered the prehospital procedures of oral and nasal intubation, cricothyrotomy, intravenous line placement, and military antishock trousers placement. The subjects were 66 males and 32 females with a mean age of 34 years. Motor vehicle crash was the most common cause of injury, followed by gunshot wounds and pedestrian injuries. The injury was fatal for 32.7% of the patients.

Findings.—Prehospital advanced airway procedures were successful in 33.7% of the patients, and at least 1 intravenous line was started in the field in 82.7%. More severely injured patients had more prehospital procedures, yet they tended to have shorter scene times. The mean scene time was 8.1 minutes, and 71.4% of the patients had a scene time of 10 minutes or less.

Conclusions.—Prehospital procedures can be done in severely injured patients with extremely short scene times in an urban emergency medical services system with strong medical control. More procedures may be spent on more severely injured patients, even though they have shorter scene times. More study is needed to determine the best priority for interventions in the field for victims of major trauma.

▶ The importance of this report lies not merely in the conclusion that in Tucson advanced life support procedures do not delay the transport of seriously injured trauma patients. Rather, Spaite et al. in their discussion point to the many simultaneous activities that a multiplicity of skilled providers can complete in the irreducible minimal period of time that must be spent at the scene with a seriously injured patient.

At the May 1992 Society for Academic Emergency Medicine meeting in Toronto, Spaite presented research identifying fully 45% of the "at-scene time interval" as spent in packaging and moving the patient to the transporting ambulance. The remaining 55% of the "at-scene interval" was spent in obtaining patient access, conducting an assessment, and therapy. In retrospect, it is likely that Tucson's emergency medical services field staffing favorably influences the packaging and moving portion of the "at-scene interval" as well. After all, many hands make light work.—S.J. Davidson, M.D.

Case and Survival Definitions in Out-of-Hospital Cardiac Arrest: Effect on Survival Rate Calculation

Valenzuela TD, Spaite DW, Meislin HW, Clark LL, Wright AL, et al (Univ of Arizona, Tucson)

JAMA 267:272–274, 1992 8–2

Introduction.—The considerable variations in case and survival definitions of out-of-hospital cardiac arrest have an effect on survival rate calculations. To determine the influence of case and survival definition, 3 different case definitions of cardiac arrest and 2 definitions of survival were applied to a consecutive sample of patients.

Methods.—Over a 22-month period, paramedics attempted the out-of-hospital resuscitation of 416 patients without a palpable pulse or spontaneous respiration. After excluding nontraumatic causes, 372 patients were eligible for the study.

Results.—Of the events, 59% were witnessed, and 30% of the victims received CPR from a bystander. Another subgroup (46% of the patients) were those who had a witnessed arrest and whose initial cardiac rhythm was ventricular fibrillation. Survival rates ranged from 6% to 38%. The lower figure was obtained when case was defined as all arrests and survival defined as alive at discharge. The higher figure was calculated with case defined as a witnessed ventricular fibrillation and survival defined as alive at admission.

Conclusion.—There is no current standard for case and survival definitions. Thus, studies relating specific variables to survival cannot be easily compared. All prehospital emergency systems should adopt the Utstein Consensus Conference for events occurring in out-of-hospital cardiac arrest.

Numerators, Denominators, and Survival Rates: Reporting Survival From Out-of-Hospital Cardiac Arrest

Eisenberg MS, Cummins RO, Larsen MP (Ctr for Evaluation of Emergency Med Services, King County Health Dept, Seattle, Wash; Univ of Washington, Seattle)

Am J Emerg Med 9:544–546, 1991 8–3

Background.—Reported survival rates of persons suffering out-of-hospital cardiac arrest range widely from 2% to 44%. This variability can be attributed to many factors, including differences in terminology. Uniform definitions have been proposed so that valid comparisons can be made among communities. As a global outcome measure, survival rates are calculated from a numerator—the outcome of the resuscitation attempt—and a denominator—the population receiving resuscitation. The effects of different definitions for the denominator were studied.

Methods and Findings.—Data from a cardiac arrest surveillance system in King County, Washington, from 1976 to 1988 were analyzed retrospectively. Survival rates were calculated by using 8 different definitions of denominators. The 8 rates for hospital discharge ranged from 16% to 49% (Fig 8–1). In the lowest survival rate, the denominator included all cases of cardiac arrest for whom emergency medical services personnel started CPR. For the highest survival rate, the denominator included all

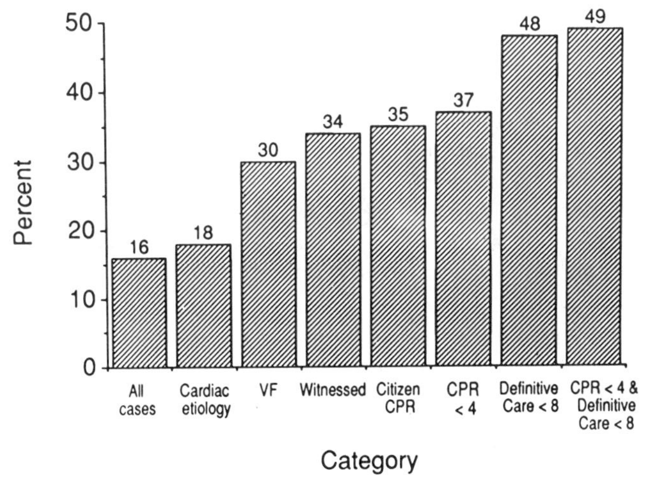

Fig 8–1.—Percent discharged from out-of-hospital cardiac arrest in King County, Washington, for different subgroups of all cardiac arrests. (Courtesy of Eisenberg MS, Cummins RO, Larsen MP: *Am J Emerg Med* 9:544–546, 1991.)

cases of presumed cardiac etiology in which the first recorded rhythm was ventricular fibrillation, the collapse was witnessed, CPR was started by bystanders within 4 minutes, and definitive care was provided within 8 minutes.

Conclusions.—The definition of cases in the denominator can markedly affect the resulting survival rate. If valid cross-community comparisons are to be made, there must be national and international agreement about definitions of denominators.

► Sudden cardiac death has been the focus of civilian emergency medical services (EMS) systems since the 1960s. Improved survival from cardiac arrest has been achieved by some EMS systems, yet broadly accepted performance standards for EMS systems' cardiac arrest survival rates have not been forthcoming. At best, EMS system managers interested in improving their system's cardiac arrest survival rate have been advised to improve the four elements of the "chain of survival": early system access, early CPR, early defibrillation, and early advanced life support.

Eisenberg et al. (Abstract 8–3) point to the absence of precise definitions and uniform reporting style as the largest obstacle inhibiting further insight into cardiac arrest survival. Without consistent definitions, a common denominator enabling the comparison of intersystem and intrasystem data (outcome results) is impossible. More importantly, the relative benefits of different system designs, means of delivering care, and other health services (organizational and operational) and clinical issues cannot be identified because knowledge of baseline system performance remains unknown.

Quality improvement activities within systems are similarly hampered. Valenzuela et al. (Abstract 8–2) point out that calculation of the cardiac arrest survival rate requires the precise definition of the numerator and denominator to ensure comparability. Most researchers advocate reporting the numerator as the number of patients discharged alive from the hospital, and many agree that the most useful denominator is the number of patients with witnessed cardiac arrest of cardiac etiology who sustain ventricular fibrillation and receive bystander CPR. Yet, consistent reporting is elusive.

The December 1990 Utstein Consensus Conference developed specific recommendations for the reporting of out-of-hospital cardiac arrest data as well as a glossary of terms in an effort to ensure comparability. The Utstein style is an important first step toward defining the common denominator in cardiac arrest survival.

The Utstein style emphasizes reporting data in a template that facilitates calculation of the cardiac arrest survival rate as well as a variety of other intermediate outcomes by using consistent combinations of numerators and denominators defined in the glossary. While some of the resulting measures may not be of interest to all EMS systems, these measures do provide important clues to EMS system managers who recognize the importance of evaluating both health services and clinical issues in improving their EMS system.—D.T. Kim, M.D.

Cause of Death in Unsuccessful Prehospital Resuscitation
Silfvast T (Helsinki Univ Central Hosp, Finland)
J Intern Med 229:331–335, 1991 8–4

Introduction.—Most available information on causes of prehospital cardiac arrest has been obtained from successfully resuscitated patients. If resuscitation is unsuccessful, the cause of death is usually estimated from a patient's documented history or is derived at autopsy. The cause of cardiac arrest in patients who could not be resuscitated was analyzed.

Patients.—During 1987 to 1988, 1,052 patients sustained prehospital cardiac arrests in Helsinki. Prehospital resuscitation was attempted in 509 patients; 381 of them had a witnessed cardiac arrest attributable to presumed coronary causes, and 128 had either an unwitnessed cardiac arrest or cardiac arrest attributable to obvious noncardiac conditions. Resuscitation was successful in 177 patients and unsuccessful in 204. An autopsy was performed on 80 (39%) of those 204 patients, and the autopsy diagnoses were then related to the initial cardiac rhythm recorded at the scene. The initial cardiac rhythm recorded in cardiac arrest was classified as ventricular fibrillation (VF), asystole, or electromechanical dissociation (EMD).

Results.—The initial cardiac rhythm was VF in 42 (53%) of the 80 autopsied patients, EMD in 28 (35%), and asystole in 10 (12%). Coronary heart disease caused the fatal cardiac arrest in 33 (78%) patients with VF, in 12 (43%) with EMD, and in 5 (50%) with asystole. Fifteen (54%) patients whose initial cardiac rhythm was EMD had a non-coronary cause of death at autopsy, including a ruptured myocardium with cardiac tamponade complicating myocardial infarction in 4 patients, massive pulmonary embolism in 6 patients, and cardiac tamponade resulting from a dissecting aortic aneurysm in 5 patients.

Conclusions.—Coronary heart disease was the cause of death in most patients with an initial cardiac rhythm of VF, whereas non-coronary causes of death were present in most patients whose initial cardiac rhythm was EMD, thus suggesting a relationship between the initial cardiac rhythm and the cause of cardiac arrest in unsuccessful resuscitation.

▶ Studies have demonstrated that the cause of death estimated from the patient's history is unreliable, yet an autopsy is an infrequently used "gold standard" in the United States. In this article from Helsinki, some interesting observations emerge, but the reader must exercise caution because of the small percentage of the sample that underwent autopsy. *True* EMD is almost invariably fatal, and yet over half of the cases of EMD were incorrectly diagnosed, even though the prehospital response team included a physician. Autopsy revealed the cause of death to be due to causes that are "potentially reversible." An organized electrical rhythm in the absence of central pulses and no heart sounds on auscultation can represent an undetectable low-flow state resulting from pulmonary emboli, cardiac tamponade, tension pneumothorax, or hypovolemia from dissection. As noted above, patients with VF are more likely to have the cause be coronary occlusion.—W.J. Koenig, M.D.

Change in Survival From Out-of-Hospital Cardiac Arrest and Its Effect on Coronary Heart Disease Mortality, Minneapolis–St. Paul: The Minnesota Heart Survey

Tillinghast SJ, Doliszny KM, Kottke TE, Gomez-Marin O, Lilja GP, Campion BC (Kaiser Permanente Med Ctr, Sacramento, Calif; Univ of Minnesota, Minneapolis; Mayo Clinic and Found, Rochester, Minn; Univ of Miami, Fla)

Am J Epidemiol 134:851–861, 1991 8–5

Background.—Most reports of reduction of mortality from cardiac arrest by emergency medical services have been descriptive in nature and have not addressed community impact in particular. An ongoing surveillance study designed to assess the effect of advanced cardiac life support services on survival from cardiac arrest was examined.

Methods.—The study area was the Minneapolis–St. Paul, Minnesota, metropolitan area, which saw the introduction of advanced cardiac life support ambulances in 1973. Ambulance and hospital emergency room records were examined for possible instances of out-of-hospital cardiac arrest from 1972, the year before the introduction of advanced life support ambulances, to 1982, by which time these services were well established. Potential cases and survival to discharge were validated by a study of hospital records. The cases were checked against death certificates for the year in which the arrest occurred and the following year.

Results.—In 1972, age-adjusted 1-year survival rates for survivors of out-of-hospital cardiac arrest for patients aged 30 to 74 years were 1.8% for men and .5% for women. In 1982, these figures had improved to 11.7% and 3.5%, respectively. Similarly, mortality rates of coronary heart disease decreased by 34.9% for men and 41.7% for women. Of this decline, improved survival from out-of-hospital cardiac arrest was thought to account for 5.4% for men and 4.3% for women.

Conclusions.—Advanced cardiac life support services resulted in a small but significant reduction in the mortality rate of coronary heart disease in the Minneapolis-St. Paul area. The decrease is along the lines of 5%. More patients may get to the hospital alive, but it is unsure whether all are benefiting equally from in-hospital care.

▶ Readers, beware of the significant limitations (discussed by the authors) of a retrospective analysis performed on a system with 10 years intervening. It is interesting to note that only 8 of 23 providers kept adequate data in 1972 as compared with 23 of 23 in 1982. We should also be humbled that while advanced life support did have a small, but significant effect on the overall decline in coronary artery disease mortality, it was only 5% of the total decline. This is not inconsistent with studies by Goldman that estimate the impact nationally at 4% of the total. Clearly, trying to decrease deaths due to coronary disease is a multidisciplinary approach that extends beyond the boundaries of emergency medical services.—W.J. Koenig, M.D.

Psychological Factors Related to Prehospital Delay During Acute Myocardial Infarction

Kenyon LW, Ketterer MW, Gheorghiade M, Goldstein S (Henry Ford Hosp, Detroit)

Circulation 84:1969–1976, 1991 8–6

Background.—Mortality rates from acute myocardial infarction (AMI) may be reduced by as much as 50% if emergency therapy is implemented within the first few hours after symptom onset. Many patients, however, delay in responding to their symptoms, thereby reducing their chances for survival. Patient factors that might explain a delay in seeking medical attention for AMI were examined.

Methods.—Patients admitted with the primary diagnosis of out-of-hospital AMI between October 1989 and January 1990 were included. The 103 subjects were interviewed after transfer from the cardiac intensive care unit to a general hospital floor. Variables studied included the length of delay, demographic and medical history factors, psychological characteristics of somatic and emotional awareness, and type A behavior.

Results.—The patients' mean age was 62 years. Nearly half (43%) had a history of cardiac problems. Only a third realized that they were having a heart attack before hospital arrival; just over 20% received prehospital thrombolytic treatment. The mean prehospital delay time was 9.0 hours. Neither type A behavior nor any demographic or medical history categories appeared to be significantly associated with a delay in seeking medical attention. Patients with low emotional awareness had a longer median delay (12.8 hours) than those with high emotional awareness (3.8 hours). Similarly, those with low somatic awareness delayed longer (7 hours) than patients with high somatic awareness (4 hours).

Conclusions.—Patients who are more capable of identifying their emotions and bodily sensations are more likely to seek early treatment for symptoms of AMI. Patients with low sensitivity to bodily processes and emotions and coronary risk factors should be educated by their physicians on the need for seeking prompt treatment for symptoms of cardiac disease.

▶ This study explores an interesting factor that should not be ignored by emergency physicians when deciding where best to devote resources aimed at reducing morbidity from AMI. Patients waiting 12 hours to seek emergency care will not benefit from prehospital thrombolysis or 12-lead ECGs.

A prior history of myocardial infarction should imply a high level of awareness, and yet studies have shown that denial in this high-risk group, as this article demonstrates, often causes extended delays in seeking medical help. Sadly, the inability of many patients to identify "what their body is telling them" may undermine our attempts at public education. Recent studies quantifying the impact of public education tend to support this thesis.—W.J. Koenig, M.D.

Comparison of Aeromedical Crew Performance by Patient Severity and Outcome

Burney RE, Passini L, Hubert D, Maio R (Univ of Michigan, Ann Arbor)
Ann Emerg Med 21:375–378, 1992 8–7

Background.—Crew composition is a continuing controversy in aeromedical transport. At the authors' center, both physician/nurse (P/N) and nurse/nurse (N/N) crews have been used since 1987 to staff 2 helicopter ambulances. Illness or injury severity and patient outcomes of patients transported by the P/N and N/N crews were compared.

Methods.—Data were obtained from the air ambulance and medical records for retrospective examination. Six hundred fifty-nine patients aged 16 years or older were studied. Illness or injury severity was measured by the Revised Trauma Score, APACHE-II, and Therapeutic Intervention Scoring System. Mortality, length of intensive care unit stay, and length of hospitalization were the outcome measures.

Findings.—Four hundred eighteen had been transported by the P/N team, and 241 had been transported by the N/N team. The 2 groups did not differ significantly in sex, Revised Trauma Score, APACHE-II, or Therapeutic Intervention Scoring System. Patients transported by the P/N team tended to be younger, with a mean age of 45.7 years as compared with 50.9 years. There were also more cardiac and trauma patients in the P/N group. Also, these patients were more likely to have been transferred from an emergency department or scene. Mortality, length of stay in the intensive care unit, and length of stay in the hospital did not differ between the P/N and N/N groups. The time spent at the scene or hospital was also comparable.

Conclusions.—There were no objective differences in patient outcomes between those transported by the P/N and by the N/N team. Small differences were found in the types of flights taken by the 2 teams, but there were no differences in objective measures of severity between groups. There was no objective evidence suggesting that 1 crew composition was superior to the other.

▶ Ten percent of hospital-based helicopter programs in the United States use an RN/physician attendant crew. It appears that the economic forces driving crew usage are stronger than the medical forces, especially in light of articles that attempt to measure outcome objectively. Physicians are not cheap, and even training programs experience difficulty in staffing air ambulance programs full-time. Despite some indication that seriously injured blunt trauma victims may experience improved survival with a physician-staffed crew (1,2), the subset of patients benefiting is very small in most programs and does not warrant full-time physician staffing in most programs. Rather than expending so much energy debating proper crew configuration, the industry would benefit from some carefully designed studies defining appropriate use of the helicopter.—W.J. Koenig, M.D.

References

1. *1992 Program Survey. J Air Med Transport*, vol. 11, no 5, May 1992.
2. Baxt WG: *JAMA* 257:3246, 1987.

Prospective Study of Manikin-Only Versus Manikin and Human Subject Endotracheal Intubation Training of Paramedics

Stratton SJ, Kane G, Gunter CS, Wheeler NC, Ableson-Ward C, Reich E, Pratt FD, Ogata G, Gallagher C (Los Angeles County Paramedic Training Inst, Torrance, Calif; Univ of California; County of Los Angeles Fire Dept; Downey Community Hosp, Downey, Calif)

Ann Emerg Med 20:1314–1318, 1991 8–8

Introduction.—Questions regarding the ethics of using animal and human subjects have led to an interest in the feasibility of training paramedics in endotracheal intubation (ETI) by means of a manikin. Individual field ETI success rates for paramedics were evaluated after they participated in a manikin-only or a manikin-plus-cadaver training program.

Methods.—The paramedic training program for Los Angeles paramedics was revised significantly in 1988. The new program consists of a 60-minute didactic and audiovisual lecture and 5 20-minutes-per-student supervised manikin practice sessions under distracting conditions. Sixty-one students were certified and 40 paramedic students were certified in an additional manikin-plus-cadaver training program. Correct tube placement was evaluated by the paramedics and hospital personnel.

Results.—During the study period, 39 paramedics in the manikin-only group and 21 in the manikin-plus-cadaver group attempted field ETI. The 2 groups were comparable in the number of encounters per paramedic. Success rates were 86% for the manikin-only group and 85% for the manikin-plus-cadaver group. Complication rates were similar for the 2 groups. Paramedics in the manikin-plus-cadaver group did believe, however, that cadaver exposure added to their ability to perform ETI.

Conclusion.—The manikin-only method of teaching ETI to paramedics appears to provide adequate training. This is an important finding in light of the limited availability of human subjects and fresh cadavers.

▶ I applaud this attempt to modify classic "skill learning." However, the authors admit that the β-error in this study makes significant comparisons difficult. In addition, I do not believe adding 3 cadaver intubations to the 100 minutes of "supervised manikin practice sessions" that all the paramedics received is a significant alteration in the teaching experience.

Currently, standard instruction in ETI for prehospital providers includes didactics, practical teaching, and ETI performed on live human subjects, preferably in a controlled setting such as the operating room. I do not believe that this study supports changing these current standards.—D.J. Cionni, M.D.

Prehospital Care Base Command

Monitoring EMS Protocol Deviations: A Useful Quality Assurance Tool

Salerno SM, Wrenn KD, Slovis CM (Strong Mem Hosp, Rochester, NY; Univ of Rochester)

Ann Emerg Med 20:1319–1324, 1991 8–9

Background.—Quality assessment and assurance in the emergency medical services (EMS) system depends upon the establishment of protocols and the education of EMS providers to follow these standards. Hospital and prehospital records were reviewed to determine common EMS protocol deviations and their potential impact on patient outcome.

Methods.—The EMS system in 2 upstate New York counties consists of 7 advanced life support ambulance services associated with 5 area hospital emergency departments. During a 2-month period, 1,246 ambulance runs were examined for protocol deviations. Deviations were then reviewed and characterized as minor, serious, or very serious. The impact of the deviation upon the patient was graded as positive, negative, or without effect.

Results.—Protocol violations were found in 199 (16%) of the runs. These deviations were judged minor in 55% of the cases, serious in 38%, and very serious in 7%. The majority of patients (89.5%) had no obvious effects, 5% improved, and 5.5% experienced complications. The EMS technicians committed 69% of the protocol deviations without the consent of medical control. The problems identified by the review included misconceptions in the use of intravenous therapy, a number of serious deviations in advanced cardiac life support protocols, and a lack of communication with medical control.

Conclusion.—Quality EMS care can be obtained only when the standards encompassed in the protocols are upheld. Reviews are useful in revealing protocol deviations and pointing out possible limitations of the protocols. An annual or semiannual review is advocated.

▶ Salerno et al. advocate monitoring of protocol deviations correlated to resultant patient outcome. If implemented as described, this methodology has the potential to assist EMS system managers and medical directors in improving overall system effectiveness. Unfortunately, this methodology is difficult to implement in many systems because the hospital record is frequently inaccessible to the EMS medical director.

Consequently, EMS systems mistakenly substitute monitoring of protocol deviations without an assessment of the impact of these deviations on patient outcomes. This misguided effort at "inspection of the defectives" focuses the EMS medical director's attention on the processes the EMS system uses to produce deviations rather than on the processes used to produce favorable results.

When hospital records are inaccessible, EMS medical directors must evaluate all prehospital records, including those without deviations. In EMS systems where insufficient resources prevent a review of all records, sampling methodologies that ensure a review of all providers in all types of cases combined with systematic data collection and analysis should supplant the usual case-by-case anecdotal review of records, especially anecdotal reviews focused only on deviations.—S.J. Davidson, M.D.

Medical Command Errors in an Urban Advanced Life Support System

Holliman CJ, Wuerz RC, Meador SA (Pennsylvania State Univ, Hershey, Pa)

Ann Emerg Med 21:347–350, 1992 8–10

Introduction.—The 4% rate of command physician errors found in the few previous studies of medical command practices have led some physicians to question the need for medical command in most advanced life support (ALS) cases. However, prompted by the complaints of paramedics in their urban emergency medical services (EMS) system, the physicians studied their rate of medical command errors and attempted to identify the most common types of errors.

Methods.—The study took place in a midsized city EMS system in which on-line medical command was provided on a rotating basis by 3 city hospitals. As part of an ongoing quality assurance program by the ALS service's medical director, all ALS run sheets for a 28-month period were examined. Those in which "true" deviations from the EMS protocols occurred were identified by a consensus of 3 physician reviewers.

Findings.—Among 3,839 ALS runs, there were 194 medical command errors in 167 runs, an overall rate of 4.4%. Seventy-six percent of these were errors of omission—failing to order a required intervention or denying a paramedic's request for an intervention. The other 24% were errors of commission—ordering a dangerous or inappropriate intervention. Six types of errors accounted for 80% of the total. The most common was failure to order a fingerstick glucose determination or intravenously administered glucose solution bolus in possible hypoglycemic alteration of mental status, followed in order by inappropriate release to basic life support, failure to order intravenous line placement, ordering an intravenous aminophylline drip when transport time was less than 5 minutes, failure to order naloxone for possible narcotic overdose, failure to order sublingual nitroglycerin for probable ischemic chest pain, and failure to order intravenously administered fluids for hypotensive patients with signs of volume depletion. Nearly half of the errors were made by 4 physicians. No deaths could be ascribed to a medical command error, although follow-up data were limited.

Conclusions.—Six common types of medical command errors in ALS cases are identified. These errors should be the focus of ongoing physician education efforts. The error rate might be decreased by quality assurance monitoring and greater reliance on protocols by paramedics.

▶ Holliman et al. report "errors" that represent a variety of relatively minor protocol deviations, mostly errors of omission, without any evidence of deleterious patient impact. This error rate may not even be due to medical command physician error because they exclusively reviewed paramedic-written run reports in evaluating medical command physician errors. All other analyses of physician on-line medical command (OLMC) services reviewed contemporaneous medical command documentation of physician analysis and decision making.

I believe that EMS medical directors should acknowledge the humanity of medical command physicians and reconfigure the system of OLMC to reduce errors. Medical command errors might be reduced if OLMC services were targeted rather than broadly required. Then, physicians would associate OLMC with critical decision making in prehospital patient care rather than regard it as a routine function intended to reinforce physician primacy in prehospital patient care.—S.J. Davidson, M.D.

Do-Not-Resuscitate Orders in the Emergency Department

Wrenn K, Brody SL (Grady Mem Hosp; Emory Univ, Atlanta, Ga)

Am J Med 92:129–133, 1992 8–11

Background.—Although the use of "do-not-resuscitate" (DNR) orders for certain patient populations has been widely discussed, there has been almost no discussion of the use of these orders in the emergency department. The nature of the decision to write a DNR order in the emergency department was assessed.

Methods.—Thirty-seven consecutive patients for whom a DNR order was written were studied prospectively. The orders were written by personnel assigned to the emergency department of a large inner city teaching hospital. In each case, data were collected on who was involved in the decision, the difficulty the family or patient had in agreeing to the order, acute and chronic problems, how often the patient could enter into the process, and final outcomes.

Findings.—House officers assigned to the emergency department initiated the DNR order in 65% of the cases. The family was involved in 89%. The family did not significantly resist the DNR order in any case. In general, patients receiving DNR orders were elderly, demented, and debilitated with multiple chronic medical problems or young with a malignancy or AIDS and had become critically ill and unstable. Only 5 patients were able to enter into the decision to have a DNR order. Physicians had discussed DNR status previously with only 14% of the patients.

Conclusions.—Because physicians are still considerably reluctant to discuss the DNR issue with patients before they become critically ill, emergency department physicians must often write DNR orders. Although the emergency department is not the best setting for discussing DNR orders, such orders can be written by emergency department physicians after consultation with the patient's family.

▶ At first, it seems that the need for "DNR" orders in the emergency center is counterintuitive. Emergency physicians and personnel are, by basic instinct, "rescuers with reflexes." Indeed, the credo of emergency medicine is "to preserve life."

Nevertheless, 60% of all deaths in America occur in the hospital, and of these, 13% occur in the emergency center. As the number of young Americans with fatal disease such as AIDS increases, the need is all too apparent.—E.H. Taliaferro, M.D.

Using Paramedics to Identify At-Risk Elderly

Gerson LW, Schelble DT, Wilson JE (Northeastern Ohio Universities, Rootstown; Akron Gen Med Ctr, Ohio)

Ann Emerg Med 21:688–691, 1992 8–12

Rationale.—One of every 4 persons older than 75 years requires help in basic physical or home-related activities. Basic needs may go unmet if appropriate services are unavailable, if those who require them are not identified, or if people are not linked with services. As initial responders to calls for medical aid, paramedics are able to identify elderly persons whose adverse physical, psychological, social, or environmental circumstances place them at risk.

Program.—As part of the routine monthly run reviews, paramedics were educated in their role as case finders and taught how to observe the home situation and record problems that appeared to require investigation. Special emphasis was placed on signs of abuse and on how to communicate effectively with the elderly.

Methods.—In a prospective nonrandomized open trial, 130 fire fighter paramedics evaluated 6,000 persons aged 60 and older. Their performance was graded by trained geriatric assessors.

Results.—The paramedics identified 197 persons as possibly having problems, and 124 of them were assessed. A problem was in fact present in all but 3 of those cases, a positive predictive value of 98%. Intervention proved useful for nearly half of those who were identified and assessed. Equal benefit was noted for patients having social, medical, and mental problems. Those with environmental problems were helped somewhat less often.

Conclusion.—Paramedics are able to identify elderly persons at risk and thereby provide an effective linkage with service agencies in the community.

▶ Using emergency medical services (EMS) systems and providers for other than emergent aspects of primary care may well be the wave of the future. This study examines a related issue and shows that EMS systems may be useful for more than the provision of acute care.

Keep your eyes open! Driven by a competitive health care market and more advanced prehospital providers and systems, involvement of EMS systems in activities such as home health care, health screening, and in-home treatment of minor emergencies is a real possibility in the not-too-distant future.—D.J. Cionni, M.D.

Effect of Standing Orders on Paramedic Scene Time for Trauma Patients

Gratton MC, Bethke RA, Watson WA, Gaddis GM (Univ of Missouri, Kansas City)

Ann Emerg Med 20:1306–1309, 1991 8–13

Introduction.—There is some controversy regarding the on-scene use of advanced life support (ALS) procedures for trauma patients. Opponents argue that rapid transport is preferable, whereas proponents feel that patients benefit from ALS at the scene. A study was done to determine whether a protocol change establishing standing orders would decrease the scene time in trauma patients.

Methods.—Beginning in July 1989 under a new protocol for the Metropolitan Ambulance Services Trust, paramedics could place intravenous lines, administer fluid boluses, and perform oral intubation with in-line stabilization before base station contact. In a retrospective review, 2 groups of physiologically unstable patients were compared. The 87 controls had been transported in the 6-month period before the initiation of standing orders. During the following 6 months, 110 patients were transported.

Results.—The 2 groups were similar in mean age, proportion of male patients, survival rate, and mechanism of injury. The standing order protocol did not affect the scene time. The mean scene times were 15.3

minutes for controls and 15.1 minutes for the revised standing order group. Patients in the 2 groups had a similar number of procedures.

Conclusion.—On-scene time was not altered by the use of standing orders. Further investigation is necessary to define the factors that do contribute to on-scene time and the relative benefits of standing orders and on-line medical contact.

▶ Gratton and colleagues' narrow conclusion seems hardly worth the effort expended. Their experiment as described altered a system policy, on-line medical command (OLMC) vs. standing orders, but sought only a presumed patient benefit—reduced scene time. Other work (1, 2) evaluating OLMC has been done. The *system* effects such as the total number of calls managed by physicians or physician time expended in OLMC are important to measure.

I have previously suggested (3) and continue to believe that OLMC must be evaluated rather than simply accepted as a routine practice. It may not be an essential requirement if effective off-line medical control through prospective and retrospective mechanisms is in place.

Emergency medical service (EMS) is a public health service. To optimize care for the community as a whole, whenever possible, EMS physicians should conduct their experiments so as to evaluate total system effects, not simply those on small experimental groups of patients. Gratton and colleagues missed an opportunity to do so herein.—S.J. Davidson, M.D.

References

1. Hoffman JR, et al: *West J Med* 153:283, 1990.
2. Erder MH, et al: *Ann Emerg Med* 28:261, 1989.
3. Davidson SJ, Erder MH: *West J Med* 154:226, 1991.

Dealing With Violent Patients in Flight

Kennedy MG (Boston Med Flight, Mass)

J Emerg Nurs 17:295–298, 1991 8–14

Introduction.—Emergency care providers must often deal with violent patients. The demands of a flight environment require extra care in managing these patients.

Discussion.—Anxiety in patients may result in violent behavior, which may be caused by ethanol intoxication or hypoxia resulting from injuries. The latter can be treated with intubation and ventilation with 100% oxygen where appropriate. Anxiety resulting from pain can be treated with morphine sulfate and patient reassurance; the effects of morphine sulfate can be easily reversed if hypotension develops. Paralytic agents can be helpful in permitting easier ventilation of combative persons; vecuronium is short-acting and can facilitate neurologic examination at the receiving facility.

Other causes of violent behavior in the flight environment can include altitude-induced hypoxia. Oxygen supplementation is recommended for all patients. The unusual aeromedical environment may be frightening to patients. Because safety is paramount in air medical transport, 4-point physical restraints should be used for patients who have demonstrated any propensity toward violent behavior. Chemical restraints such as benzodiazepines, narcotics, and smooth-muscle relaxants may be necessary.

Conclusion.—Prevention is the key to ensure safe transport of violent patients. Thorough patient evaluation is necessary, reassurance is extremely helpful, and appropriate restraint should be applied. All patients should receive supplemental oxygen, and nasogastric or orogastric tubes should be placed when appropriate, with suction available. If the crew doubts the safety of the flight, the patient should not be transported by air.

▶ This is a very commonsense article. The basic tenets are prevention and anticipation. Absolute patient control is mandatory for the safety of the crew and the patient during flight. Time may not permit an in-depth interview with the patient to assess mental stability or the level of anxiety. The crew must assume the worst. Reassurance should be given before lift-off, and the patient should be appropriately restrained with good intravenous access in case chemical restraints must be given. Communication with the pilot is also important in case an emergency landing is in order until the situation is under control.—J.T. Amsterdam, M.D.

Air Travel and Oxygen Therapy in Cardiopulmonary Patients
Gong H Jr (Univ of California, Los Angeles)
Chest 101:1104–1113, 1992 8–15

Background.—Persons with cardiopulmonary disorders often choose to travel by air. Several technological advances have enhanced these persons' ability for air travel. The acute responses of cardiopulmonary patients to altitude hypoxia and methods for providing adequate oxygenation during commercial flights were studied, along with clinical information, practical guidelines, and procedures for patients requiring supplemental O_2 during air travel.

Responses to Altitude Hypoxia.—The compensatory responses to acute hypoxia that occur in normal individuals may also occur to varying degrees in patients with cardiopulmonary disorders. The drop in altitude oxygenation in patients with pre-existing pulmonary disorders relies mainly on the person's mechanism for hypoxemia, the rate of ascent, the duration at final altitude, and the final altitude achieved, which determines the maximum ambient partial pressure of oxygen (PO_2) and inspired PO_2. Hypoventilation, ventilation-perfusion mismatching, shunting, diffusion impairment, low mixed venous PO_2, or combinations of these may be the mechanisms of hypoxemia and result in an unpredictable net effect on gas exchange at altitude.

In-Flight Emergencies.—Cardiopulmonary and neurologic disorders are the most frequent causes of major in-flight morbidity and mortality. The incidence of in-flight exacerbations of pulmonary disorders appears to be very low. However, the number of at-risk travelers and preventable in-flight events and the role of O_2 therapy during these events are not known. Flight-related medical illnesses probably occur more often than reported or believed.

In-Flight Oxygen Therapy.—Policies governing supplemental O_2 during travel are diverse and can be frustrating to travelers. Patients need to plan far ahead and obtain advice from health care professionals and airline special services. United States air carriers require a physician's prescription stating the duration of in-flight O_2 use and flow rate at 8,000 ft. Patients need to remember that airlines do not provide O_2 for use in terminals. However, patients do not need to bring their O_2 equipment as checked luggage if comparable equipment can be arranged at the destination. Patients should always learn the air carrier's policy on in-flight O_2 use and confirm that O_2 will be available during the entire trip.

Conclusions.—Air travel today is relatively convenient, safe, and affordable. United States air carriers generally recognize and accept that in-flight O_2 therapy is safe and manageable, but many problems still exist in obtaining and using supplemental O_2.

▶ This is an important article to have on hand for emergency physicians practicing in emergency departments near major airports. For instance, one pearl buried in this article is "Cottrell estimated that a preflight Pa_{O_2} of 70 mm Hg would be required to maintain an adequate Sa_{O_2} at 6,214 feet." Therefore, when advising cardiopulmonary patients seeking consultation regarding the need for in-flight oxygen, a logical starting point is to obtain a room-air blood gas determination.—E.H. Taliaferro, M.D.

7.5% Sodium Chloride/Dextran for Resuscitation of Trauma Patients Undergoing Helicopter Transport

Vassar MJ, Perry CA, Gannaway WL, Holcroft JW (Univ of California, Davis Med Ctr, Sacramento)

Arch Surg 126:1065–1072, 1991 8–16

Introduction.—Animal models of hemorrhagic shock have shown that very small volumes of 7.5% hypertonic sodium chloride combined with 6% dextran 70 (HSD) are effective in rapid resuscitation. The solution's physiologic actions may result partly from rapid expansion of plasma volume by an osmotic fluid shift from the intracellular to the intravascular space. A prospective, double-blind trial was undertaken to compare prehospital HSD resuscitation of trauma patients with conventional resuscitation using isotonic fluids.

Methods.—Studied were 166 severely injured patients with systolic pressures of 100 mm Hg or less who were being transported to the emergency department (ED) by the Life Flight Service. In prehospital resuscitation, the patients received 250 mL of either HSD or lactated Ringer's solution followed by conventional isotonic fluids. Blood pressures on arrival to the ED and overall survival were compared for the 2 groups.

Results.—Patients receiving HSD needed less fluid before hospitalization and arrived in the ED with higher systolic blood pressures. Sixty-four percent of the HSD group survived to hospital discharge as compared with 59% of the group given lactated Ringer's solution. Survival rates for patients with severe head injuries were 32% with HSD and 16% with lactated Ringer's solution, although differences in actuarial survival did not attain statistical significance. The use of HSD was not associated with any adverse side effects.

Conclusions.—Prehospital administration of HSD to severely injured patients can increase blood pressures more than lactated Ringer's solution can. There is also a tendency toward improved survival in patients with severe head injuries.

► The prehospital multicenter trial (1) with patients receiving HSD reached very similar conclusions: the prehospital administration of a 250-cc bolus of HSD appears to be safe in hypotensive trauma patients but does not improve survival. A subset of patients who are taken to surgery following penetrating trauma do appear to have improved survival, but caution should be used in any system seriously evaluating the aggressive use of hypertonic fluids to restore blood pressure in trauma victims. While we are all interested in therapeutic modalities that could be implemented in the prehospital phase of care, current evaluation (in Houston) of minimal fluid resuscitation in the hypotensive trauma victim prior to definitive surgery may cause a paradigm shift in our thinking about the prehospital care of these patients.—W.J. Koenig, M.D.

Reference

1. Mattox KL, et al: *Ann Surg* 213:482, 1991.

Field Therapy

Safety of Pre-Hospital Therapy With Morphine Sulfate

Bruns BM, Dieckmann R, Shagoury C, Dingerson A, Swartzell C (Stanford Univ Hosp, Calif; San Francisco Gen Hosp)

Am J Emerg Med 10:53–57, 1992 8–17

Objective.—The safety of morphine sulfate (MS) in the prehospital environment has not previously been adequately documented. The safety of using prehospital MS in an urban emergency medical services system was assessed in a prospective observational study.

Study Design.—During a 6-month study in San Francisco County, paramedics assessed patients for ischemic chest pain, pulmonary edema, or both; made contact with the base hospital; and when the base physician or mobile intensive care nurses concurred with the paramedic's assessment, administered 2- to 4-mg doses of intravenous MS according to treatment protocols. Field paramedics and emergency department (ED) physicians recorded clinical assessments and patient responses to therapy. Safety was evaluated by determining the accuracy of paramedic field assessment vs. ED physician diagnosis, appropriateness of prehospital MS therapy, and therapeutic complications.

Outcome.—Paramedics administered MS to 84 patients. When compared with ED physician's diagnoses, paramedics' assessments were considered accurate in 65 patients, an accuracy rate of 77%. Paramedics correctly recognized ischemic chest pain but missed physical findings of pulmonary edema in 5 patients and accurately diagnosed pulmonary edema but missed ischemic chest pain in 4 patients. For these 9 patients the paramedics' assessments were considered inaccurate, but the judgment to give MS was considered appropriate. Hence, the rate of appropriate MS field use was 88%. In the remaining 10 patients, the ED physicians' diagnoses included conditions other than ischemic chest pain or pulmonary edema and the paramedics' assessments were considered inaccurate and the management inappropriate. Overall, respiratory depression or hypotension during MS therapy in 5 patients developed a complication rate of 6%. Only 1 patient received MS inappropriately, a complication rate of 10%; the other 4 received MS appropriately, for a complication rate of 5%.

Conclusion.—In a system with on-line medical direction, paramedics can safely administer MS. The observed incidence of complications is low among patients who received MS appropriately or inappropriately.

▶ Although I believe that "paramedics can safely administer MS", this article does not convince me of that fact.

A more pertinent question raised by the authors is that of efficacy: "the benefit of morphine sulfate to the ultimate outcome of patients treated for ischemic chest pain and pulmonary edema in the field is not clear." Recent work by Wuerz and Meador (1) has made us acutely aware that some of the things we do in the field may not only lack efficacy but may actually be harmful. Proof of the safety and efficacy of prehospital advanced life support procedures, therapies, and drugs is sorely needed. It is time that we start basing what we do on need and proven efficacy rather than using the technical imperative.—D.J. Cionni, M.D.

Reference

1. Wuerz RC, Meador SA: *Ann Emerg Med* 21:669, 1992.

Cervical Spine Movement During Airway Management: Cinefluoroscopic Appraisal in Human Cadavers

Hauswald M, Sklar DP, Tandberg D, Garcia JF (Univ of New Mexico, Albuquerque)

Am J Emerg Med 9:535–538, 1991 8–18

Introduction.—Although airway management in trauma patients should minimize the risk of further injury to the cervical spinal cord, the relative safety of various procedures of airway management is not known. Different airway maneuvers were tested on 8 human cadavers shortly after death to determine their effects on cervical spine movement.

Methods.—The cadavers were subjected to 4 groups of airway procedures: ventilation with a bag-valve-mask device, oral endotracheal intubation, guided oral intubation over a lighted stylet and flexible laryngoscope, and nasal intubation with and without a fiber-optic bronchoscope. All procedures were performed with the cadaver in the supine position secured by a hard cervical collar and with the head taped to a backboard. Cinefluoroscopy was performed continuously to record anteroposterior cervical spine movement.

Results.—The mean maximum cervical spine displacement was 2.93 mm for mask procedures, 1.55 mm for oral procedures, 1.65 for guided oral procedures, and 1.20 for nasal procedures. Whereas mask ventilation resulted in significantly more cervical spine displacement than the other procedures studied, differences observed among the other procedures were not significant.

Conclusion.—Oral and nasal methods of endotracheal intubation result in less cervical spine movement in flaccid persons than mask ventilation does. Clinicians should use the method with which they are most experienced and skillful.

▶ The key to immobilization of the cervical spine during all airway maneuvers is to minimize movement. This study shows that with each of the techniques there is some movement. Cadavers certainly differ from intoxicated and combative adults. Therefore, when the cervical spine must be immobilized as much as possible, a controlled rapid-sequence induction with good in-line immobilization should be strongly considered. See also Abstract 2–23.)—J.T. Amsterdam, M.D.

Spinal Immobilization on a Flat Backboard: Does It Result in Neutral Position of the Cervical Spine?

Schriger DL, Larmon B, LeGassick T, Blinman T (Univ of California, Los Angeles)

Ann Emerg Med 20:878–881, 1991 8–19

Background.—Proper procedure for spinal immobilization of trauma victims requires maintaining the neck in a neutral position. Some physicians advocate placing the occiput directly against a stiff backboard, whereas others suggest that padding be added. Here, physicians studied the amount of occipital padding required to achieve the neutral position which was defined as the normal anatomic position of the head and torso when standing and looking straight ahead.

Methods.—Measurements of height, weight, occipital offset, and head, neck, and chest circumferences were obtained in 100 healthy young adult volunteers without histories of back disease. Subjects were measured in both the standing and supine positions. Three trained observers independently measured occipital offset in the first 30 subjects. The remaining subjects were measured by only 1 observer. A univariate linear regression model was used to determine whether either the same individual measures or combined indices could accurately predict occipital offset.

Results.—The amount of occipital offset necessary to achieve the neutral position varied from 0 to 3.75 in.; the mean was 1.5 in. The mean occipital offset was significantly greater for men than for women. Easily obtained body measurements did not accurately predict occipital offset.

Conclusions.—Immobilization on a flat backboard would have placed 98% of these study subjects in relative cervical extension. Occipital padding would have increased the percentage of patients placed in the neutral position that would increase patient comfort during transport to the hospital. The amount of occipital padding required to achieve the neutral position varies with individuals and cannot be predicted by easily obtained body measurements.

▶ Much of the care and treatment rendered in the prehospital setting is based on in-hospital research or anecdotal experiences. Consequently, it is refreshing to see research that is aimed at better defining the prehospital practice of spinal immobilization, which is as fundamental to prehospital care as the ABCs.

I agree with the authors that the ability of the skilled observers to accurately determine the "correct" amount of padding needed to maintain the "neutral" position probably could not be reproduced in the field, and if one were to consider occipital padding, a standard amount would have to be used.

I strongly support the conclusion that the study "should not be generalized to populations other than that studied." Some prehospital programs have already incorporated occipital padding into their training. It is imperative that instructors clearly emphasize its possibly limited applicability. (See also Abstract 8–18.)—M.K. Bourn, R.N., M.S.N., E.M.T.P., with D.J. Cionni, M.D.

Prehospital Thrombolysis in Acute Myocardial Infarction: The Belgian Eminase Prehospital Study (BEPS)

BEPS Collaborative Group (Genval, Belgium)

Eur Heart J 12:965–967, 1991 8–20

Introduction.—Thrombolytic therapy is most effective when given soon after the onset of symptoms of acute myocardial infarction (AMI). Various programs have been designed to educate the public and emergency medical personnel on the importance of early intervention. The feasibility of prehospital thrombolysis was investigated.

Methods.—Six centers in Belgium took part in the study. Eligible patients were under the age of 75 years, arrived within 4 hours after the onset of typical chest pain, and showed ECG evidence of an evolving AMI. General practitioners at participating centers were informed of the availability of prehospital thrombolysis by a mobile intensive care unit (MICU) team. Consenting patients were administered intravenous eminase in the MICU.

Results.—Sixty-two patients, 52 men and 10 women, took part in the study. An initial diagnosis of suspected AMI was confirmed in 60 patients by a rise in creatine kinase isoenzyme levels and ECG findings. The mean time between the onset of pain and arrival of the MICU was 70 minutes, including 13 minutes between the call and the arrival of the MICU at the patient's home. The mean time between the onset of pain and the administration of eminase was 95 minutes, a time gain estimated to be 50 minutes over the initiation of thrombolysis in the emergency department. Four patients experienced ventricular fibrillation, and 1 had cardiogenic shock during the prehospital period. Two patients died during hospitalization.

Conclusion.—Prehospital treatment advanced the start of thrombolysis by nearly an hour. Further studies may confirm the beneficial effects of prehospital thrombolysis on short- and long-term mortality.

▶ Some facts appear to be emerging from the increasing volume of literature on the prehospital administration of thrombolytics:

1. The number of patients who meet the criteria for field administration is a small percentage of chest pain patients accessing 911 for their chest pain.
2. Trained paramedics can accurately identify acute myocardial infarction in the field and safely identify the appropriate candidates for thrombolytic therapy.
3. In the *short*-transport time systems where the studies have originated, there is a reduction in time to administration of thrombolytics that is attribut-

able to transmission of the 12-lead ECG to the receiving hospital. There is a smaller incremental time benefit when the paramedics actually administer the medication in the field.

4. As noted by the authors of this Belgian study, it is imperative that studies carefully analyze the beneficial impact on cardiac function of the additional minutes gained. While the "time is muscle" concept is important, the benefits of each incremental step should be evaluated before systems go to great expense to carry this modality to their patients in the field.—W.J. Koenig, M.D.

▶↓ Public policy and medical research are inextricably linked. Often, research results drive development of law. In Pennsylvania, a strong emergency medical service (EMS) law requires specific prehospital clinical trials demonstrating safety and efficacy before any drug or device, whether newly Food and Drug Administration approved or historically broadly utilized, is approved by the commonwealth's division of EMS for addition to the prehospital armamentarium. Thus, Pennsylvania-based EMS researchers project selection, driven by this legal requirement, results in the evaluation of various drugs and devices specifically for prehospital use. The following articles, both from Pennsylvania sites (Abstracts 8–21 and 8–22), report on prehospital studies of commonly employed emergency department diagnostic or therapeutic modalities.

Intravenous Adenosine in the Prehospital Treatment of Paroxysmal Supraventricular Tachycardia

McCabe JL, Adhar GC, Menegazzi JJ, Paris PM (Univ of Pittsburgh; Mercy Hosp, Pittsburgh, Pa; Ctr for Emergency Medicine of Western Pennsylvania)
Ann Emerg Med 21:358–361, 1992 8–21

Background.—Paroxysmal supraventricular tachycardia (PSVT), a dysrhythmia, occurs commonly in the prehospital setting. The clinical efficacy and safety of intravenous adenosine administration for PSVT was assessed in the field.

Methods.—Thirty-seven adults with a diagnosis by paramedics of PSVT were studied prospectively. Adenosine, 6 mg, was given by rapid intravenous bolus. A 12-mg bolus was given if the patient did not respond within 2 minutes and repeated once if needed. If there was still no effect, the paramedics contacted the medical command physician for further instruction.

Findings.—Electrocardiographic tracing review showed that 26 patients, or 70%, were in PSVT. Eleven had rhythms other than PSVT. Five of these had atrial fibrillation, 4 had sinus tachycardia, and 2 had ventricular tachycardia. Eighty-eight percent of the patients with PSVT converted to sinus rhythm after adenosine was given. Seven of 11 patients with hypotension at presentation were in PSVT and became hemodynamically stable on conversion with adenosine. The 4 patients with hypotension and non-PSVT rhythms had no blood pressure changes after adenosine was administered. None of the 9 patients subsequently found to have wide-complex tachycardia had hemodynamic compromise after adenosine administration. Adverse effects were infrequent, mild, and transient.

Conclusions.—Adenosine is effective and safe in the prehospital treatment of clinically diagnosed PSVT. In most cases, it terminated PSVT. It is also helpful in diagnosing other primary atrial dysrhythmias.

▶ This article is the first study of the safety and efficacy of adenosine use by paramedics in the field. Prehospital providers have had few options for the treatment of PSVT and have relied upon vagal maneuvers, electrical cardioversion of the unstable patient, and rapid transport. Verapamil has been used by paramedics in some systems, but its negative inotropic and vasodilator properties may worsen hypotension or congestive heart failure in the field.

Adenosine has been recognized as a safe and effective anti-arrhythmic agent and is now widely used in the hospital to convert PSVT. Its side effects are mild and transient and usually resolve without intervention. When administered for rhythms other than PSVT, including wide-complex tachyarrhythmias, it rarely results in hemodynamic compromise or deterioration of the rhythm; this makes it an excellent choice in the field where a 12-lead ECG is unavailable and where the rhythm misidentification rate may be higher. This study suggests that adenosine can also be used safely and effectively by paramedics in the prehospital arena.

Adenosine may be a useful agent in the prehospital treatment of unstable PSVT. Its use in stable patients, particularly if the transport time is brief or the diagnosis is uncertain, should be balanced against the high cost of the drug and the risk of further patient deterioration during transport. (See also Abstract 3–20).—Carol A. Hart, M.D. (EMS Fellow), with S.J. Davidson, M.D.

An Evaluation of Pulse Oximetry in Prehospital Care

Aughey K, Hess D, Eitel D, Bleecher K, Cooley M, Ogden C, Sabulsky N (York Hosp, Pa)

Ann Emerg Med 20:887–891, 1991 8–22

Background.—The use of pulse oximetry in patients in the emergency room has become common. There have been no studies assessing the accuracy of pulse oximetry in the field, however.

Methods.—Thirty patients were studied in the prospective, cross-sectional, prehospital comparison of pulse oximetry oxygen saturation (Spo_2) and arterial oxygen saturation. A pulse oximeter with a digital probe was used to measure Spo_2 in the field. Arterial blood gases were determined during oximeter use, and oxygen saturation (Hbo_2) was measured by CO oximetry.

Results.—No significant differences were found between SpO_2 and HbO_2. The 2 were strongly correlated. The bias between SpO_2 and $HbO_2$was −.3, with a 2.4 precision. When SpO_2 was 88% or above, HbO_2 was always 90% or above. The mean carboxyhemoglobin content was 1.3%. The mean methemoglobin concentration was .9%. No significant differences were found between heart rate measurements by pulse oximetry and ECG.

Conclusions.—Pulse oximetry is accurate enough to be useful in the field when SpO_2 is more than 88%. It is potentially useful in patients with clinical signs of acute hypoxemia and those receiving interventions that may produce acute hypoxemia. More research is needed to assess the accuracy of pulse oximetry in increased carboxyhemoglobin and methemoglobin states and very low saturations.

▶ Pulse oximetry, which is most useful in monitoring trends, may be inaccurate in a single reading. Nonetheless, Aughey and colleagues have demonstrated a level of reliability that confirms the utility of pulse oximetry in the field. However, inexperienced or insufficiently trained paramedics may forget that the pulse oximeter's report on oxygen saturation is not the whole story and that early respiratory failure may be manifested by carbon dioxide retention only, even while oxygenation is relatively well preserved.

Recently, a massively obese pickwickian patient with early right-sided heart failure who complained of breathlessness had a pulse oximeter–measured oxygen saturation of 97%. The paramedics, who did not look forward to carrying this patient down 2 narrow flights of stairs, encouraged the patient to walk down with them. Upon getting out to the porch, the patient collapsed in cardiac arrest. Certainly, paramedics should not walk a breathless patient, yet the normal pulse oximeter result probably contributed to a false sense of security that led them to do so.

Too often, when emergency medical service (EMS) medical directors introduce new devices or treatments, we fail to consider the psychological and sociologic impacts of the new device on the field providers. Spaite has publicly acknowledged that past EMS research has been flawed as a result. Certainly, implementation of EMS research results should consider the potential for unintended outcomes and consider methods to minimize deleterious consequences.—S.J. Davidson, M.D.

Prehospital Transcutaneous Cardiac Pacing for Symptomatic Bradycardia

Hedges JR, Feero S, Shultz B, Easter R, Syverud SA, Dalsey WC (Oregon Health Sciences Univ; Emergency Med Services System, Olympia, Wash; Univ of Cincinnati, Ohio; Albert Einstein Hosp, Philadelphia, Pa)

PACE 14:1473–1478, 1991 8–23

Introduction.—Transcutaneous cardiac pacing (TCP) has been shown to improve patient outcome when used within 10 minutes of the onset of cardiovascular compromise. Prehospital studies of TCP, however, have been limited. The importance of the initial hemodynamic status and prehospital TCP upon survival of patients with symptomatic bradycardia was investigated.

Methods.—The study setting was a countywide emergency medical services (EMS) system that has been in operation since 1974. Paramedics respond to approximately 120 episodes of cardiovascular collapse each year, about half of which involve a primary bradyasystolic rhythm. Data from 2 TCP trials were pooled.

Results.—Twenty-seven of 51 eligible patients received TCP. The paced and nonpaced groups were similar in mean age, sex distribution, initial rhythms, and mean times from collapse until treatment and a paceable rhythm. Four patients who survived to leave the hospital were all in the paced group. All of these patients had CPR within 1 minute of symptom onset, paramedic arrival within 4 minutes, and pacing within 13 minutes of symptom onset. Emergency department arrrival with a palpable pulse was greater in the paced group (26%) than in the nonpaced group (13%).

Conclusion.—Results suggest that TCP does benefit patients with bradycardia who have a palpable pulse when first evaluated. Because of the high cost and small number of patients likely to benefit, TCP will be most effective in EMS systems with rapid response times, long transport times, and a high proportion of cardiac patients.

▶ Prehospital TCP has recently received a lot of attention. The findings of Hedges et al. mirror the findings of work done by myself (1) and current industry thinking, that is, TCP in the prehospital arena is probably not helpful for bradyasystolic cardiac arrest but may be beneficial in hemodynamically significant bradycardia.

The authors' caution regarding widespread implementation based on equipment and training costs is currently not valid. Monitor/defibrillator/pacer devices are quickly becoming standard for the provision of advanced life support and are replacing the stand-alone pacers used in these studies. In addition, compact video programs are currently available for training.—D.J. Cionni, M.D.

Reference

1. Cionni DJ, et al: *Prehospital Disaster Med* 6:372, 1991.

A Field Comparison of the Pharyngeotracheal Lumen Airway and the Endotracheal Tube

Bartlett RL, Martin SD, McMahon JM Jr, Schafermeyer RW, Vukich DJ, Hornung CA (Richland Mem Hosp, Columbia, SC; Springhill Mem Hosp, Mobile, Ala; Carolinas Med Ctr, Charlotte, NC; University Med Ctr, Jacksonville, Fla;

Dorn Veterans Hosp, Columbia, SC)
J Trauma 32:280–283, 1992 8–24

Background.—Intubation with an endotracheal tube (ET) is still the treatment of choice for airway management. However, variation in skill and proficiency and technical limitations in the prehospital setting often require alternative ways to control the airway. One alternative is the pharyngeotracheal lumen (PtL) airway. The ease and efficacy of the PtL airway and the ET in field conditions were compared in a multicenter study.

Methods.—One hundred eleven victims of cardiac arrest were studied prospectively. The ET and PtL were alternated as the airway of first choice. The PtL airway, a tube within a tube (Fig 8–2) can be placed in either the trachea or the esophagus to control the airway.

Findings.—The PtL airway was significantly easier to use, as determined by the time needed to intubate the patient and the number of attempts needed to place the device. Arterial blood gas determinations, measured first on arrival at the hospital and again 15 minutes later, did not differ significantly between the 2 airway devices. The first arterial blood gas values during PtL ventilation were $Paco_2$, 58 mm Hg; Pao_2, 163 mm Hg; and pH, 7.15. The first arterial blood gas values during ET ventilation were $Paco_2$, 53 mm Hg; Pao_2, 156 mm Hg; and pH, 7.16. There were no adverse effects.

Conclusions.—As measured by arterial Pco_2, the ability of the PtL airway to deliver effective ventilation is comparable with that of the ET.

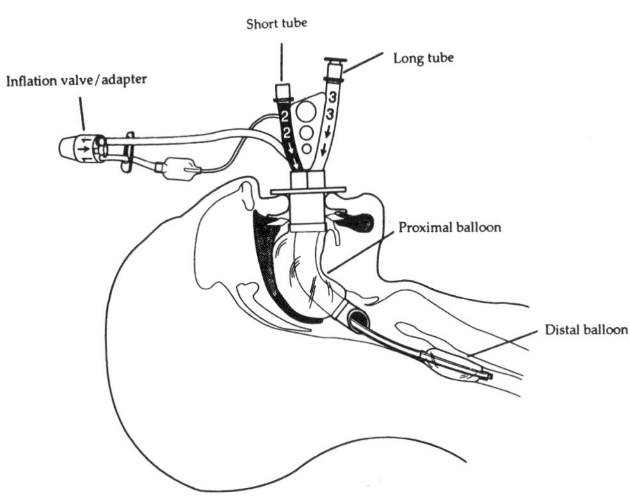

Fig 8–2.—Diagram of the pharyngeotracheal lumen airway. (Courtesy of Bartlett RL, Martin SD, McMahon JM Jr, et al: *J Trauma* 32:280–283, 1992.)

The PtL airway is an effective alternative when ET airway control cannot be achieved.

▶ I agree that the PtL airway is a better airway than the esophageal obturator airway, easier to insert than an ET, and just as efficacious as an ET when used correctly.

My adulation stops there, however, and I have some concerns regarding the authors' summary conclusion. They suggest the use of the PtL as an alternative method of airway management for "rescue personnel" not permitted by regulations to use the ET. The fact is that some rescue personnel are not permitted to perform endotracheal intubation because of a lack of training or cognitive ability. The authors themselves state that "the retention of PtL placement skills is related more to the operator's cognitive abilities rather than the maintenance of motor skills" and that "misidentification of the tube location and possible rupture" are possible complications. I completely agree with *these* statements. Typically, advanced airway management (I would consider the use of a PtL advanced airway management) is reserved for those with advanced training. Therefore, I believe that use of the PtL should currently be reserved for those prehospital providers with advanced training.

I was also intrigued by the fact that the majority of the study patients arrived at the receiving hospitals hypercapnic. It reminds me of the ventilatory rate still recommended by my mentor when ventilating a patient in cardiac or respiratory arrest: "bag the be-geesus out of them."—D.J. Cionni, M.D.

Triage/Injury and Illness Prevention

Impact of Physician Experience on Triage of Emergency Room Patients With Acute Chest Pain at Three Teaching Hospitals

Ting HH, Lee TH, Soukup JR, Cook EF, Tosteson ANA, Brand DA, Rouan GW, Goldman L (Harvard Univ, Boston; Yale Univ, New Haven, Conn; Univ of Cincinnati, Ohio)

Am J Med 91:401–408, 1991 8–25

Introduction.—It has previously been suggested that physicians in training may be less accurate in diagnosis than more experienced physicians. For patients with acute chest pain arriving at the emergency room, diagnostic errors can have drastic clinical and legal consequences. This issue was investigated by testing the effect of physician experience on the initial evaluation affecting triage of patients with acute chest pain.

Methods.—Data were gathered prospectively on 7,857 patients who came to the emergency rooms of 3 teaching hsopitals between 1984 and 1986. Patients were diagnosed with acute myocardial infarction, unstable angina, or other diagnosis. Multivariate logistic regression analyses, corrected for hospital site and 20 clinical variables, were used to assess the odds ratios for admission to the coronary-care unit and hospital in association with incremental increases in physician experience.

Results.—Fourteen percent of patients had acute myocardial infarction, 32% had acute ischemic heart disease, and 4% had a life-threatening complication. Physicians with more experience were more likely to admit patients to the coronary care unit and hospital. This increased admission rate was similar for patients with and without life-threatening conditions. Receiver opeating characterisitic (ROC) curve regression analyses showed that as physicians gained more experience they moved along a single ROC curve rather than shifting to a new or better ROC curve.

Conclusion.—This large, prospective multicenter study provides evidence that increasing physician experience leads to a lower threshold for admitting to the hospital all patients with and without acute myocardial infarction, acute ischemic heart disease, or major complications. This increased diagnostic sensitivity does not appear to be accompanied by detectable improvements in diagnostic accuracy. It is unclear whether the lower threshold for hospital admittance represented improved quality of care. Less experienced physicians did not have decreased diagnostic ability in the circumstances evaluated here.

▶ This article demonstrated that in the teaching hospitals evaluated, as residents increased in training level, they were more apt to admit patients with chest pain to a monitored environment, yet their accuracy in predicting true cardiac disease did not improve. It is difficult to say whether this improved patient care. With a single miss, not only may the outcome for the patient be poor, but the settlement in court may be quite high. Clearly, there needs to be a high index of suspicion for patients with chest pain. Younger ages must be considered every year; risk factors must be carefully assessed. In addition, the admitting physicians must better appreciate the input of the emergency physician and further evaluate such patients once a myocardial infarction is ruled out as the cause of chest pain.—J.T. Amsterdam, M.D.

Family Presence During Cardiopulmonary Resuscitation: Foote Hospital Emergency Department's Nine-Year Perspective

Hanson C, Strawser D (Foote Hosp, Jackson, Mich)

J Emerg Nurs 18:104–106, 1992 8–26

Introduction.—In 1982, Foote Hospital in Jackson, Michigan, at the urging of the hospital chaplain and a group of emergency department (ED) physicians and nurses, initiated a program in which family members remained present to support the patient during efforts at resuscitation. Although the program encountered resistance at first, it has come to be widely accepted in the ED and community. Nine years of experience with this program are evaluated.

Program Description.—The experience took place at a 500-bed urban community hospital that has 53,000 ED patients per year. The idea was prompted by 2 incidents in which family members insisted on being present during resuscitative efforts; later, a survey of the families of recently deceased patients disclosed that 72% wished they could have been present during resuscitation. The family is prepared in the grieving room by a nurse and the chaplain and told that they can be with the patient if they wish. The family member is escorted to the code room, if authorized by the physician. He or she sometimes needs encouragement to enter the room, and they are asked to leave if invasive procedures become necessary. Room is made at the bedside, and the family member is encouraged to touch and speak to the patient. The chaplain stays with the family at all times, continues support if death is pronounced and helps them through the difficult decisions that follow.

Evaluation.—In a survey of 47 family members, 76% stated that being present in the room helped them adjust to the death. Sixty-four percent believed that their presence helped the patient, and many remarked on how much effort went into saving the patient's life. An informal survey of nurses revealed that their initial fears about the program were unjustified. Family members rarely disrupted the resuscitative efforts. The family's presence did sometimes make it more difficult for the nurses to control their emotions; this was viewed as both a positive and negative aspect. Seventy-one percent of staff members endorsed the program despite the extra stress it entailed.

Discussion.—A policy of allowing family members to remain present during resuscitative efforts in the ED should be considered. The authors have extended their program to families of trauma patients, children in cardiac arrest, and homicide victims. To help staff members in dealing with the most upsetting of these situations, their hospital is considering the implementation of critical-incident stress debriefing teams.

▶ The key to the success of the program at Foote Hospital is the tight control of family member visits to the code room. Family members are not present during the first hectic minutes as the patient is quickly assessed and invasive procedures carried out. Although this visiting process is not standard practice at my institution, I think that there is a place for it and it should not be rejected out of hand.—E. Ruiz, M.D.

A Population-Based Study of Motorcycle Injury and Costs

Braddock M, Schwartz R, Lapidus G, Banco L, Jacobs L (Connecticut Childhood Injury Prevention Ctr, Hartford, Conn)

Ann Emerg Med 21:273–278, 1992 8–27

Background.—Several studies have shown that many injured motorcyclists are uninsured and that a significant portion of their medical costs is paid by public funds. However, most such studies described the experiences of a single trauma center, which may not be representative of the whole population at risk for motorcycle injuries. A population-based injury and acute-care cost profile for fatal and nonfatal motorcycle collisions in Connecticut was examined.

Methods.—Death certificates, hospital discharge data, and police accident reports were studied. Data were obtained for the years 1985 through 1989.

Findings.—One hundred twelve deaths from motorcycle injuries were identified on Connecticut death certificates, for an annual death rate of 1.2 per 100,000 persons. The highest death rates occurred among men aged 20 to 24 years. Motorcyclists not wearing helmets were 3.4-fold more likely to die than those wearing helmets. About 2,361 motorcycle-related hospital discharges resulted in an annual hospitalization rate of 24.7 per 100,000 persons. Twenty-two percent of all injuries involved the head, neck, or spine. The total costs exceeded $29 million. Twenty-nine percent of hospitalized patients did not have insurance. Forty-two percent of the cost was not reimbursed to the hospitals.

Conclusions.—Motorcycle injuries significantly contribute to mortality, morbidity, and medical costs in the state of Connecticut. A uniform helmet law would save about 10 lives and prevent more than 90 nonfatal injuries in that state annually, with an associated cost savings of $5.1 million.

▶ This is a very well done study that should be reading for every state that does not have mandatory motorcycle helmet laws (see also Abstracts 8–28 and 8–29). Besides being irresponsible, the failure to wear a motorcycle helmet is placing a burden on the rest of society that we should not accept. The injuries are simply too significant for people not wearing motorcycle helmets to allow this behavior anywhere.

One aspect of this study that I particularly like is the fact that it was a population-based injury study. All too often, studies are conducted at a single center wherein you have an isolated example of patients who may or may not be reflective of the entire population. We clearly need more large population-based studies such as this to help shape injury control policies.—W.H. Spivey, M.D.

The Impact of Motorcycle Helmet Use

Offner PJ, Rivara FP, Maier RV (Brooke Army Med Ctr, Fort Sam Houston, Tex; Univ of Washington, Seattle)

J Trauma 32:636–641, 1992 8–28

Introduction.—There is overwhelming evidence that head injuries are responsible for most motorcycle trauma deaths and that the use of motorcycle helmets effectively reduces the risk of head injury. However, mandatory helmet use laws are opposed by special interest motorcycle groups that claim that such laws are an infringement of their personal freedom. Furthermore, detractors argue that the majority of motorcycle trauma injuries occur in body regions other than the head. The impact of motorcycle helmet use on the morbidity and cost of motorcycle trauma was studied after controlling for nonhead injuries by calculating an Injury Severity Score (ISS) for each patient that did not include head injury.

Results.—During a 5-year period, 425 patients with a mean age of 27.3 years were admitted with motorcycle trauma to a regional level I trauma center. Eighty-nine percent of the trauma patients were male, and 11% were female. Of the 425 patients, 164 (39%) were wearing helmets when the accident occurred, and 261 (61%) were not. The mortality rates were 9.1% in helmeted riders and 7.7% in nonhelmeted riders. The difference was statistically not significant. The overall mortality rate was 8.2%. Only 38% of the helmeted riders suffered head injuries as compared with 66% of those who did not wear a helmet. This difference was statistically highly significant. Similarly, helmeted patients were less likely to require endotracheal intubation, required shorter stays in the intensive care unit (ICU), and required shorter rehabiliation. Multiple regression analysis revealed that the total cost of acute hospital care for helmeted patients was 40% lower than it was for patients who did not wear a helmet. Those benefits were lost as the nonhead injuries became more severe, which suggests that helmets are most effective in less severe collisions. However, because riders who are injured in less severe collisions account for more than 80% of all motorcycle accident victims, the benefit of wearing a motorcycle helmet remains significant.

Conclusions.—After controlling for nonhead injuries, the beneficial impact of wearing a motorcycle helmet remains indisputable because it limits the occurrence of head injury, the need for intubation, the length of ICU stay, and the need for rehabilitation when injury occurs.

▶ It seems hard to believe that yet another rather sophisticated study is necessary to drive home the fact that helmet use saves lives and "all the pros wear helmets" (see also Abstract 8–29). By excellent statistical analysis, the authors have been able to answer the concern of those who object to mandatory helmet legislation. Their concern is that while perhaps protecting the head, helmet usage promotes more severe nonhead injuries. Their data refute this and clearly show that unhelmeted riders dig into the public pocketbooks and have significantly increased mortality and morbidity. As the cost of care continues to escalate in public concern, so too must helmet usage.—D.K. Wagner, M.D.

A Prospective Study of the Impact of Helmet Usage on Motorcycle Trauma

Kelly P, Sanson T, Strange G, Orsay E (Univ of Illinois, Chicago)

Ann Emerg Med 20:852–856, 1991 8–29

Background.—In Illinois, one of the few states without a mandatory motorcycle helmet law, motorcycle crashes account for nearly 13% of motor vehicle fatalities but fewer than 2% of motor vehicle crashes. This prospective, multicenter study defined the effect of helmet use on the morbidity, mortality, and health care costs of motorcycle crashes.

Methods and Results.—The subjects were 398 victims of motorcycle crashes seen less than 24 hours after the injury from April through October. These patients were drawn from 8 Illinois institutions, including urban, rural, teaching, and community hospitals. Approximately 15% of patients were wearing helmets and 85% were not. The Injury Severity Score was about 12 in non-helmeted patients vs. about 7 in helmeted patients. Approximately 42% of nonhelmeted patients had head and neck injuries vs. 24.1% of helmeted patients. Glasgow Coma Scores were 14.51 in helmeted and 13.73 in nonhelmeted patients. Only 1 of the 26 patients who died was wearing a helmet, and not wearing a helmet was a major risk factor for increased severity of injury. Health care costs were 23% higher for the nonhelmeted group—about $7,200 vs. $5,900.

Conclusions.—In motorcycle accident victims, wearing a helmet can decrease the severity of injury and the incidence of head injuries. Health care costs also tend to be higher in patients who do not wear helmets, not including indirect and rehabilitation costs.

▶ Emergency physicians need to speak out when necessary to promote both bicycle and motorcycle helmet laws. Every bit of research in this area has reached a conclusion similar to this article. The lack of adequate laws costs you, the working citizen, big time. Write your legislator today.—R.M. McNamara, M.D.

Reporting Alcohol-Impaired Drivers: Results From a National Survey of Emergency Physicians

Chang G, Astrachan B, Weil U, Bryant K (Harvard Med School, Boston, Mass; Univ of Illinois, Chicago; Yale Univ, New Haven, Conn)

Ann Emerg Med 21:284–290, 1992 8–30

Background.—Alcohol has been implicated in at least half of traffic fatalities, thus prompting the recommendation that emergency room physicians report drunk drivers assessed by them. Little is known about physicians' perceptions of the usefulness of reporting such patients or their willingness to do so. An exploratory study was done to ascertain physicians' opinions on the mandatory reporting of alcohol-impaired drivers encountered in the emergency department to the police or authorities from the Division of Motor Vehicles.

Methods.—Two thousand four hundred sixty-four physicians were selected randomly from the American College of Emergency Physicians listing and sent anonymous survey forms. The one-time-only questionnaires elicited demographic information and attitudes toward mandatory reporting and alcohol treatment.

Findings.—The survey response rate was 43%. Seventy-eight percent of the respondents said that they agreed with mandatory reporting. More than half indicated strong agreement. Through canonical discriminant analysis, the complex factors affecting attitude toward mandatory reporting were identified. Most of the physicians who endorsed mandatory reporting apparently believed that alcoholism is a treatable illness. Concerns about confidentiality appeared to moderate commitment to reporting for some of the respondents.

Conclusions.—Seventy-eight percent of the respondents to this survey agreed that patients treated for injuries sustained as a result of driving while under the influence of alcohol should be reported to authorities. Thus, emergency room physicians appear to support mandatory reporting of alcohol-impaired drivers encountered in the course of clinical work. However, these results are only preliminary and must be interpreted cautiously.

▶ This paper suffers from the same problem that most surveys have, i.e., it has a low response rate. Furthermore, the people who are most likely to respond are those who have the strongest feelings about this subject. They are also most likely to be the ones who feel that emergency physicians should actively intervene and report intoxicated drivers.

Regardless of the weaknesses, this study does point out that most emergency physicians do recognize that this is a problem and feel that it is our responsibility to intervene. I found it somewhat disturbing, however, to review the reasons given for not reporting patients to authorities. Many emergency physicians feel that this is a legal problem, not a medical one, and others express concern that if the patient were tested and not warned by physicians to get treatment, the physicians could later be held legally liable if anything happened to the patient. It never ceases to amaze me for what you can be held liable today. See also Abstract 8–31.—W.H. Spivey, M.D.

The Effect of Legal Drinking Age on Fatal Injuries of Adolescents and Young Adults

Jones NE, Pieper CF, Robertson LS (Hunter College, New York, NY; Duke Univ, Durham, NC; Nanlee Research, Branford, Conn)
Am J Public Health 82:112–115, 1992 8–31

Background.—Raising the legal drinking age (LDA) reduces the number of young drivers involved in fatal motor vehicle crashes. The effect of LDA on other types of fatal injuries among adolescents and young adults was studied.

Methods.—Data were collected from all 50 states and the District of Columbia for the years 1979 through 1984. Injury death rates were determined for persons aged 15 to 24. Categories of death examined included motor vehicle driver, motorcyclist, pedestrian, unintentional injury excluding motor vehicles, suicide, and homicide.

Results.—Higher LDAs were associated with reduced death rates for motor vehicle drivers, pedestrians, unintentional injuries excluding motor vehicle injuires, and suicide. The effect of LDA varied among categories and age groups, but the overall benefits of a drinking age of 21 were clear. The suicide rate, for example, was found to be 9.7% greater among persons of a given age who can drink legally than among persons of the same age who cannot.

Conclusion.—Raising the LDA to 21 years postpones legal access to alcohol among pre-LDA adolescents, prevents traumatic deaths that occur with earlier legal access, and delays the onset of heavy drinking and its associated fatal injuries. An LDA of 21 years may thus have a significant positive impact.

▶ Alcohol, which remains our national drug of choice, continues to cause mayhem on our streets. In addition to the well-publicized toll of alcohol-related motor vehicle fatalities, the authors note associations with non–automobile-related fatal trauma, accidents, and suicides. While national attention is frequently focused on other recreational drugs, we need to continue educational efforts directed at the risks associated with the use of alcohol, including the negative health effects separate from those related to drunk driving.—R.M. Rutstein, M.D.

Emergency Center Operations

An Analysis of Emergency Physicians' Cumulative Career Risk of HIV Infection

Wears RL, Vukich DJ, Winton CN, Fluskey LL, MacMath TR, Li S (Univ of Florida, Jacksonville; Univ of North Florida, Jacksonville)
Ann Emerg Med 20:749–753, 1991 8–32

Background.—The risk of becoming infected with HIV from any single exposure is generally thought to be small. However, repeated exposure to very small risks can add up to a relatively large cumulative risk. A study was done to determine point and range estimates of the cumulative career risk of occupationally acquired HIV infection by emergency physicians and to determine whether the efficacy of universal precautions is seriously lessened by prolonged risk over time.

Methods.—Eight scenarios were developed for high vs. low prevalence of HIV, no precautions vs. universal precautions, and prevalence increasing to a steady state vs. peaking and then declining. Monte Carlo estimation of the mathematical models of cumulative risk was done.

Results.—Assuming that HIV seroprevalence increases to a steady-state level, the median estimate of cumulative risk of HIV infection over a 30-year career in a high-prevalence area when universal precautions were not used was 1.4%. For low-prevalence emergency departments

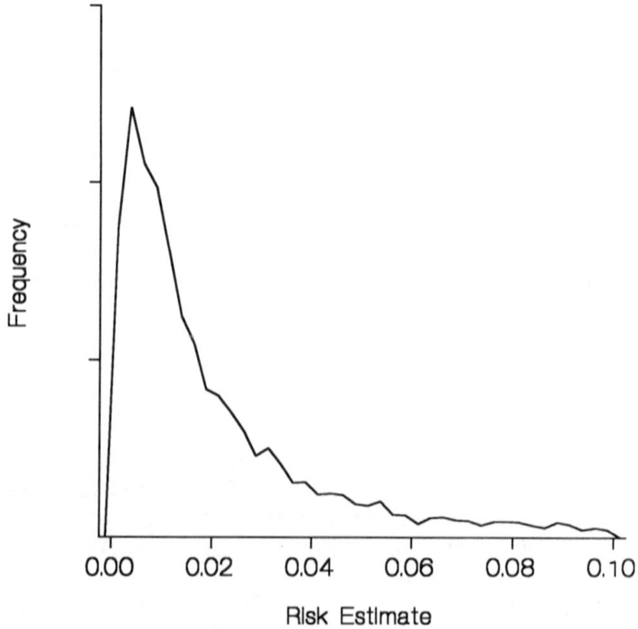

Fig 8–3.—Distribution of risk estimates for the high-prevalence emergency departments assuming prevalence rises to a steady state and universal precautions are not used. The 25th, 50th, and 75th percentiles of these estimates are .006, .014, and .033, respectively. The mean is .040. (Courtesy of Wears RL, Vukich DJ, Winton CN, et al: *Ann Emerg Med* 20:749–753, 1991.)

under those conditions, the median was .1%. Universal precautions, with a presumed efficacy of about 40% reduced the risk by approximately 30% (Fig 8–3).

Conclusions.—The cumulative risk of occupationally acquired HIV infection in emergency physicians is not trivial. Universal precautions, although their efficacy is somewhat lessened by repeated exposure over time, still seem to reduce the risk. Knowing the magnitude of the risk should be useful in making decisions about the implementation of preventive measures.

▶ Occupationally acquired HIV infection is something we all *think* about but never really *worry* about because we use universal precautions and therefore assume that the risk is small (1).

However, this paper, which looks at the cumulative risk of HIV infection over an entire career as an emergency physician, reveals that the risk is "not trivial," but neither is it cause for hysteria. Also, it should heighten the awareness of all emergency physicians to be steadfast in our methods of universal precautions with every patient we encounter.

This increasing level of risk for emergency physicians may have important implications, such as more difficult/more expensive access to disability insurance, guaranteed health insurance, and life insurance. It may also play a role in discouraging medical students from studying the specialty of emergency medicine or encouraging practicing emergency physicians to find "lesser-risk" venues of patient care.—J.J. Kelly, D.O., F.A.C.E.P.

Reference

1. Marcus R: N *Engl J Med* 319:1118, 1988.

Health Care Access Problems of Medically Indigent Emergency Department Walk-In Patients

Pane GA, Farner MC, Salness KA (Univ of California Irvine, Orange)

Ann Emerg Med 20:730–733, 1991 8–33

Background.—Many indigent and uninsured patients are forced to seek emergency and basic health services in an emergency department (ED) because they do not have access to health care anywhere else. Because the characteristics of walk-in emergency patients have not been well studied, the extent of health care access problems experienced by a representative sample of stable walk-in ED patients was assessed.

Methods.—The authors' urban level I trauma center and teaching hospital treats approximately 38,000 emergency patients per year. Stable walk-in ED patients were given an access-to-health care survey while waiting in the triage area. Pregnant women of more than 20 weeks' gestation and patients with an acute medical emergency requiring immediate attention were excluded from the study. It took 48 days to reach the study quota of 1,000 patients, and 94% of those eligible agreed to participate. The survey was available in English and Spanish and was administered by a bilingual investigator who occasionally assisted with its completion as needed.

Results.—Eighty percent of the patients were less than 40 years old, 52.3% were Hispanic, 68.3% had an annual income of less than $10,000, 7.3% were homeless, and 37.4% were employed. Twenty-five percent of the patients used the ED as their routine source of health care, and 83.2% had public aid/self-pay insurance status. During the past year, 33.3% had delayed seeking needed medical care, 12.6% had been refused care by a health care provider, and 7.3% had been refused care at an ED. Public aid/self-pay insurance status was significantly associated with routine use of the ED for health care, an annual income of less than $10,000, refusal of care by a health care provider, refusal of care at an ED, and delay in seeking health care. An annual income of less than $10,000 was significantly associated with routine use of the ED and delay in seeking health care.

Conclusions.—Low-income and uninsured patients are significantly more likely to use the ED as their routine source of health care and delay seeking needed health care than are higher-income and fully insured patients. It appears that the nation's health care system is not accessible to a large segment of the U.S. population.

▶ The authors develop data that serve to validate a common perception among emergency physicians, namely, that the emergency center provides the primary access port to the health care system for economically disadvantaged individuals and that such individuals are likely to have advanced conditions at the time of access. While health care policy planners continue to emphasize the necessity of a broader national primary-care network, it is apparent that for the foreseeable future, emergency centers will continue to serve this function to a large segment of the population. Consequently, it is essential that individual institutions plan appropriately to absorb the breadth of concerns that a predominantly primary-care practice produces. If properly organized and spread across the entire spectrum of patients coming to the emergency center, the actual costs per encounter can be reduced and efficiencies of care developed.—D.K. Wagner, M.D.

Emergency Departments and Crowding in United States Teaching Hospitals

Andrulis DP, Kellermann A, Hintz EA, Hackman BB, Weslowski VB (Natl Public Health and Hosp Inst, Washington, DC; Univ of Tennessee, Memphis)

Ann Emerg Med 20:980–986, 1991 8–34

Objective.—The true extent of crowding in hospitals and emergency departments was investigated by mailing questionnaires to member institutions of the National Association of Public Hospitals and the Council of Teaching Hospitals. Respondents were hospital administrators and emergency department directors at 239 member institutions, all non-VA, general acute-care centers.

Findings.—Three fourths of the hospitals reported an increase in emergency department visits over the past 3 years. Mean holding times for patients admitted to the hospital were 3½ hours for a floor bed and nearly 3 hours for a bed in the intensive care unit (ICU). Half the hospitals reported maximum waiting times of 10 hours or longer for floor beds and 7 hours or longer for ICU beds. The hospitals had attempted to deal with crowding in a variety of ways: limiting access to certain types of patients, transferring patients to other hospitals, and ambulance diversion.

Implications.—Currently emergency department visits may reach 90 million nationwide. Many of those who visit emergency departments may find ready access to high-quality care difficult to find. Crowding may be a particular problem in metropolitan areas, but it is a truly pervasive problem throughout the country.

► These investigations, as well as other research on operational emergency department issues (see Abstract 8–37), are strategic for the health of emergency medicine and the sanity of all of us who will practice emergency medicine into the 21st century. We must be able to objectively track and monitor the crucial issue of overcrowding and systematically attack it on a multilevel basis before "America's medical safety net" becomes American's next domestic crisis.—J.J. Kelly, D.O., F.A.C.E.P.

The Emergency Department as a Pathway to Admission for Poor and High-Cost Patients

Stern RS, Weissman JS, Epstein AM (Harvard Med School; Harvard School of Public Health, Boston, Mass)

JAMA 266:2238–2243, 1991 8–35

Background.—The function of the emergency department (ED) as a route to hospital admission may be especially important from the perspective of reimbursement and public health. The link between socioeconomic status and admission from the ED, as well as the association between this route of admission and hospital resource use, was studied.

Methods.—The study included 20,089 patients admitted to 5 hospitals over a 6-month period. Through structured interviews, the proportion of patients in the various socioeconomic and disease groups that entered by way of the ED was ascertained. Length of stay and charges for those patients were then compared with those of patients admitted through other pathways.

Findings.—The overall proportion of patients admitted through the ED was 51%. When compared with other patients, the elderly and those of lower socioeconomic status were more likely to be admitted through the ED. Odds ratios were 1.87 for the elderly, 2.38 for those of lower income, 1.47 for those of lower occupational status, and 1.69 for those of lower educational level. Patients admitted through the ED stayed 27% longer and incurred 13% higher charges than other patients, even after adjustment for diagnosis-related group (DRG), severity according to DRGSCALE, and socioeconomic status and exclusion of outliers. The magnitude of these effects varied somewhat at the different hospitals, but insurance status was strongly associated with ED use at all hospitals.

Conclusions.—Patients of low socioeconomic status are more likely to be admitted to the hospital through the ED, and patients admitted in this way use more resources than other patients in the same DRG. Increasing the availability of ED services is likely to lead to more hospitalizations of patients in the lower socioeconomic groups; such hospitals may be at a significant financial disadvantage under per-case reimbursement systems. Some system to compensate hospitals for these extra costs may help preserve access to care for disadvantaged patients and ensure the viability of the hospitals.

► These data are not surprising. Even in a system with citywide neighborhood clinics for indigent patients, such facilities are often so overburdened that appointments are several weeks away. The patients come to the ED instead and are admitted thorough the ED rather than the clinic. It is interesting that the authors found higher costs and longer stays among those patients admitted through the ED. Unfortunately, the reimbursement system for these patients does not account for their increased costs. In order to survive, how do hospitals manipulate the system to offset increased costs? Limiting ED admissions may create further barriers for medically underprivileged patients. Increasing reimbursement for patients admitted through the ED may create a setting where admissions are funneled through the ED. Neither is a solution. The authors recommend increased compensation for hospitals with a higher proportion of admissions through the ED, but a defined plan where this system is not abused, i.e., the ED becomes the admitting office, is important. Any answers? (See also Abstract 8–37.)—J.M. Mitchell-Savinsky, M.D.

Appropriateness of Patient Transfer From a Nursing Home to an Acute-Care Hospital: A Study of Emergency Room Visits and Hospital Admissions

Bergman H, Clarfield AM (Sir Mortimer B Davis-Jewish Gen Hosp, Montreal; McGill Univ, Montreal, Canada)

J Am Geriatr Soc 39:1164–1168, 1991 8–36

Background.—Although little research has been done on this subject in Canada, many physicians believe that a large proportion of transfers of patients from nursing homes to acute-care hospitals are inappropriate. To examine this issue, a study was undertaken of all transfers from a public nursing home near Montreal to acute-care hospitals.

Methods.—From 1981 to 1983, records of all patients transferred were examined for the cause of the transfer, the diagnosis made in the emergency room (ER) or hospital, the length of acute-care hospital stay, and the outcome of the hospital visit. Transfers were considered appropriate if they resulted in hospital admissions, if the ER physician deemed that the problem required diagnostic and therapeutic procedures not available in the nursing home, or if the severity of the condition were such that death occurred in the ER.

Results.—Of 112 residents in this 80-bed nursing home, 102 transfers of 55 residents occurred during the 3-year study period. Of these 102 transfers, 17% resulted in direct admission, 34% resulted in hospital admission via the ER, 4% resulted in death in the ER, and 45% resulted in a return to the nursing home without hospital admission. In the last category, only 7 of the 46 cases could have been given a diagnosis and treated exclusively in the nursing home. A total of 93% of all transfers studied were considered medically appropriate.

Conclusion.—In this Canadian nursing home during the study period, most of the transfers of residents to acute-care hospitals were appropriate.

► This article addressed a problem familiar to all emergency physicians and is particularly interesting because the results of the Canadian study are compared with similar studies done in the United States. The article points out that the U.S. studies show a much greater proportion of inappropriate transfers to the emergency department from nursing homes and that this is probably partly due to the fact that in Canada, patients in nursing homes can be seen as often as needed and the physician will be paid. In contrast, in the United States, frequent physician visits to these patients are not encouraged by the payment system. This is certainly a major problem to be confronted in the United States as our patient population in long-term care facilities increases. As we struggle with the problem of health care financing in the United States, we must consider that certain dollars are better spent in preventing an illness or treating it in its early stages than waiting until the patient is "really sick."

If we truly believe that many transfers could be prevented, we need to carefully scrutinize the data for opportunities to improve the current system of health care for nursing home patients in the United States.—E.J. Lucid, M.D.

Patients Who Leave a Public Hospital Emergency Department Without Being Seen by a Physician: Causes and Consequences

Baker DW, Stevens CD, Brook RH (Univ of California, Los Angeles; Univ of California-Los Angeles, Torrance)

JAMA 266:1085–1090, 1991 8–37

Background.—Emergency departments at public hospitals are supposed to provide a safety net for patients who truly need medical care and cannot receive it elsewhere. Because of overcrowded conditions, however, many individuals leave the facility without having seen a physician. This study assessed whether patients who sought care at a public hospital emergency department and left without seeing a physician needed immediate medical attention and whether they obtained care after leaving.

Methods.—During a 2-week period, physicians studied all adult ambulatory patients who registered at the emergency department at Harbor-UCLA Medical Center between 7 A.M. and 11 P.M. who subsequently left without seeing a physician. The study group also included a 20% random sample of those who waited to see a physician. Subjects completed a self-reported health status questionnaire, available in Spanish and English. Physicians used the triage nurse's assessment and a retrospective physician's acuity rating to assess the urgency of the problem and then created a 4-level acuity measure to classify the 32 most common complaints.

Results.—Patients who left without seeing a physician reported that they had waited 6.4 hours before leaving. Those who saw a physician waited 6.2 hours. There were no differences between groups in the chief complaint, assessment of the triage nurse, physician's acuity ratings, or self-reported health status. However, 46% of those who left should have had immediate medical attention, and 29% warranted care within 24 to 48 hours. Eleven percent of those who did not see a physician were hospitalized the following week, and 3 patients required emergency surgery. Nine percent of those who did see a physician were hospitalized. Nearly half (49%) of patients who left had not seen a physician at the 1-week follow-up.

Conclusions.—Patients who leave emergency departments without seeing a physician may be in danger unless triage criteria are sensitive for detecting life-threatening disease. In this study, the 4-level acuity scale classified 17 of 19 patients who left but subsequently needed hospitalization as patients requiring prompt medical attention. Implementation of such triage criteria may help provide faster access to care for those who truly need it, but the criteria should be evaluated prospectively before implementation.

▶ The subject of waiting time in the emergency center is of increasing importance as more patients are turning to the emergency center for care due to failure of other areas of the health care system. The impact of waiting times on patient welfare is of great concern.

This study looked at patients presenting between 7 A.M. and 11 P.M. only. The high incidence of patients leaving who needed immediate attention (46%) is of special concern. This would indicate that the department studied is overcrowded with true emergencies. Nevertheless, the authors emphasize a need for better ambulatory care services to blunt the overcrowding by seeing less seriously ill patients.

Waiting times in this study appear to be adversely affecting the welfare of the emergency patient population by limiting emergency care to patients who truly need it. More resources need to be devoted to the emergency department in question as well as improving alternative sites for ambulatory care. Our institutional experience has not yet reached this severity. Patients leaving our department due to prolonged waiting times seem to be those with lower acuity levels. (See Abstract 8–38.) J.E. Clinton, M.D.

Consequences of Queuing for Care at a Public Hospital Emergency Department

Bindman AB, Grumbach K, Keane D, Rauch L, Luce JM (San Francisco Gen

Hosp; Univ of California, San Francisco)
JAMA 266:1091–1096, 1991 8–38

Background.—Emergency departments at public hospitals are becoming increasingly crowded. Some patients wait for a long time, and others leave without ever having received care. The length of time waiting for care at a public hospital emergency department was studied to determine what amount of time was sufficiently discouraging to cause patients to leave without seeing a physician and whether their leaving adversely affected their health and subsequent use of health care services.

Methods.—For 1 week, all patients waiting for emergency care at San Francisco General Hospital were surveyed. A follow-up survey was performed 7 to 14 days later. English-, Spanish-, or Cantonese-speaking patients older than 18 years of age were eligible for inclusion. The survey, written in the subject's native language, took less than 15 minutes to complete. Responses of patients who left without seeing a physician were compared with those of patients who did see a physician.

Results.—Eighty-five percent of the survey participants saw a physician; 15% left without having seen one. There were no significant differences in demographic characteristics between the groups. The longer patients had to wait, the more likely they were to leave. At follow-up, patients who left without having seen a physician were twice as likely to report that the pain or seriousness of the condition was worse than were patients who did see a physician. Four percent of patients who left without receiving medical attention required subsequent hospitalization, and 27% returned to an emergency department.

Conclusions.—Many patients who visit an emergency department may have relatively minor problems that will resolve without complications whether or not they see a physician. In the survey, many also expressed a willingness to defer care for a few days if they could receive a clinic appointment. However, some patients fare poorly if they do not receive emergency department care. Unfortunately, it is difficult to predict which patients who leave without seeing a physician will get worse.

► The subject of waiting times in the emergency center is of increasing importance as more patients are turning to the emergency center for care due to failure of other areas of the health care system. The impact of waiting times on patient welfare is of great concern.

The methodology, analysis, and conclusions reached seem sound. The authors do not overstate their findings. The notsurprising finding that patient elopement increases with waiting times is clear. Since elopement is greatest in the lowest-acuity patients, the phenomenon's impact on patient outcome is difficult to assess.

Trends in waiting time and patient walkout statistics need frequent monitoring by emergency center managers. Measures to decrease waiting times need to be focused on the peak periods of patient demand, which often occur at odd hours in public hospitals. An emergency department computerized patient-tracking system can be an excellent tool, allowing these data to be used most effectively.—J.E. Clinton, M.D.

Gangs, Drugs, and Homicide in Los Angeles

Meehan PJ, O'Carroll PW (Centers for Disease Control, Atlanta, Ga)
Am J Dis Child 146:683–687, 1992 8–39

Background.—Gang involvement in the narcotics trade is widely believed to be responsible for a high percentage of homicides among youths in Los Angeles. This assumption needs to be critically examined because it has direct relevance to homicide prevention program design.

Methods.—All homicides recorded in a police data base from 1986 to 1988 in Los Angeles were analyzed. Detailed data from police files were then studied. The association between gang homicide victimization and victim cocaine use for all 1987 homicides was also examined. In addition, narcotics arrest histories for gang homicide victims were compared with histories for other homicide victimas.

Findings.—Gang-motivated homicides were found to be less likely than other homicides to involve narcotics. Narcotics-motivated homicides were less likely than others to involve a gang member. In 1987, victims of gang-motivated homicides were less likely than other homicide victims to have detectable blood cocaine levels. Young victims of gang-motivated homicide were no more likely to have a history of narcotics arrests than were victims of other types of homicide.

Conclusions.—If gang activity and narcotics trafficking are related to increased homicide risk, this relationship accounts for a small percentage of the risk. It was recommended that gang activity and narcotics trafficking or use be considered separate, important risk factors for homicide instead of interrelated cofactors.

▶ There are some difficulties and ambiguities in the data collection and analysis that is the heart of this article, which may cast its conclusions into doubt. Anyone who has a serious interest in these issues owes it to himself to read the "Materials and Methods" section in detail. If the authors' conclusions are correct, however, they call into question the conventional wisdom regarding the relationship of illicit drugs to gang violence.—J. Schoffstall, M.D.

Preformatted Charts Improve Documentation in the Emergency Department

Humphreys T, Shofer FS, Jacobson S, Coutifaris C, Stemhagen A (Univ of Pennsylvania, Philadelphia; Hosp of the Univ of Pennsylvania, Philadelphia)
Ann Emerg Med 21:534–540, 1992 8–40

Introduction.—Complete documentation is a particular challenge in the emergency department (ED), a high-volume, high-acuity setting in which patient care demands compete with administrative responsibilities. A study was conducted to determine whether the use of programmed charts could improve documentation in the ED and to assess any effect on clinical outcomes.

Methods.—Charts were specially designed for obstetric and gynecologic examinations in the ED. For each patient of childbearing age with gynecologic complaints of abdominal pain, bleeding, or vaginal discharge, the ED physician was provided with a programmed or blank chart in randomized fashion. Charts were examined for the presence of documentation criteria for patient history, physical examination, laboratory studies, diagnosis, and discharge instructions for common categories of patient complaints. Outcome scores of 0% to 100% were based on the persistence of complaints at a follow-up interview. Ninety-nine programmed charts and 30 blank charts were evaluated; another 30 blank charts were excluded because of illegibility.

Results.—Documentation of the history, physical examination, and laboratory studies was 81% on programmed charts and 71% on blank charts. The greatest benefit was in documentation of the patient history — 75% complete for the programmed charts and 60% complete for the blank charts. The improvement in documentation was not significantly related to patient outcome measures or to satisfaction with the quality of care. The use of programmed charts was related to patient satisfaction with the physician's explanation of the problem.

Conclusions.—The use of programmed charts in the ED can facilitate documentation, thus increasing the physician's time with the patient. The greatest improvements in the quality of documentation were in the areas of history and physical examination. Patient outcome or quality of care is not reliably indicated by the quality of documentation alone.

► It has been recognized previously that formatted data collection sheets improve not only data collection but diagnostic accuracy as well (1). This study reinforces that idea. With the arrival of practice guidelines (2), charts preformatted with specific guideline criteria have the potential for improving documentation and decreasing medicolegal risk. Whether they will improve outcome is less clear. They did not in this study, but outcome measures were poorly done (admitted patients were dropped from the study, for example), and the group studied was relatively small.

There are some disconcerting things in this study that should give us pause. Fully half of the handwritten charts had to be dropped from the study because they were completely illegible. The group with the worst chart documentation was the attending physicians. Even the preformatted charts were incomplete almost 20% of the time.

The handwritten ED chart is a dinosaur. It is time-consuming and laborious to document in a manner legible, reimbursable, and defensible in court, and as a result, it is often written very poorly. Preformatted charts may help, but dictated and typed charts, perhaps with automatic real-time computerized quality assurance checks are the wave of the future.—J. Schoffstall, M.D.

References

1. de Dombal FT, et al: *BMJ* 302:1495, 1991.
2. Davidson SJ: *Ann Emerg Med* 19:943, 1990.

Emergency Department Record Keeping and the Potential for Injury Surveillance

Runyan CW, Bowling JM, Bangdiwala SI (Univ of North Carolina, Chapel Hill; North Carolina Dept of Environment, Health and Natural Resources)

J Trauma 32:187–189, 1992 8–41

Background.—Successful design of injury prevention measures requires an understanding of the occurrence and circumstances of injuries. This understanding necessitates good record keeping on injured persons. Emergency departments are an important source of data that can be used to develop injury prevention measures. A survey was done to examine record-keeping practices in emergency departments.

Methods.—A self-administered questionnaire was mailed to emergency department directors in 129 North Carolina hospitals. A repeat mailing to nonrespondents was done 3 to 4 weeks later. Telephone interviews were conducted with hospitals still not responding. The overall response rate was 98%.

Findings.—Only 41% of lower-volume facilities included a measure of injury severity in their emergency department records. Sixty-two percent of the higher-volume emergency departments had such a measure. Forty percent of the lower-volume facilities and 37% of higher-volume ones recorded coded diagnostic data on their patients. Fewer than 20% in each group recorded external causes of injury. Generally, higher-volume emergency departments collected more data than did lower-volume facilities.

Conclusions.—This survey revealed great variability in the types of data that would be available to researchers attempting to study emergency department records. The absence of information about the external cause of injury was notable.

Value of Radiograph Audit in an Accident Service Department

Thomas HG, Mason AC, Smith RM, Fergusson CM (John Radcliffe Hosp, Oxford, England)

Injury 23:47–50, 1992 8–42

Background.—In the accident service (A/S) department of 1 hospital, all trauma radiographs are reported by an experienced radiologist and those that were misinterpreted by the casualty officer are presented at a daily clinicoradiologic conference. The value of this practice was reviewed over a 6-month period.

Data Analysis.—For the 25,798 patients seen at the A/SA department 16,246 radiographs were requested and reported. Among these, 456 (2.8%) were considered to have been potentially misinterpreted, including 167 missed fractures (1%), 55 suspected fractures (.3%), and 72 false positive diagnoses of fracture (.4%). A total of 114 patients (.7%) were recalled for further assessment or imaging and treatment, but fewer than 50% of patients with missed or suspected fractures required changes in their prescribed course of treatment. All 72 false positive diagnoses were appropriately treated, and no changes in management were required. Incorrect diagnoses more commonly involved the ankle, wrist, foot, elbow, and hand; fractures of the fingers were the most comonly missed diagnoses in children. A review of the more serious injuries stressed the significance of fractures of the upper or lower ribs with possible underlying neurovascular, lung, or upper abdominal organ trauma; correct interpretation of axial or lateral shoulder radiographs, especially when dislocation is suspected; and adequate views of C1 to T1 for injuries of the cervical spine.

Discussion.—It appears that a daily radiograph audit in the A/S is beneficial to patient care and can significantly reduce the risk of litigation.

▶ This British review looks at the accuracy of radiograph interpretation by physicians staffing a trauma emergency department. Patients who were evaluated for nontraumatic conditions were excluded in this study. Of all radiographs taken, only 1% had fractures missed by the casualty officer. One curiosity is that skull radiographs were the third most commonly ordered study (see Abstract 2–11), preceded by ankle and wrist radiographs. Audits in the United States demonstrate great expertise in the interpretation of radiographs by emergency physicians. Although radiology support is helpful for quality control, such support is not always essential for the interpretation of plain radiographs when experienced emergency medicine physicians are reviewing radiographs.—E.J. Reisdorff, M.D.

Medical Problem Solving and Uncertainty in the Emergency Department

Sklar DP, Hauswald M, Johnson DR (Univ of New Mexico, Albuquerque)
Ann Emerg Med 20:987–991, 1991 8–43

Objective.—The diagnostic processes employed by experienced and novice emergency physicians were examined at the emergency department of a county university medical center in a large southwestern urban area. Forty-eight patient encounters by 8 attending and senior resident physicians were compared with 81 encounters by 40 junior residents and senior medical students.

Study Design.—The study participants developed a diagnostic impression after reviewing the patient's chief complaint, nurse triage notes, and the vital signs. Tests were then chosen and a final impression formulated when the results became available. The clinicians also marked a visual analogue scale to indicate their degree of certainty about their diagnoses.

Results.—The novices performed essentially as well as the experienced clinicians in developing an initial differential diagnosis. Both groups became more certain when making a final diagnosis, but the experienced clinicians indicated a greater increase in certainty than the novices. The experienced clinicians deviated from the conventional history-physical-laboratory sequence much more often than did the novices.

Conclusions.—Expert decision making in the emergency setting is characterized by moderate initial diagnostic uncertainty, a flexible strategy of laboratory testing, and a substantial increase in diagnostic certainty by the time a final impression is offered.

▶ For some reason, medical education articles have been noted to cause headaches 100% of the time in this reviewer. The bottom line of this study is that grizzled veterans learn to be cautious about establishing an impression on the basis of a chief complaint, vital signs, and a brief nurse's note and to be very confident that they were able to come up with the right diagnosis despite exhibiting deviant behavior.—R.M. McNamara, M.D.

9 Toxicology

Poisonings

Complete Heart Block After Flumazenil

Herd B, Clarke F (North Tees Gen Hosp, Cleveland, Ohio)

Hum Exp Toxicol 10:289, 1991 9–1

Introduction.—The benzodiazepine competitive antagonist flumazenil is often used for the treatment of benzodiazepine sedation, especially in patients for whom it is desirable to avoid ventilation. In an elderly patient, the use of flumazenil was associated with complete heart block. This association has not been previously reported.

Case Report.—A 79-year-old woman was admitted while deeply unconscious, apparently because of an overdose of paracetamol and temazepam. Because her blood oxygen tension was 6.4 kPa and her carbon dioxide tension was 4.8 kPa, she was treated with oxygen. She was administered acetylcysteine and also received 500 μg of fluamzenil over a period of several minutes. One minute after the injection, complete heart block developed with a low-volume pulse of about 15 to 20 beats per minute. The patient vomited without ill effect, and her heart rate increased to 30 to 50 beats per minute with a first-degree block. After receiving atropine, she reverted to sinus rhythm at a rate of 95 beats per minute; her systolic blood pressure was 90 mm Hg, and her oxygen tension was 16 kPA. Later her heart rate fell, and she was again administered atropine; her blood pressure increased to 120/70 mm Hg. An ECG showed no alterations when compared with one recorded before the overdose. Levels of cardiac enzymes were normal. Her transaminase level was only minimally and transiently elevated. Her serum paracetamol level 11 hours after the presumed overdose was 1,028 mg/L. Her serum nifedipine level was never determined because of a serum storage error. After her treatment was complete, the patient also admitted taking atenolol and nifedipine. Her recovery was uneventful.

Discussion.—No good explanation for the sudden onset of bradycardia was proposed, although temporal factors in part make it unlikely that it was caused by atenolol and nifedipine. Patients receiving flumazenil should be closely monitored.

► Flumazenil is a new drug, and unexpected side effects should be watched for closely, but in this case, the patient's bradycardia is much more likely to have resulted from the combination of a β-blocker and a slow calcium channel blocker.—W.P. Burdick, M.D.

Severe Oral Phenytoin Overdose Does Not Cause Cardiovascular Morbidity

Wyte CD, Berk WA (Detroit Receiving Hosp, Mich)

Ann Emerg Med 20:508–512, 1991 9–2

Introduction.—The possibility of cardiovascular complications from phenytoin overdose has led physicians to care for patients in a monitored setting at substantial cost. Circulatory complications have, however, been rare in fatal cases; neurologic complications have predominated.

Objective.—Fifty-seven patients seen in a 2-year period with a peak phenytoin concentration of 40 μg/mL or above were studied. The mean age was 44 years. Six patients had a history of heart disease. The mean peak phenytoin level was 49.4 μg/mL.

Findings.—Blood pressure at admission was slightly higher than at discharge. No dysrhythmia or high-grade atrioventricular block was seen in the 36 patients having ECG monitoring. Half of the patients had ECG abnormalities, but these were not closely related to the presence of toxic drug levels. The PR interval was not consistently related to the blood phenytoin concentration. No patient required treatment for hemodynamic disorder, and there were no deaths.

Conclusion.—It is not necessary to routinely care for stable patients with severe phenytoin overdose in a monitored setting.

▶ This retrospective chart review of 57 patients admitted for significant oral phenytoin overdoses makes the point that significant cardiovascular complications are not related to an oral overdose of this agent, but rather have been described exclusively in the context of rapid parenteral administration. It is probably the case that stable patients with toxic phenytoin levels may be observed in the hospital setting outside of the critical care unit. Of interest, the authors review in some detail the data regarding the relative roles of propylene glycol, which is the diluent used with parenteral forms of phenytoin, vs. phenytoin itself as the principal cause of cardiac toxicity in the rapid intravenous infusion model. They conclude that it is probably the propylene glycol moiety that is the most cardiac toxic. The authors further comment that a phenytoin overdose may still result in significant CNS toxicity, particularly in lowering the pre-existing seizure threshold, and note the danger of morbidity related to accidents occurring as a result of ataxia and poor judgment stemming from phenytoin-induced neurologic toxicity. Therefore, an in-hospital observation period would still be prudent to recommend for those patients with significant toxic levels and evidence of CNS involvement.—F.M. Henretig, M.D.

Clinical Characteristics of Angiotensin-Converting Enzyme Inhibitor-Induced Angioedema

Roberts JR, Wuerz RC (Mercy Catholic Med Ctr; The Med College of Pennsylvania, Philadelphia)

Ann Emerg Med 20:555–558, 1991 9–3

Background.—Angiotensin-converting enzyme (ACE) inhibitors are widely used in the treatment of hypertension and congestive heart failure. Although the ACE inhibitors have a relatively good clinical safety profile, the potential for severe life-threatening angioedema as a result of airway compromise has only recently been recognized. Two patients suddenly experienced severe life-threatening angioedema associated with enalapril and captopril therapy.

Case Report 1.—A 60-year-old woman was seen in the emergency department (ED) with tongue swelling of sudden onset. She was unable to speak clearly and could not swallow her saliva. The patient had been taking enalapril for about 2 years for essential hypertension. At examination, she was in moderate respiratory distress and showed mild diaphoresis without cyanosis. She was given epinephrine subcutaneously and cimetidine, methylprednisolone, and diphenhydramine intravenously but did not respond. Because of increasing respiratory difficulty, blind nasotracheal intubation was performed, and she was admitted to the intensive care unit where she was treated with dexamethasone and humidified oxygen. The swelling gradually decreased and she was extubated on the third hospital day and discharged 5 days later with a warning not to use ACE inhibitors. No further follow-up was available.

Case Report 2.—A 49-year-old man who had been taking captopril for hypertension for more than 1 year came to the ED because of increasing edema of the face and lips over the previous 8 hours. Tongue swelling rapidly developed during the next hour, and he began to experience hoarseness and increasing shortness of breath. He was treated with intravenously administered diphenhydramine and methylprednisolone, but there was no improvement. After shrinkage of the nasal mucosa, successful blind nasotracheal intubation was performed, and he was treated with intravenous corticosteroids. The patient improved over the next 18 hours and was extubated and discharged with a final diagnosis of captopril-induced angioedema.

Comments.—A review of the literature revealed 227 reported cases of this severe complication of ACE inhibitor therapy. Accentuated bradykinin activity is thought to be the major etiologic factor rather than an immunogenic process. Angioedema may suddenly occur even after the drug has been well tolerated for a long period of time. Once angioedema develops, patients should be monitored aggressively and treated immediately because it is a potentially fatal complication.

▶ Angioedema is the most common reason patients with reactions to ACE inhibitors come to emergency centers. Characteristically, this edema is of rapid progression, usually facial in nature and progressive from one side to the opposite side. Patients often describe watching their "face blow up" while looking at themselves in the mirror. Despite significant edema, in our experience, clinical airway obstruction has been uncommon. The authors, however, show that this can, in fact, occur and provide guidelines for its management. Close observation of these patients is mandatory, and as the authors note, occasional control of the airway is essential.—D.K. Wagner, M.D.

Seizure Following Brief Exposure to the Insect Repellent *N,N*-Diethyl-m-Toluamide

Lipscomb JW, Kramer JE, Leikin JB (Rush-Presbyterian-St Luke's Med Ctr, Chicago, Ill)

Ann Emerg Med 21:315–317, 1992 9–4

Background.—Concern over Lyme disease has augmented the use of insect repellents to prevent tick bites. The most effective repellent, N,N-diethyl-m-toluamide (DEET), is effective against ticks but is absorbed through the skin and has caused a number of adverse dermatologic and systemic reactions.

Case Report.—A 5-year-old boy had a major motor seizure while napping at day camp. He was in good health, although assessment a year earlier had shown mildly delayed motor skills and coordination as well as behavioral problems. That morning Muskol (95% DEET) had been applied to virtually his whole body, and OFF had been applied later. Diazepam was given intravenously but respiratory arrest necessitated intubation and ventilatory assistance until the next morning. Two doses of activated charcoal were given and the boy's skin was washed. An electroencephalogram on day 3 showed changes of diffuse encephalopathy with occasional epileptiform discharges in the right posterior region. No further seizures occurred. The urine contained .003 μg/mL of DEET at 9 to 30 hours of hospitalization.

Implications.—Exposure to DEET was relatively brief in this case. Seizures developed without the prodromal features mentioned in previous reports. The use of DEET is very widespread, but toxicity should be considered in a patient who has seizures or encephalopathy after having applied the material. High-concentration formulations and total-body application should be avoided in children.

▶ This report is a reminder that DEET can cause seizures and toxic encephalopathy. One of the problems is that DEET is a very effective insect repellant and there just are not many substitutes that seem to control insects as well. We need the pharmaceutical industry to work on safer alternatives. The authors point out that although millions of doses of DEET are used each year, toxicity is rare. My advice to parents is to apply DEET sparingly and to avoid total-body applications. Second, I recommend Avon's "Skin So Soft" cream, which often provides excellent repellent activity.—S. Wason, M.D.

Fatal Rodenticide Poisoning With Brodifacoum

Kruse JA, Carlson RW (Detroit Receiving Hosp, Mich)

Ann Emerg Med 21:331–336, 1992 9–5

Background.—The increased prevalence of rodents resistant to warfarin has led to the development of the hydroxycoumarin anticoagulant brodifacoum. A man attempted to commit suicide by ingesting d-CON Mouse-Prufe II.

Case Report.—A 25-year-old man consumed 4 boxes of d-CON Mouse-Prufe II. Each box contained 42 g of bait consisting of .005% brodifacoum. Nine days later he entered the hospital with syncope, hematochezia, gross hematuria, epistaxis, anemia, and a severe coagulopathy. Radiography showed pleural, pericardial, and mediastinal bleeding. He was treated with vitamin K and fresh frozen plasma and later discharged on a regimen of oral phytonadione. His coagulopathy recurred and required multiple plasma transfusions and prolonged treatment with oral phytonadione. Fifteen weeks after he was discharged, he again sought medical attention for additional brodifacoum ingestion. Initially, his neurologic status was normal. However, he suddenly became comatose in the emergency department soon after emesis was induced with syrup of ipecac. Computed tomography of the brain showed a subarachnoid hemorrhage that resulted in brain death within 24 hours.

Conclusions.—This is the second reported case of fatal human poisoning from brodifacoum. It illustrates that specific identification of the toxic agent can be of critical importance in managing a poisoned patient. The incorrect assumption that rodenticide-induced coagulopathy was pathognomonic for warfarin poisoning led to repeat hospitalization with a major bleeding episode. The extended half-life of brodifacoum necessitates long-term treatment and monitoring. Phytonadione, not menadiol, must be used to reverse coumarin-induced coagulopathy. By raising intracranial pressure, the induction of vomiting may have played a role in precipitating the fatal intracranial hemorrhage in this case.

► Somewhere in the annals of medical literature, a review that we wrote got buried (1). Our conclusions were that accidental "lick or taste" ingestions of superwarfarins is unlikely to result in morbidity or mortality. Deliberate ingestions, often involving numerous packets, do result in prolonged bleeding that, on occasion, as this report suggests, can be fatal.—S. Wason, M.D.

References

1. Katona B, Watson S: *J Emerg Med* 7:627, 1989.

Acute Fluoxetine Overdose: A Report of 234 Cases

Borys DJ, Setzer SC, Ling LJ, Reisdorf JJ, Day LC, Krenzelok EP (Hennepin Regional Poison Ctr, Minneapolis, Minn; Minnesota Regional Poison Ctr, St Paul; North Texas Poison Ctr, Dallas; Univ of Pittsburgh, Pa)

Am J Emerg Med 10:115–120, 1992 9–6

Background.—Little is known about the toxicity of the antidepressant fluoxetine. A prospective, multicenter study was done to develop a toxicity profile of the initial signs and symptoms in persons with acute fluoxetine overdoses.

Methods.—The cases reported to 1 of 4 American Association of Poison Control Centers' regional poison control centers were studied. All patients studied had ingested an overdose of fluoxetine. A standard data collection form was used to obtain information on patient age, current medications, dose, coingested drugs, initial symptoms, vital signs, ECG abnormalities, outcomes, and fluoxetine levels.

Findings.—Eighty-seven patients ingested fluoxetine alone, and 147 ingested it with ethanol or other drugs. Sixty-seven adults and 20 children took fluoxetine alone. Symptoms in adults were tachycardia in 15 cases, drowsiness in 14, tremor in 5, vomiting in 4, and nausea in 4. Thirty patients had no symptoms. Twelve adults had total fluoxetine levels of 232 to 1,390 ng/mL.

Conclusions.—Symptoms developing after an acute overdose of fluoxetine are apparently minor and of short duration. The only intervention necessary for patients with an acute fluoxetine overdose is aggressive supportive care.

▶ When compared with the significant toxicity seen with an overdose of the tricyclic antidepressants (TCAs), fluoxetine is a relatively safe drug. Fluoxetine especially lacks significant CNS or cardiac toxicity, and it has no anticholinergic effects. Fluoxetine's safety is probably related to its mechanism of action. While the TCAs block the uptake of norepinephrine and serotinin, fluoxetine selectively inhibits only the uptake of serotonin. Occasional deaths have been reported with fluoxetine alone or when ingested with multiple other drugs, so it pays to be clinically cautious—enough of anything can be dangerous (1). Fluoxetine levels are not readily available, but they are of no clinical value anyway. There is no specific antidote for fluoxetine toxicity, and serum alkalization—the first line of treatment of TCA toxicity—appears to have no value. One shortcoming of this study is that it investigated only cases that were reported to the poison center network—sicker patients may have been missed.—J.R. Roberts, M.D.

Reference

1. Kincaid RL, et al: *J Anal Toxicol* 14:327, 1990.

Cyanide Toxicity From Acetonitrile-Containing False Nail Remover
Geller RJ, Ekins BR, Iknoian RC (Fresno Community Hosp and Med Ctr, Fresno, Calif)
Am J Emerg Med 9:268–270, 1991 9–7

Background.—Acetonitrile is a widely available 2-carbon aliphatic nitrile used as a solvent remover of acrylic sculptured fingernails that are bonded to the natural nail with durable glues. Its toxicity is not widely appreciated, however. A patient with cyanide toxicity from acetonitrile-containing false nail remover was studied to stress the need for careful monitoring and aggressive treatment in such patients.

Case Report.—A 3-year-old boy was brought to the emergency room 30 minutes after ingesting acetonitrile. He showed no symptoms. Prompt gastric lavage was done with activated charcoal administration. Hours later, he began to show signs of clinical toxicity. Mental status abnormalities and vomiting preceded a generalized seizure. Sodium thiosulfate was administered, and the boy had an uneventful recovery. A blood cyanide level obtained just after presentation in the emergency room but reported after the child was sent home revealed significant exposure. During the boy's hospitalization, cyanide toxicity was inferred from his history of ingestion and a significant absence of venous blood hemoglobin desaturation.

Conclusions.—Even small amounts of acetonitrile can be harmful. Signs of toxicity are delayed. All acetonitrile ingestions should therefore be considered dangerous. Patients should be observed and assessed repeatedly for at least 24 hours. When cyanide level determinations are not available, lethargy, vomiting, seizures, and the lack of normal venous blood hemoglobin desaturation provide clues to cyanide toxicity.

Cyanide Poisoning From a Cosmetic Nail Remover
Losek JD, Rock AL, Boldt RR (Medical College of Wisconsin, Milwaukee)
Pediatrics 88:337–340, 1991 9–8

Background.—Acetonitrile is the principal chemical in Super Nail Nail Off, a product used to remove sculptured fingernails. When inhaled or ingested, acetonitrile is metabolized to cyanide. Several deaths from inhalation of acetonitrile have been reported, and there has been 1 death from ingestion.

Case Study.—A 23-month-old boy who was previously healthy was examined by emergency physicians 12 hours after having ingested approximately 60 mL of Super Nail Nail Off. The patient had vomited 3 times 6 hours after ingestion but otherwise did not appear ill. After physical examination, which was within normal limits, the boy received oxygen and was admitted to the hospital. Twenty-four hours postingestion, the boy became unresponsive and had staring episodes. Because his oxygen saturation was low, he received amyl nitrite, which did not change his condition. Arterial blood gas analyses showed the following values: pH, 7.43; partial pressure of carbon dioxide, 26.4 mm Hg; partial pressure of oxygen, 167.6 mm Hg; HCO_3, 17 mEq/L; and oxygen saturation, 99%. His lactic acid concentration was 50.1 mg/dL, with a methemoglobin level of .7 g/dL. Physicians administered activated charcoal with magnesium citrate and intravenous sodium thiosulfate every 4 hours. After 2 doses of sodium thiosulfate, the lactic acid level had decreased to within normal range, and his arterial blood gas values were pH, 7.42; partial pressure of carbon dioxide, 33.8 mm Hg; partial pressure of oxygen, 435.8 mm Hg; HCO_3,21.8 mEq/L; and oxygen saturation, 99.9%. During his hospital stay, the patient received sodium thiosulfate every 4 hours for 5 doses. The patient's level of consciousness returned to normal, and pulse oximeter readings were up to 98% while he was breathing room air. The patient was discharged on the third day of hospitalization. Laboratory reports later revealed that his whole-blood cyanide levels were 2.1 μg/mL 12 hours after ingestion and 3.8 μg/mL 25 hours after ingestion.

Conclusions.—Acetonitrile is a component of a number of cosmetic fingernail products available to the general public. Since 1991, these products have been packaged in childproof containers because they contain a potentially lethal amount of acetonitrile. However, these products should not be mistaken for nail-polish removers containing acetone.

► These 2 cases (Abstracts 9–7 and 9–8) remind us that acetonitrile artificial nail removers are not the same as benign acetone-based nail polish removers and that substances whose inactive parent compounds are only later transformed into toxic metabolites can appear misleadingly innocuous at the time of ingestion (see also Abstract 9–26). Thus, although the onset of most cyanide toxicity is extremely rapid, the delayed presentation in these cases is pharmacologically predictable. Because of efforts to ensure safe packaging, this particular ingestion will probably remain rare, but emergency physician familiarity with it is still important because of its potential seriousness and the probability that appropriate intervention can be effective.—J.R. Hoffman, M.D.

Effects of Calcium Channel Blocker Overdose-Induced Toxicity in the Conscious Dog

Schoffstall JM, Spivey WH, Gambone LM, Shaw RP, Sit SP (Med College of Pennsylvania, Philadelphia; Janssen Research Found, Spring House, Pa)

Ann Emerg Med 20:1104–1108, 1991 9–9

Objective.—There is little information on the cardiovascular effects of an acute overdose of slow calcium channel blockers. In a nonblinded, controlled animal study, the effects of nifedipine, diltiazem, and verapamil overdoses on systemic hemodynamics and cardiac output distribution were examined.

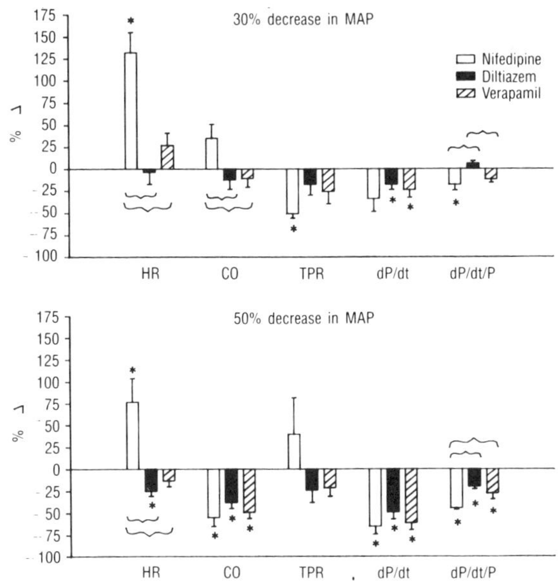

Fig 9–1.—Global hemodynamic parameters expressed as percent change from baseline when subjects' blood pressure decreased 30% from baseline (*top*) and 50% from baseline (*bottom*). Column labels dP/dt/P represents dP/dt normalized to MAP. Starred points are significantly different from baseline. Brackets indicate significant differences between drug groups. (Courtesy of Schoffstall JM, Spivey WH, Gambone LM, et al: *Ann Emerg Med* 20:1104–1108, 1991.)

Methods.—Nineteen unanesthetized chronically instrumented mongrel dogs were studied before and after intravenous infusion of .03, .1, .3, 1, and 3 mg of the study drugs per kilogram. Diltiazem and verapamil were also given at a dose of 10.0 mk/mg of drug per kilogram. Infusion was stopped when the mean arterial pressure (MAP) decreased 50% from the preinfusion value.

Results.—When MAP declined 30% from baseline (moderate toxicity), 1.43 mg of nifedipine per kilogram decreased total peripheral resistance by 51%, increased cardiac output by 35%, and increased the heart rate by 132% (Fig 9–1). Coronary blood flow increased 93%, and iliac blood flow increased 45%, while mesenteric and renal blood flows did not change significantly. At equivasodepressor doses (1.43 to 4.43 mg of drug per kilogram), diltiazem and verapamil caused less peripheral vasodilation and reflex tachycardia. When MAP decreased 50% (severe toxicity), all 3 drugs decreased cardiac output and caused redistribution of cardiac output favoring the coronary bed. The heart rate remained elevated with nifedipine but fell with diltiazem and verapamil. The latter 2 drugs also caused high-grade atrioventricular block resulting in bradycardia. Myocardial contractility was significantly lower for nifedipine than for diltiazem at moderate toxicity and lower for nifedipine than diltiazem or verapamil at severe toxicity.

Implications.—In the conscious dog, moderate-level hypotension induced by calcium channel blockers is associated with disparate effects on systemic hemodynamics, probably resulting from differential reflux sympathetic activation. At a more severe level, the toxic effects of these drugs are similar and manifested predominantly by their actions on the slow calcium channel. Hence, the therapeutic interventions required for nifedipine poisoning may differ from those appropriate for poisoning with diltiazem or verapamil. The shock state in nifedipine toxicity may be due to negative inotropy coupled with relative hypovolemia secondary to an increase in venous capacitance and may be reversed by a combination of crystalloid therapy and inotropic agents. Because the fall in cardiac output in diltiazem or verapamil overdose is mainly due to the decline in heart rate, a pacemaker may provide the best initial therapy.

▶ It is hoped that these animal studies of the toxicity of these commonly used calcium channel blocking agents will aid in the management of overdosage in humans. In addition, the cause of iatrogenic overdosage will be better understood so that we will be able to avoid this cause of toxicity.—G.V. Anderson, M.D.

Accidental and Intentional Poisonings With Ethylene Glycol in Infancy: Diagnostic Clues and Management

Saladino R, Shannon M (The Children's Hosp, Boston, Mass)

Pediatr Emerg Care 7:93–96, 1991 9–10

Introduction.—Ethylene glycol is a potentially lethal poison that is readily available in automobile antifreeze and windshield de-icer fluids. Of all glycol exposures, 48% occur in children 17 years or younger.

Case Reports.—Two children, both girls, aged 3 and 8 months, were seen with CNS depression and metabolic acidosis. The first child demonstrated the difficult nature of the diagnosis of an occult accidental ingestion. In this patient, complications included hematuria, seizures, and transient renal failure due to acute tubular necrosis. The patient's serum ethylene glycol level was 222 mg/dL, and analysis of the water used to mix her formula revealed 29% ethylene glycol. In the second patient, the accidental finding of breakdown products of ethylene glycol, glycolic acid, and glycine in her blood served as a clue for further investigation of a suspected intentional poisoning with ethylene glycol.

Discussion.—Ethylene glycol is rapidly absorbed from the gastrointestinal tract and reaches peak blood levels 1 to 4 hours after ingestion with a half-life of 2.5 to 3 hours. The metabolic products of ethylene glycol, including glycolic acid, glycoxylic acid, and oxalate, are largely responsible for the metabolic acidosis of ethylene glycol poisoning (Fig 9–2). Target-organ cellular damage involves the kidney, brain, myocardium, pancreas, and blood vessel walls. Deposition of calcium oxalate crystals

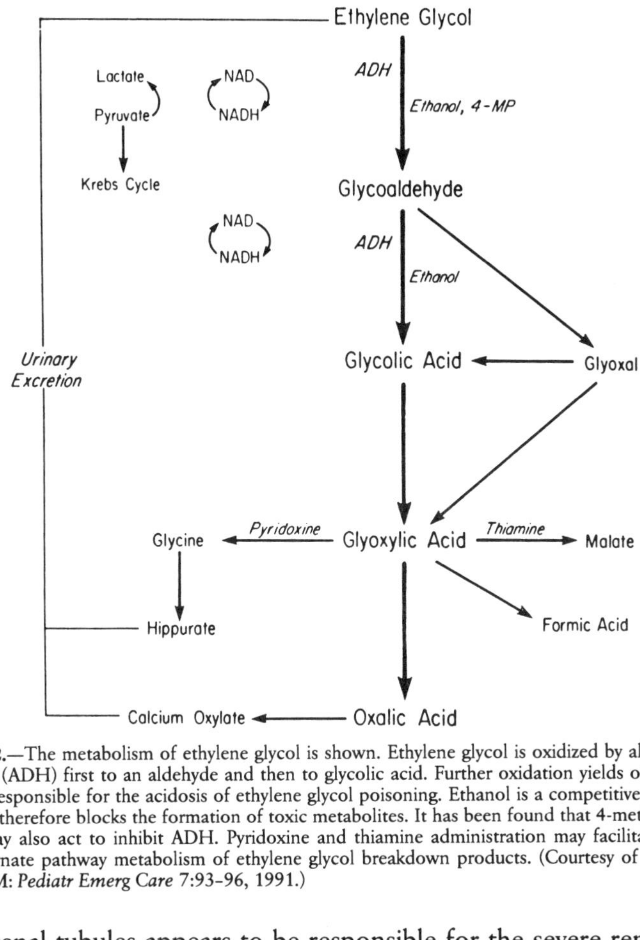

Fig 9–2.—The metabolism of ethylene glycol is shown. Ethylene glycol is oxidized by alcohol dehydrogenase (ADH) first to an aldehyde and then to glycolic acid. Further oxidation yields other organic acids, all responsible for the acidosis of ethylene glycol poisoning. Ethanol is a competitive inhibitor of ADH and therefore blocks the formation of toxic metabolites. It has been found that 4-methyl pyrazole (4-MP) may also act to inhibit ADH. Pyridoxine and thiamine administration may facilitate the indicated alternate pathway metabolism of ethylene glycol breakdown products. (Courtesy of Saladino R, Shannon M: *Pediatr Emerg Care* 7:93–96, 1991.)

in the renal tubules appears to be responsible for the severe renal injury that accompanies ethylene glycol poisoning.

Conclusions.—The clinical course of ethylene glycol poisoning is varied and includes inebriation, hematuria, cardiorespiratory compromise, and neurologic effects. The diagnosis should be suspected in a patient who is inebriated without the odor of ethanol or has a metabolic acidosis with a widened anion gap, an osmolal gap, or calcium oxalate crystalluria. Treatment requires correction of fluid and electrolyte disturbances and consideration of ethanol therapy and hemodialysis to reduce the levels of ethylene glycol and its metabolites. Ethanol has an affinity for the hepatic enzyme that is 100-fold greater than that of ethylene glycol. Ethanol is a competitive inhibitor of alcohol dehydrogenase and blocks the formation of toxic metabolites; the nontoxic parent compound is renally excreted. Ethanol therapy is indicated in the presence of serum ethylene glycol levels greater than 20 mg/dL and acidemia regardless of the level.

► Ethylene glycol is another of the very few intoxications truly associated with major morbidity and mortality if appropriate, aggressive therapy is not rapidly instituted. But such therapy can commence only if the diagnosis is suspected, and this can sometimes be one of the most difficult diagnoses to make. The authors point out those clinical settings that should arouse suspicion: intoxication without an alcohol odor (but when the two are co-ingested, this can be misleading, especially since the formation of toxic matabolites may be temporarily delayed), severe and persistent anion-gap acidoses, especially with an osmolal gap (although paradoxically this latter finding is worse in the presence of the parent compound and decreases just at the time the acidosis, caused by metabolites, becomes more and more pronounced), and crystalluria (although this, too, is frequently absent). Thus, there must be a truly high index of suspicion and sometimes empirical institution of therapy in clinically unstable patients when there are any of the features of ethylene glycol poisoning. This is also one of the few poisonings where confirmatory toxicologic analysis is occasionally of great value.

While ethanol is useful in delaying production of the toxic metabolites, it should not be thought of as the mainstay of therapy. Hemodialysis is the key here and should be used in all but the most trivial ethylene glycol poisonings, regardless of ethanol (or when it becomes available, 4-MP) therapy.—J.R. Hoffman, M.D.

Very Severe Self-Poisoning Lithium Carbonate Intoxication Causing a Myocardial Infarction

Perrier A, Martin P-Y, Favre H, Muller AF, Urban P, Chevrolet J-C (Hôpital Cantonal Universitaire, Geneva, Switzerland)

Chest 100:863–865, 1991 9–11

Background.—Lithium is frequently prescribed for patients with manic-depressive illness despite its side effects and narrow therapeutic margin. Although acute lithium poisoning is relatively uncommon, its occurrence is life-threatening. The patient who survives may have permanent neurologic and renal sequelae. This report describes a patient with very severe lithium intoxication who had 1 of the highest plasma lithium levels ever reported.

Case Report.—A 46-year-old man who had been taking lithium carbonate for 10 years for manic-depressive disease was admitted to the hospital in a comatose condition. The patient's pulse was 84 beats per minute, and his blood pressure was 100/60 mg Hg. He had ocular incoordination, diffuse hypertonia, and increased deep-tendon reflexes. There was no Babinski sign or clonus. The patient's lithium plasma level was 14.6 mmol/L, which confirmed the diagnosis of voluntary lithium intoxication. The patient underwent intubation and gastric lavage. He required 4 courses of protracted hemodialysis to lower the lithemia to nontoxic ranges. There was a rebound increase after each course. The patient remained comatose for a total of 7 days. Other prolonged neurologic manifestations included hyperreflexia and fluctuating focal signs. He also developed hypotension, cardiovascular collapse, nephrogenic diabetes insipidus, and diarrhea. Less-common features were acute myocardial infarction without coronary artery lesions and thrombocytopenia. The patient eventually recovered completely.

Discussion.—The occurrence of a myocardial infarction, thrombocytopenia, and requirement for prolonged and repeated hemodialysis was probably related to unusually high plasma lithium levels. Lithium clearance is directly correlated with urinary flow, so rehydration should be begun early to re-establish normal renal function. Theoretically, more-frequent short-lasting sessions of hemodialysis could have been more useful than the prolonged procedures.

▶ Case reports by definition describe events that are so unusual as to be clinically meaningless for most of us most of the time. Thus, neither the apparent myocardial infarction associated with lithium overdose nor the "complete recovery" despite such high levels is particularly worth remembering. The case does remind us, however, that unlike the vast majority of overdoses, lithium intoxication (which, by the way, is more frequently a "therapeutic toxicity" related to changes in lithium dose or the introduction of new medications [e.g., for vomiting, diarrhea, or congestive heart failure] than to single large ingestion) is a true life threat that must be treated aggressively. Early and prolonged dialysis is critical, and renal "consultants" must be taught that the decision to institute dialysis should be based far more on the patient's clinical condition than merely the level of lithium in the blood.—J.R. Hoffman, M.D.

Anaphylactic Reactions to a Psyllium-Containing Cereal

James JM, Cooke SK, Barnett A, Sampson HA (Johns Hopkins Hosp, Baltimore, Md)

J Allergy Clin Immunol 88:402–408, 1991 9–12

Background.—Occupational allergy to psyllium, characterized by rhinitis, wheezing, and gastrointestinal distress, has been previously studied in pharmaceutical and health care workers. A study of 20 of 24 women reporting allergic reactions to the psyllium-containing cereal Heartwise (Kellogg Co., Battle Creek, Mich) is examined. The allergic symptoms and supporting immunologic evidence for the allergic reactions are studied.

Methods.—Twenty of 24 patients reporting to the Kellogg Company allergic reactions to Heartwise cereal from 1989 to 1990 were studied by history and laboratory investigations. Histories were obtained by questionnaire and telephone surveys, and sera were tested for antibodies to fractionated psyllium antigens.

Results.—All patients evaluated were female with a median age of 53 years, and 14 of the 20 were nurses. Twelve women reported atopic symptoms, but 18 had laboratory data suggesting atopy. Only 3 women denied prior exposure to psyllium. Eleven of 15 subjects who had previously dispensed psyllium-containing laxatives had experienced nasal congestion and itching, watery itchy eyes, chest tightness, or coughing while dispensing these products. Four of 7 patients who had previously taken psyllium-containing laxatives experienced nausea and abdominal cramping. After 2 to 30 minutes of ingesting less than 1 cup of cereal, patients experienced allergic reactions. The most common symptoms included wheezing, tightness in the throat or chest, urticaria, itching or tingling in the mouth, and nasal congestion/pruritis; other associated symptoms included vomiting and diarrhea. All women required medical treatment, including 55% who were treated in an emergency room. Nearly three quarters of the women received antihistamines, and more than 20% received epinephrine and corticosteroids. In all subjects, specific IgE and IgG antibodies to various protein fractions of psyllium were detected.

Conclusion.—Susceptible individuals with occupational exposure to psyllium dust seem to be at high risk of reacting to ingested psyllium products. Other prior exposures to psyllium, including dispensing or ingesting bulk laxatives containing psyllium, seemed to sensitize these individuals to ingestion of Heartwise.

▶ This is one more unusual circumstance where knowing the association between a specific occupational exposure and a particular and potentially dangerous response (anaphylaxis) can be useful.—J.R. Hoffman, M.D.

Anaphylaxis From Administration of Intravenous Thiamine

Stephen JM, Grant R, Yeh CS (Tufts/New England Med Ctr; Tufts Univ, Boston, Mass)

Am J Emerg Med 10:61–63, 1992 9–13

Introduction.—The routine administration of intravenous thiamine hydrocholoride (vitamin B_1) to patients at high risk of thiamine deficiency, such as chronic alcoholics and other malnourished patients, is widespread. Although rare, intravenously administered thiamine can cause potentially fatal anaphylactic reactions.

Case Report.—A 32-year-old man who had ethanol intoxication was evaluated for left shoulder pain and numbness caused by slipping on ice. Thiamine hydrocholoride, 100 mg, was administered intravenously. Within 2 minutes the patient complained of intense pruritus, and the infusion was stopped. The patient then experienced hypotension, light-headedness, anxiety, intense erythema, respiratory distress, and substernal chest pain. The patient improved with aggressive therapy.

Conclusion.—In view of the large number of patients treated with thiamine who do not have side effects, it appears that thiamine is relatively safe. However, although rare, thiamine-induced anaphylaxis can be life-threatening, and 9 deaths have been reported in the foreign literature.

▶ A simple rule of thumb should be used when administering drugs to patients: anyone can be allergic to any drug, and the nurse or physician administering a drug should be prepared to treat anaphylaxis or other allergic reactions. This extremely rare reaction to thiamine, given the millions of doses that are given annually, should reinforce that rule.—E.J. Otten, M.D.

Crack/Cocaine Abuse

Cocaine-Associated Chest Pain

Zimmerman JL, Dellinger RP, Majid PA (Baylor College of Medicine, Houston, Tex)

Ann Emerg Med 20:611–615, 1991 9–14

Introduction.—Although the development of acute myocardial infarction (MI) is a well-documented complication of cocaine abuse, the more frequent occurrence of cocaine-associated chest pain without MI has received less attention in the literature. The clinical and ECG features of cocaine abusers who came to the emergency department (ED) with chest pain and were admitted to the coronary care unit were analyzed.

Patients.—During a 4-month period, 48 long-term cocaine abusers aged 17 to 51 years had to be admitted because of chest pain. There were 34 men and 14 women with a mean age of 29 years. None of the patients had a previous history of diabetes mellitus, MI, or a significant family history of coronary artery disease. The route of cocaine abuse was smoking in 29 patients (59%), intravenous injection in 16 patients (32%), smoking plus intravenous injection in 3 patients (6%), and not recorded in 1 patient. Twenty-two patients had abused cocaine for more than a year, and the mean duration of cocaine abuse was 5 years. In 13 patients chest pain developed within 1 hour after cocaine abuse.

Findings.—Initial ECGs were available for all 48 patients. Eight patients (16%) had normal ECGs. Five patients (10%) had sinus tachycardia as the only ECG abnormality. Sixteen patients (33%) had repolarization abnormalities consisting of upward-coved ST-segment elevation and T-wave abnormalities. Follow-up ECGs were available for 31 patients, 10 of whom had persistent repolarization abnormalities. Three patients (6%) sustained acute MIs.

Conclusions.—Long-term cocaine abusers with chest pain and persistent abnormalities on follow-up ECGs may well have chronic myocardial changes that are causing the ischemia.

▶ This paper adds to the growing literature on cocaine-associated chest pain. This was a retrospective study design of 48 long-term cocaine users admitted to the hospital because of severe chest pain. Three of these patients (or 6%) were found to have sustained acute MI. The etiology of MI in cocaine-associated cardiac events is not entirely clear, although factors related to increased myocardial oxygen demand, coronary vasospasm, and platelet aggregation with thrombus formation are all among the possibilities that have been proposed, and all make pathophysiologic sense, given the intense vasoconstriction and platelet activation that is known to be associated with cocaine. There are also now numerous biopsy studies of patients who have died of cocaine-induced cardiac pathology that show so-called contraction bands of myocardial necrosis, which may reflect small-vessel chronic vasculitis changes. This is a confusing and complicated body of literature, and the dilemma facing the emergency medicine practitioner in evaluating cocaine-using patients with acute chest pain is considerable. Although the incidence of MI is low, a liberal approach to hospitalization for those patients with any ECG abnormalities and/or clinical features of ischemic chest pain probably ought to be encouraged. Unfortunately, the majority of cocaine users who come to the ED with chest pain will have additional worrisome features such as shortness of breath, diaphoresis, or palpatations, and furthermore the majority of such patients will have abnormal ECGs. An elevated creatine phosphotinase level is almost universal in patients with cocaine toxicity, and a single determination in the emergency center will not rule in/out acute MI with any accuracy. One possible way to rule out myocardial ischemia may be to use bedside echocardiography to assess wall motion, but this is only in the initial stages of investigation. My reading of the literature would suggest that there are no specific features of the cocaine abuser with chest pain that can be identified acutely in the ED and reliably predict or exclude MI. Therefore, if cardiac criteria for thrombolysis are present, thrombolytics should be used.—F.M. Henretig, M.D.

Plasma Cocaine and Tetracaine Levels Following Application of Topical Anesthesia in a Swine Laceration Model

Terndrup TE, Mariani PJ, Walls HC, Spear RM, Karatay CM (State Univ of New York; Onondaga County Health Dept, Syracuse, NY)

Am J Emerg Med 9:539–543, 1991 9–15

Background.—The combination of .5% tetracaine, .05% epinephrine, and 11.8% cocaine (TAC) is increasingly used as a topical anesthetic for lacerations. However, questions remain as to the extent of systemic absorption of the components of TAC and their physiologic effects.

Whether plasma levels of the components could be measured after TAC application to swine was determined.

Methods.—After an overnight fast and anesthetization, 10 domestic swine underwent tracheostomy with mechanical ventilation and femoral venous and arterial cannulation. Stage 3 anesthesia was maintained by intermittent thiopental and pancuronium. The heart rate (HR), arterial pressure, and plasma cocaine and tetracaine levels were measured periodically during 180 minutes. Half of the animals received TAC, 5 mL, applied for 15 minutes to a standardized facial laceration. Plasma samples were analyzed for cocaine and tetracaine by gas chromatography and mass spectroscopy.

Results.—Dunnett's multiple-range test showed significant changes in HR and mean arterial pressure. After 10 minutes, all animals in the experimental group showed measurable plasma cocaine levels, but none had measurable tetracaine. Experimental and control animals showed no differences in HR or arterial pressure changes.

Conclusions.—The standard TAC solution applied to lacerations appears to result in measurable plasma cocaine levels but not tetracaine. The levels observed are of a magnitude to cause physiologic effects in humans. Achieving consensus as to the best topical anesthetic for use in the emergency department will require more research into the anesthetic formulation, timing, and technique of application.

▶ This is a reasonable attempt to develop a pharmacokinetic model of cocaine absorption and elimination. It is evident that sufficient cocaine is absorbed from topical application to a laceration to potentially cause noticeable changes in cardiovascular physiology.—G.V. Anderson, M.D.

Cocaine Adsorption to Activated Charcoal In Vitro

Tomaszewski C, Voorhees S, Wathen J, Brent J, Kulig K (Denver Gen Hosp, Colo; AnalytiTox, Inc, Englewood, Colo; Univ of Colorado, Denver; Morrison, Colo)

J Emerg Med 10:59–62, 1992 9–16

Background.—Activated charcoal (AC) is commonly used after cocaine ingestion. However, the ability of AC to bind with this drug has not been established. Whether AC adsorbs cocaine at the ranges of pH that may be encountered in the gastrointestinal tract was determined.

Methods.—A stock solution of cocaine was prepared, and varying concentrations of powdered AC were added to cocaine samples and filtered. A sample of each filtrate was added to 1 mL of methanol and analyzed by high-pressure liquid chromatography for cocaine content.

Findings.—Cocaine adsorption to charcoal for AC:drug ratios of 1:1 was 40%; 2.5:1, 92%; and 5:1, 99% at pH 1.2. At pH 8, these values were 78%, 98%, and 99%, respectively. All means were significantly different from the control at each pH level. In addition, cocaine adsorption was significantly greater at pH 8 than at pH 1.2 at the AC:drug ratio of 1:1.

Conclusions.—Activated charcoal avidly binds cocaine. As the proportion of AC increased, so did cocaine adsorption. More than 90% of cocaine was adsorbed at AC:cocaine ratios of 2.5:1 and above, regardless of the pH. Therefore, with the doses of AC commonly used in clinical practice—50 to 100 g—there may be more than enough AC to adsorb a potentially lethal cocaine dose.

▶ This study provides in vitro data to support the empirical use of AC after cocaine ingestion. In fact, the findings are much in line with other drugs that adsorb to AC. At the practical level, we are often faced with "body stuffers" who ingest crack cocaine (wrapped or unwrapped) to avoid arrest. Our practice has been to recommend whole-bowel irrigation of these patients. As it turns out, there are no data to support the efficacy of whole-bowel irrigation for cocaine. Perhaps these studies will follow soon.—S. Wason, M.D.

Neurovascular Complications of Cocaine Abuse

Peterson PL, Roszler M, Jacobs I, Wilner HI (Wayne State Univ; Detroit Receiving Hosp, Detroit)

J Neuropsychiatry Clin Neurosci 3:143–149, 1991 9–17

Background.—An estimated 5 million Americans abused cocaine regularly in 1985, and in 1986, 15% of the population reportedly had used it at least once. Neurovascular complications have not been examined in a large prospective group of patients from a single institution.

Patients.—More than 30,000 admissions to Detroit Receiving Hospital, an inner-city emergency trauma center, were reviewed. The patients studied were 45 years of age or younger and were admitted with an acute neurologic deficit that lasted at least 24 hours and appeared to result from vascular pathology. Those using cocaine intravenously at the time of the event were excluded. The 33 patients, who had 35 acute neurovascular events related to cocaine abuse, represented 3% of the cocaine-related admissions.

Findings.—Thirteen of the 33 patients admitted intravenous drug abuse, but 10 of them reported that they no longer used intravenous drugs; all had changed to crack cocaine. A majority of patients were hypertensive when admitted, but only 1 required treatment. Eighteen patients had ischemic infarcts, and 15 had hemorrhagic neurovascular events. One patient had a recurrent infarct and died. Five patients with hemorrhage died in the hospital, and 1 died after a recurrent event.

Discussion.—A great majority of these neurovascular events were related to the abuse of crack cocaine. Young persons with such events should be asked about the use of cocaine and should have urine screening for cocaine metabolites. Those who have a hemorrhagic event related to cocaine abuse should undergo angiography.

▶ While it is difficult to base sweeping conclusions on this information (due to some problems with the study design), several points to remember are worth stressing. Acute neurologic events in young people should raise suspicion of cocaine use, although in at least the majority of cases this will not be the etiology. Unlike the situation with cocaine-related coronary ischemia/infarction, there is rarely any significant delay between cocaine use and the onset of neurologic symptoms. About half these patients will have bland infarcts, and half will have hemorrhage. As in other series, the vasculitis described with amphetamines does not appear to occur; on the other hand, the incidence of aneurysms and arteriovenous malformations among those with hemorrhage was extraordinarily high in this report. Finally and perhaps most important for emergency physicians, the marked prevalence of hypertension at the time of patient presentation reminds us of the predominant α-adrenergic overdrive caused by cocaine and suggests that phentolamine (a titratable α-adrenergic blocker) may have an important role to play in selected cocaine users with acute or evolving neurologic findings.—J.R. Hoffman, M.D.

Association Between Life-Threatening Cocaine Toxicity and Plasma Cholinesterase Activity

Hoffman RS, Henry GC, Howland MA, Weisman RS, Weil L, Goldfrank LR
(New York City Dept of Health, NY; Vanderbilt Univ, Nashville, Tenn)
Ann Emerg Med 21:247–253, 1992 9–18

Background.—Many researchers have suggested, without any clinical evidence, that patients with plasma cholinesterase deficiency, either genetic or acquired, are more susceptible to the adverse effects of cocaine. Whether there is an association between life-threatening manifestations of cocaine toxicity and plasma cholinesterase activity in a cohort of cocaine-intoxicated patients was determined.

Methods.—One hundred eighty-seven patients seen in the emergency department on 191 consecutive occasions were enrolled in the prospective study. All had signs and symptoms consistent with cocaine intoxication. The electrometric method was used to determine plasma cholinesterase activity. Cocaine-positive patients were stratified into 1 of 2 groups: life-threatening and non–life-threatening toxicity. Cocaine-negative patients served as controls.

Findings.—The mean plasma cholinesterase activity for those in the life-threatening and non–life-threatening groups was 682 and 904 Michel units/L, respectively. In the control group, this value was 1,058 Michel units/L. The differences among these 3 groups were significant.

Conclusions.—Life-threatening manifestations of cocaine intoxication and reduced plasma cholinesterase activity are associated. Further research is needed to clarify the nature of this relationship.

▶ Since cocaine is hydrolyzed to a nontoxic metabolite by cholinesterase, it seems logical that patients deficient in this enzyme may manifest toxicity more readily. Serial blood cocaine or metabolite levels were not measured in this study, but the increased side effects were presumably due to higher cocaine levels persisting for a longer period of time. Another clinical manifestation of a lower serum cholinesterase level is sensitivity to succinylcholine, another drug metabolized by this enzyme. The critically ill cocaine user may experience prolonged respiratory and muscle paralysis if succinylcholine is used therapeutically. Low cholinesterase levels may explain why infants have seizures when exposed to exhaled crack cocaine smoke or after swallowing small amounts of cocaine. Currently, cholinesterase levels cannot be analyzed fast enough to help the clinician, but it is intriguing to speculate on a possible antidote role if some form of cholinesterase could be administered to patients in a toxic condition. Another potentiator of cocaine toxicity is alcohol. When used together, ethanol and cocaine combine to form cocaethylene, a compound with a longer half-life and probably more toxic profile than the parent cocaine itself. Finally, some ingenuous, cost-conscious, and pharmacologically astute cocaine users have been reported to inject themselves with small quantities of organophosphate insecticides (such as RAID) to inactivate their own cholinesterase and get a more intense high from a smaller amount of cocaine (1).—J.R. Roberts, M.D.

Reference

1. Aaron CK, et al: *Vet Hum Toxicol* 31:375, 1989.

Rhabdomyolysis Associated With Cocaine Abuse

Nolte KB (Univ of New Mexico, Albuquerque)

Hum Pathol 22:1141–1145, 1991 9–19

Background.—Rhabdomyolysis associated with exposure to environmental toxins or drug abuse has been reported. Recent clinical reports have described rhabdomyolysis associated with cocaine abuse but have not presented detailed autopsy findings. The pathologic abnormalities in 2 patients who died of cocaine-associated rhabdomyolysis were assessed.

Case 1.—A 31-year-old man with a 10-year history of drug abuse was hospitalized after being found disoriented and combative. His clinical course was characterized by a progressive rhabdomyolysis, azotemia, and disseminated intravascular coagulation. He was successfully resuscitated from asystole on the fifth day of hospitalization but died on the seventh hospital day. Skeletal muscle showed necrosis without evidence of vasculitis, polarizable foreign crystals, or other specific lesions. Death was attributed to hyperpyrexia with rhabdomyolysis resulting from cocaine use.

Case 2.—A 35-year-old Hispanic man with a history of drug abuse was hospitalized after being found unresponsive. Diaphoresis, muscular rigidity, and combative behavior were observed. He was successfully resuscitated from a cardiac arrest in the emergency room, and the subsequent clinical course was characterized by anoxic encephalopathy, rhabdomyolysis, temperatures to 104.4°F, and anterior cardiac ischemia detected by ECG. On the fourth hospital day, a urine specimen contained myoglobin in a concentration greater than 1 ng/dL, and vital support was withdrawn. Death was attributed to anoxic encephalopathy after cardiopulmonary arrest resulting from cocaine toxicity with rhabdomyolysis as a contributory condition.

Discussion.—The mechanism of cocaine-associated rhabdomyolysis is unknown but may include ischemia resulting from vasoconstriction, direct toxicity, hyperpyrexia, increased muscle activity from agitation or seizures, or adulterants added by the vendor. In unexplained cases of rhabdomyolysis, cocaine toxicity should be suspected. The presence of cocaine in the blood may be prolonged when rhabdomyolysis is associated with acute renal failure.

▶ Rhabdomyolysis is well known to occur with many drug overdoses (especially heroin, phenycyclidine, and amphetamines), and it is also seen as a sequela of prolonged coma from the sedative/hypnotics (1, 2). Some degree of rhabdomyolysis and an elevated creatine phosphokinase (CPK) level are almost universal findings in serious cocaine toxicity, and they should be suspected in any cocaine-abusing patient with coma, seizures, hyperpyrexia, hypotention, or severe agitation. Patients with rhabdomyolysis, acute renal failure, liver dysfunction, and disseminated intravascular coagulation (DIC) have a high mortality rate—almost 50% (3). Most clinical laboratories do not routinely test for myoglobin directly. At the bedside, one can test urine with a dipstick, and if the dipstick is positive for blood and there is an absence of erythrocytes on microscopic analysis of urine sediment, myoglobinuria can be assumed. This easy test should be done routinely because even significant myoglobinuria will not discolor the urine. In some cases of serious rhabdomyolysis, however, the myoglobinuria will be missed (the serum half-life of myoglobin is short because it is rapidly cleared). The CPK level will remain elevated for days, so do not forget to order the CPK level even if the urine test is negative. Once rhabdomyolysis or myoglobinuria is documented, forced alkaline diuresis should be instituted immediately. However, even early therapy will not always stave off renal failure. Rhabdomyolysis will release tissue thromboplastin and activate the coagulation cascade. This mechanism is thought to be responsible for the DIC seen with severe cocaine toxicity.—J.R. Roberts, M.D.

References

1. Kendrick WC, et al: *Ann Intern Med* 86:381, 1977.

2. Koffler A, et al: *Ann Intern Med* 85:23, 1976.
3. Roth D, et al: *N Engl J Med* 319:673, 1988.

Passive Inhalation of Free-Base Cocaine ('Crack') Smoke by Infants

Mirchandani HG, Mirchandani IH, Hellman F, English-Rider R, Rosen S, Laposata EA (Office of the Med Examiner, City of Philadelphia; Jeanes Hosp, Philadelphia; Univ of Pennsylvania)
Arch Pathol Lab Med 115:494–498, 1991 9–20

Background.—Cocaine is a commonly abused substance in the United States. Regardless of the route of administration, a variety of medical complications are associated with cocaine use in adults. One of these complications is sudden death. A series of infants who died unexpectedly and who were found to have traces of cocaine and/or its metabolites was reported.

Methods.—Records at the Philadelphia Medical Examiner's Office from 1987 through 1989 were reviewed to search for cases of infant death in which toxicologic analysis showed the presence of cocaine or benzoylecgonine. In all cases identified, complete autopsies had been performed. Also, a medical examiner or staff member of the Philadelphia Sudden Infant Death Syndrome Center visited each scene.

Findings.—Sixteen cases were identified. The infants were 7 girls and 9 boys aged 2 weeks to 7 months. Most had been found unresponsive in bed or on the sofa. Autopsy findings had been unremarkable in 7 cases. Pulmonary vascular congestion and edema were noted in 6. Cocaine or benzolylecgonine was found in the blood of 12 infants, in the brain in 3, and in the kidney in 2. One baby had cocaine in the liver as well as in the blood. Scene investigation documented that most of these infants had been exposed to the smoke from crack cocaine shortly before death. In only 2 cases did the care givers deny a history of drug use.

Conclusions.—The route of cocaine administration in these infants appears to have been the passive inhalation of crack smoke. The cocaine may have contributed to the deaths of these babies. Thus, infants and children in environments in which crack is smoked may inhale cocaine and potentially suffer from its adverse effects.

▶ Crack cocaine is responsible for thousands of deaths in this country annually, either directly through toxicity or indirectly through crime. It is known that a single, low dose of cocaine can cause fatal arrhythmias. Now it has been indicted as a cause of unexpected infant death through a mechanism of passive inhalation of crack cocaine smoke. It is postulated that the infant's exposure to cocaine may be prolonged and increase the risk of cardiac arrhythmias undetected by autopsy because they have less plasma cholinesterase activity. Routine drug screens may be indicated in infants after cardiac arrest.—E.J. Otten, M.D.

Therapeutic Techniques

Efficacy of Flumazenil in Acute Alcohol Intoxication: Double Blind Placebo-Controlled Evaluation

Lheureux P, Askenasi R (Erasme Univ Hosp, Brussels, Belgium)

Hum Exp Toxicol 10:235–239, 1991 9–21

Background.—Flumazenil is a benzodiazepine (BZD) antagonist used as an antidote for pharmacologic and toxic effects of BZDs. Some observations and uncontrolled studies have suggested that it could improve impairment of consciousness related to pure ethanol intoxication. This study evaluates the efficacy of flumazenil, at a dose usually active in BZD overdose, in patients with alcohol-induced coma.

Methods.—Eighteen patients admitted to an emergency department with coma related to acute alcohol (ALC) intoxication were randomized and treated blindly with intravenous placebo or 1 mg of flumazenil. A modified Glasgow Coma Scale was used to observe the evolution of consciousness. The clinical response was compared with the effect observed in patients with pure BZD overdose.

Results.—In 18 patients with ALC intoxication, 1 mg of flumazenil was not more effective than placebo in improving consciousness. Flumazenil appeared to be very active in the BZD-sedated group. Higher doses of flumazenil improved consciousness in 5 of 11 ALC-intoxicated patients who had not initially improved. At the dose usually active against BZD sedation, flumazenil did not improve CNS depression induced by ALC intoxication.

Conclusion.—Results showed that 1 mg of flumazenil administered to patients in an alcohol-induced coma was no more effective than placebo in improving consciousness. Previous reports of the efficacy of low doses of flumazenil may have corresponded to a spontaneous evolution. Better responsiveness was observed at higher doses of flumazenil, but placebo-controlled studies should be performed.

▶ Flumazenil is likely to become a very useful diagnostic and therapeutic antidote in comatose or lethargic patients. It is helpful to note that it does not arouse patients with ethanol-induced coma. There are upregulated γ-aminobutyric acid receptors in the brains of alcohol-habituated rats that are felt to be receptors for endogenous BZD antagonists; these have been used to explain alcohol "withdrawal" seizures (1). It is not clear how this finding correlates to the noncontrolled observation of arousal response to higher flumazenil doses, although it will be interesting to note whether future research with flumazenil reveals a higher incidence of seizures in alcoholics treated with this drug.—W.P. Burdick, M.D.

Reference

1. Peris J, et al: *Alcohol Clin Exp Res* 16:311, 1992.

Intravenous Acetylcysteine in Paracetamol Induced Fulminant Hepatic Failure: A Prospective Controlled Trial

Keays R, Harrison PM, Wendon JA, Forbes A, Gove C, Alexander GJM, Williams R (King's Coll, London, England)

BMJ 303:1026–1029, 1991 9–22

Introduction.—Acetylcysteine is an effective treatment for the prevention of hepatitis if given within 10 hours of a paracetamol overdose. Recent evidence has suggested that it also may be of benefit when administered from 10 to 36 hours after an overdose. A prospective study was undertaken to examine the effects of intravenous acetylcysteine on the outcome of patients with fulminant hepatic failure after a paracetamol overdose.

Methods.—Fifty patients were randomized to received either acetylcysteine, 150 mg/kg over a 15-minute period followed by 50 mg/kg over a period of 4 hours and then 100 mg/kg over a 16-hour period, or equivalent amounts of 5% dextrose. The patients, ranging in age from 16 to 60 years, also received intensive liver care. None had previously received acetylcysteine treatment. Paracetamol overdoses had occurred at least 33 hours prior to admission to the liver failure unit.

Results.—Twelve of the 25 patients who received acetylcysteine survived, significantly more than the 5 of 25 control patients who survived. Ten of the 25 patients who received acetylcysteine developed clinical signs of cerebral edema, significantly fewer than the 17 of 25 control patients who had edema. Both groups of patients had similar grades of encephalopathy and severity of liver failure as judged by prolongation of the prothrombin time. Twelve of 25 patients who received acetylcysteine developed hypotension requiring adrenaline or noradrenaline, significantly fewer than the 20 of 25 control patients who required inotropic support. All patients tolerated acetylcysteine well, with no hypersensitivity reactions seen.

Conclusion.—These findings provide evidence that intravenous acetylcysteine is a safe and effective treatment for patients with fulminant hepatic failure after a paracetamol overdose. Although it did not result in improvements in liver function as indicated by prolongation of the prothrombin time, it improved survival and was not associated with adverse reactions.

▶ The findings of this study show that intravenous acetylcysteine (IVA) significantly improves survival in patients with fulminant hepatic failure after a paracetamol overdose. Intravenous acetylcysteine has been used in Britain for years (over 10 to my knowledge) but is not Food and Drug Administration approved in this country. Apparently, IVA enhances tissue oxygen consumption in fulminant hepatic failure. The depression of myocardial contractility induced by oxygen free radicals can be prevented by IVA, which is a scavenger of oxygen free radicals. Certainly, given the morbid prognosis associated with fulminant hepatic failure secondary to a paracetamol overdose, it would be useful to have IVA in this country for treating such patients. The article does not address whether such results can be achieved with oral therapy so long after the ingestion.—J.T. Amsterdam, M.D.

Pharmacologic Interventions After an LD_{50} Cocaine Insult in a Chronically Instrumented Rat Model: Are Beta-Blockers Contraindicated?

Smith M, Garner D, Niemann JT (Univ of California, Los Angeles; Harbor-UCLA Med Ctr, Torrance)

Ann Emerg Med 20:768–771, 1991 9–23

Background.—The systemic effects of cocaine are mediated by altered synaptic transmission. The drug blocks the presynaptic uptake of catecholamines, and its effects on dopaminergic function may underlie the euphoria and addiction consequent to cocaine use. Increased levels of catecholamine at neural synapses are thought to cause the cardiovascular complications of cocaine use.

Objective.—Drug treatment of acute cocaine toxicity was investigated in instrumented conscious rats given a median infective dose of cocaine intravenously (1.4 mg/100 g body weight).

Treatments.—Administration of a saline placebo was compared with the intravenous bolus injection of .5 mg/100 g of diazepam, .2 mg/100 g of chlorpromazine, 1 mg/100 g of propranolol, 3 mg/100 g of labetalol, and .1 mg/100 g of verapamil.

Results.—Tonic-clonic seizure activity followed the intravenous injection of cocaine. None of the drugs significantly improved survival when compared with placebo. None of the animals given propranolol survived, and only 1 of 10 given labetalol survived.

Conclusion.—These findings fail to suggest a single effective antidote for cocaine overdose. β-blockade may adversely affect survival in the setting of life-threatening cocaine toxicity.

▶ Statistically, the results of this study are limited by the fact that comparisons were made among 6 groups of only 10 animals each. However, the results caution in the use of β-blockade for cocaine-poisoned patients. In humans, esmolol infusion in 7 patients with cocaine-induced tachycardia or hypertension was of no benefit and actually may have worsened some of the group (1). A very interesting study demonstrated potentiation of the adverse cardiac effects of cocaine by propranolol in stable patients undergoing cardiac catheterization (2). Propranolol increased coronary vascular resistance and decreased coronary sinus flow even further than what was seen with preceding intranasal cocaine.—R.M. McNamara, M.D.

References

1. Sand IC, et al: *Am J Emerg Med* 9:161, 1991.

2. Large RA, et al: *Ann Intern Med* 112:897, 1990.

Hyperbaric Oxygen Toxicity: Role of Thromboxane

Jacobson JM, Michael JR, Meyers RA, Bradley MB, Sciuto AM, Gurtner GH (Johns Hopkins Univ; Univ of Maryland, Baltimore; Univ of Utah, Salt Lake City; New York College of Medicine, Valhalla)

J Appl Physiol 72:416–422, 1992 9–24

Background.—Much is known about the treatment of normobaric O_2 toxicity, but fairly little is known about the pathophysiology or treatment of hyperbaric O_2-induced lung injury. The role of thromboxane on hyperbaric O_2 toxicity was explored.

Methods.—Nine groups of rabbits were studied. Two groups were exposed to room air. One normoxic control group was studied at 1 atmosphere absolute (ATA), and the other was exposed to room air at 4 ATA. Seven groups were exposed to 100% O_2 at 4 ATA for 1 hour. One of these was untreated; 1 was pretreated with superoxide dismutase (SOD) and catalase; 1 was pretreated with normal saline, the vehicle used in groups given antioxidant enzymes; 1 was pretreated with polyethylene glycol (PEG)-conjugated SOD and PEG-catalase; 1 was pretreated with the antioxidant butylated hydroxyanisole; 1 was pretreated with indomethacin; and 1 was pretreated with UK 37, an inhibitor of thromboxane synthase.

Results.—When compared with the normoxic control group, 1-hour room air exposure at 4 ATA did not significantly affect pulmonary arterial pressure, lung weight gain, or transfer rates for the aerosolized compounds. Exposure to 100% O_2 for 1 hour at 4 ATA caused pulmonary hypertension with the pulmonary arterial pressure increased to more than 100 mm Hg. In addition, hyperbaric O_2 greatly raised the concentration of thromboxane B_2 in alveolar lavage fluid and dramatically augmented lung weight gain and the transfer rate for aerosolized ^{99m}Tc-diethylenetriaminepentaacetic acid and Fluorescein isothiocyanate-dextran. Hyperbaric O_2 had no effect on the pulmonary content of malondialdehyde. Saline treatment did not prevent hyperbaric O_2-induced lung injury. Butylated hydroxyanisole completely blocked the increase in alveolar thromboxane B_2, pulmonary arterial pressure, lung weight gain, and transfer rates for aerosolized molecules. Polyethylene glycol–PEG-catalase pretreatment eliminated the hyperbaric O_2-induced increase in pulmonary arterial pressure and lung injury. Treatment with unconjugated SOD and catalase did not decrease pulmonary hypertension or lung injury. Treatment with the unconjugated enzymes did not prevent a marked increase in the transfer rate for ^{99m}Tc-diethylenetriaminepentaacetic acid. Pretreatment with indomethacin or UK 37 eliminated the increase in pulmonary arterial pressure, lung weight gain, and enhanced movement of aerosolized particles across the alveolar capillary membrane.

Conclusions.—Indomethacin and UK 37, an inhibitor of thromboxane synthase, entirely eliminate the pulmonary hypertension and edema. Stimulation of thromboxane synthesis may be a major mechanism by which hyperbaric O_2 causes lung injury in rabbits.

▶ This study suggests that thromboxane (TxB_2) plays a crucial role in the development of hyperbaric oxygen toxicity. While this hypothesis is sound and supported by other researchers, the actual measurement of TxB_2 levels in this paper is documented in only 2 rats (the butylatal hydroxyanisole–treated group). There are no charts or graphs to display one of the primary conclusions of the study, which is that decreased levels of TxB_2 are protective and elevated levels are associated with lung injury.

It is noted that 6 animals had seizures during hyperbaric exposure and were dropped from the study. There is no mention of which group(s) they were a part. Does this represent a protective effect by a particular combination of anti-oxidants, or does it reflect a direct correlation between CNS toxicity and a given drug? In clinical hyperbaric medicine, the most common manifestation of oxygen toxicity is seizures. In practice, pulmonary toxicity is a greater problem for patients receiving normobaric oxygen at an FiO_2 greater than 50% for prolonged periods of time. Perhaps data from this study would be more applicable to this group of patients.—H.D. Unger, M.D.

Rectal Ulcer With Massive Haemorrhage Due to Activated Charcoal Treatment in Oral Organophosphate Poisoning

Mizutani T, Naito H, Oohashi N (Univ of Tsukuba; Tsukuba Med Ctr, Tsukuba City, Japan)

Hum Exp Toxicol 10:385–386, 1991 9–25

Introduction.—Activated charcoal administration now serves as a nonspecific therapy for any poisoning. This lifesaving treatment had produced few complications to date. A patient treated with activated charcoal to counter the effects of ingested organophosphate insecticide and who then had massive intestinal bleeding related to the charcoal therapy was studied.

Case Report.—A 42-year-old woman had had psychotic disorders for 2 decades. She was seen in the emergency room after ingesting the insecticide fenitrothion 3 hours previously. Although comatose, she received 50 g of activated charcoal plus magnesium sulfate treatment every 4 to 6 hours for 50 hours. She also received intravenously administered dinoprost trometamol for 2 continuous weeks to prevent constipation. On the tenth hospital day, the patient passed several charcoal masses, followed by bloody stools, Endoscopic testing demonstrated a bleeding rectal ulcer that ultimately required an anal stretch procedure and surgical hemostasis to achieve full recovery.

Conclusions.—The complication of massive intestinal bleeding caused by ulceration has not been reported in patients undergoing activated charcoal treatment for poisoning. This study should alert physicians to the possibility of the complication of massive rectal bleeding occurring in this type of patient. Early and intense treatment of the constipation that often accompanies activated charcoal use is recommended to prevent such events.

▶ This unusual complication from the administration of charcoal probably could have been avoided if the patient had not received over 500 g of charcoal in combination with magnesium citrate and atropine. The patient also had melena, which could be secondary to a rectal ulcer. Perhaps the patient had an underlying problem that was exacerbated by the cathartics and charcoal.—E.J. Otten, M.D.

Elevated Blood Cyanide Concentrations in Victims of Smoke Inhalation

Baud FJ, Barriot P, Toffis V, Riou B, Vicaut E, Lecarpentier Y, Bourdon R, Astier A, Bismuth C (Université Paris 7; Service Médical de la Brigade des Sapeurs-Pompiers Créteil; Université Paris 6; Institut National de la Santé et de la Recherche Médicale Unité 275, Palaiseau; Hôpital de Bicêtre, France)
N Engl J Med 325:1761–1766, 1991 9–26

Objective.—Death from smoke inhalation results from unknown toxic gases. Hydrogen cyanide may play a role in addition to carbon monoxide; however, its contribution is not established because of delays in measuring blood cyanide concentrations. Blood samples obtained at the scene of a fire were measured to determine the importance of cyanide concentrations in victims of fire.

Methods.—The study sample comprised 109 victims of residential fires from whom blood samples were obtained before any treatment was given. There were 59 men and 50 women with a mean age of 33 years. The cyanide concentrations of the blood samples were compared with those of 40 patients with drug intoxication, 29 with carbon monoxide intoxication, and 45 trauma victims. To evaluate the metabolic effect of smoke inhalation, plasma lactate levels were also measured at admission in 39 patients without severe burns.

Findings.—In the 66 fire victims who survived, the mean blood cyanide concentration was 21.6 μmol/L; in the 43 victims who died, the blood cyanide concentration was 116.4 μmol/L. Both of those levels were higher than the 5 μmol/L level in the 114 controls. Seventy-four percent of the patients who died had cyanide concentrations above 40 μmol/L, and 46% had levels above 100 μmol/L. Blood cyanide and carbon monoxide concentrations were significantly correlated; admission plasma lactate concentrations correlated better with the cyanide concentration than the carbon monoxide concentration. Cyanide intoxication—

cyanide concentration over 40 μmol/L—was sensitively indicated by a plasma lactate concentration over 10 mmol/L.

Conclusions.—Cyanide poisoning may occur in victims of residential fires. On hospital admission, an increased plasma lactate concentration may indicate cyanide toxicity in patients who are not severely burned. Hydroxocobalamin is a promising antidote to severe cyanide inhalation.

▶ Smoke inhalation is the cause of death in most fires. The smoke contains carbon monoxide, hydrogen cyanide, and other toxins, depending on the material that is burning. This paper, from Paris, provides good correlation between the severity of smoke inhalation and the victim's cyanide level. Unfortunately, we in the United States must use the potentially harmful nitrite-thiosulfate antidote and do not have access to hydroxocobalamin, a drug that may in the future be given to fire victims at the scene by prehospital personnel and save many lives.—E.J. Otten, M.D.

Carbon Monoxide Poisoning in Children Riding in the Back of Pickup Trucks

Hampson NB, Norkool DM (Virginia Mason Clinic, Seattle; Virginia Mason Med Ctr, Seattle)

JAMA 267:538–540, 1992 9–27

Introduction.—Exposure to motor vehicle exhaust gases poses a significant potential injury to human beings. Such exposure often occurs accidentally because of a lack of awareness of the risk posed by some activities. Data on children poisoned with carbon monoxide while traveling in the back of pickup trucks were reviewed.

Methods.—The records of all pediatric patients who were treated for carbon monoxide poisoning with hyperbaric oxygen in 1986 to 1991 were reviewed retrospectively. The characteristics of the poisoning incident and clinical patient outcome were noted. Those episodes that occurred during travel in the back of a pickup truck were selected and clinical follow-up was conducted by telephone interview 2 to 55 months after treatment.

Results.—Of the 68 children treated for accidental carbon monoxide poisoning, 20 rode in the back of pickup trucks, 17 rode under a rigid closed canopy on the rear of the truck, and 3 rode beneath a tarpaulin. The average carboxyhemoglobin level was 18.2%. Loss of consciousness occurred in 15 patients, other symptoms included headache, lethargy, nausea, combativeness, confusion, blurred vision, ataxia, conjunctival irritation, somnolence, disorientation, and weakness. One child died, another had permanent neurologic deficits, and 18 had no recognizable sequelae. In all pickup trucks involved, the exhaust system had a previously known leak or a tail pipe that exited at the rear rather than at the side of the truck.

Conclusion.—There is a potential risk of carbon monoxide poisoning in passengers in the back of pickup trucks. These episodes occur when there is a leaking exhaust system or a tail pipe exiting beneath the rear bumper of the pickup truck. Allowing riders in the back of pickup trucks should be avoided, if not totally restricted.

▶ It is well known that exhaust fumes contain carbon monoxide and that if you can smell exhaust gases, you are probably being exposed to carbon monoxide. Not only pickup trucks but also station wagons with rear windows that open and any vehicle with a defective exhaust system may lead to carbon monoxide poisoning of the occupants of the vehicle. Many trauma deaths are caused by individuals riding in the back of pickup trucks. This should be reason enough to outlaw this practice even without the risk of carbon monoxide poisoning.—E.J. Otten, M.D.

Optimal Patient Position for Transport and Initial Management of Toxic Ingestions

Vance MV, Selden BS, Clark RF (Good Samaritan Regional Med Ctr, Phoenix, Ariz)

Ann Emerg Med 21:243–246, 1992 9–28

Purpose.—In patients taking oral poisons, many factors influence the gastric empyting rate and thus the drug absorption rate. One controllable factor is positioning, but previous studies have failed to assess its effects on drug absorption. The effects of various body positions on drug absorption were compared in a model of acetaminophen overdose.

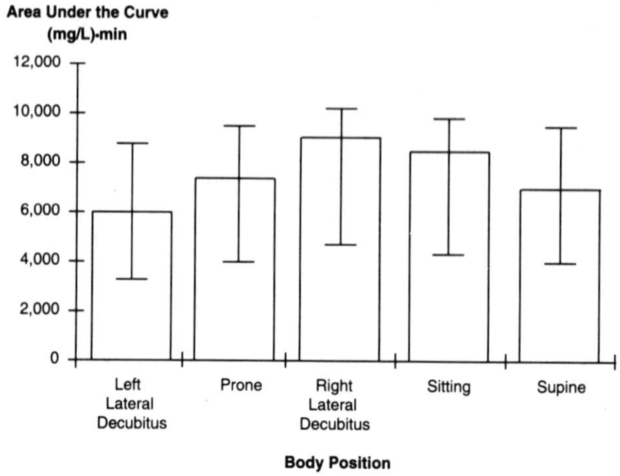

Fig 9–3.—Total area under the curve for each body position for the duration of the study. (Courtesy of Vance MV, Selden BS, Clark RF: *Ann Emerg Med* 21:243–246, 1992.)

Methods.—Twelve healthy volunteers with no concurrent use of medications affecting gastrointestinal function participated. Body positions evaluated were the left and right lateral decubitus, supine, prone, and sitting. After fasting, each subject took acetaminophen, 80 mg/kg, in the form of 160-mg children's caplets, a mean of 39 per trial. Subjects then remained in the assigned position for 2 hours, during which time acetaminophen levels were measured every 15 minutes. Total drug absorption was evaluated by calculating a 2-hour area under the curve (AUC) for each subject trial.

Results.—The lowest AUC was with the left lateral decubitus position, although it was not significantly lower than that for the supine position. Both of these AUCs, however, were lower than those for the prone, right lateral decubitus, and sitting positions (Fig 9–3).

Conclusions.—Placing a patient in the left lateral decubitus position appears to minimize initial drug absorption, although not significantly more so than the supine position. However, since the left lateral decubitus position has other advantages as well, notably preventing aspiration, orally positioned patients should be positioned this way for prehospital and initial emergency department management. Further benefits would probably be gained by placing the patient in this position after the administration of activated charcoal.

▶ The left lateral decubitus (LLD) position prevents stomach contents from entering the duodenum via a simple gravity effect. Since most drugs are poorly absorbed in the stomach and must pass into the small intestine before entering the systemic circulation, it is not expected that this position may hamper drug absorption. The coingestion of potent anticholinergic drugs has also been thought to delay systemic absorption by delaying gastric emptying. It is not clear whether this positioning could be of significant clinical value during a short ambulance ride, but the authors correctly also suggest that the LLD position be used while patients are being treated in the emergency center.—J.R. Roberts, M.D.

10 Sports Medicine

Sports-Related and Non-Sports-Related Sudden Cardiac Death in Young Adults

Burke AP, Farb A, Virmani R, Goodin J, Smialek JE (Armed Forces Inst of Pathology, Washington, DC; Office of the Chief Med Examiner, Baltimore, Md)

Am Heart J 121:568–575, 1991 10–1

Background.—Many younger athletes who die during exercise have hypertrophic cardiomyopathy and anomalous coronary arteries, whereas most over 35 years of age have severe atherosclerosis. To ascertain which conditions are preferentially seen in exercising individuals, exercise and non-exercise-related sudden deaths were compared.

Methods.—All cases of natural, unexpected cardiac death in people aged 14 to 40 years that occurred in the state of Maryland over an 8-year period were reviewed. Exercise-related deaths were defined as those with symptoms occurring during or within 1 hour of engaging in sports and with death occurring within 24 hours. Each sudden death was matched for age, sex, and race to 3 non-exercise-related deaths in random fashion.

Results.—Of 690 sudden cardiac deaths, 34 were sports related, an incidence of 5%. Nine patients had severe atherosclerosis as the cause of death, 8 had hypertrophic cardiomyopathy with asymmetry, and 6 died of unknown causes; 2 of the latter patients had tunnel arteries (table).

Exercise-Related Deaths: Distribution of Race/Sports

Cause of death (n)	*Black*	*White*	*Sport*
Severe atherosclerosis (9)	1	9	Running (5) Other (4)
Hypertrophic cardiomyopathy (8)	6	2	Basketball (7) Swimming (1)
Anomalous coronary arteries (4)	2	2	Basketball (2) Baseball (1) Soccer (1)
Others (13)	6	7	Basketball (5) Running (4) Other (4)

(Courtesy of Burke AP, Farb A, Virmani R, et al: *Am Heart J* 121:568–575, 1991.)

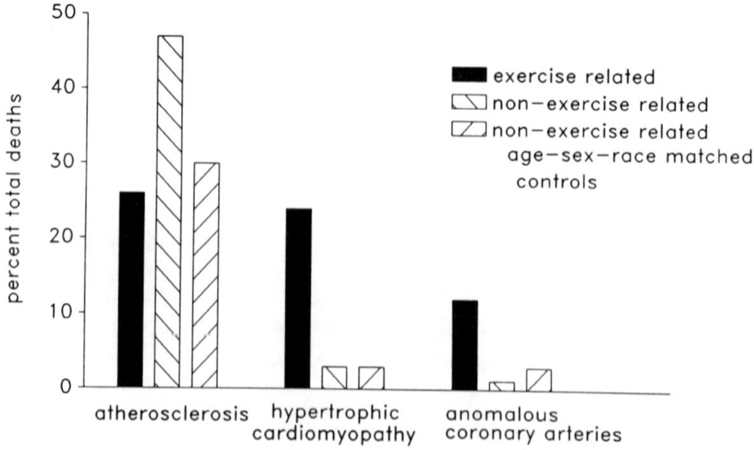

Fig 10–1.—Comparison of sports-related vs. nonsports-related deaths (atherosclerosis, hypertrophic cardiomyopathy, and anomalous coronary arteries). (Courtesy of Burke AP, Farb A, Virmani R, et al: *Am Heart J* 121:568–575, 1991.)

Other causes of death included coronary artery anomalies, idiopathic concentric left ventricular hypertrophy, myocarditis, arrythmogenic right ventricle, and Kawasaki disease. When compared with controls, exercise-related deaths were more likely to result from hypertrophic cardiomyopathy (Fig 10–1). The incidence of severe atherosclerosis was no different between the 2 groups when matched controls were considered. The mean age of subjects with hypertrophic cardiomyopathy was 24 years vs. 32 years for those with severe atherosclerosis.

Conclusions.—In younger people with hypertrophic cardiomyopathy, exercise may result in sudden cardiac death. Of all exercise-related sudden cardiac deaths, the younger victims are usually black and have hypertrophic cardiomyopathy, and the older ones are usually white and have severe atherosclerosis. This information may be useful in counseling athletes and in setting up preventive screening programs.

▶ This is an interesting and timely article because of the popularity and importance of exercise in the United States. It is not surprising that the mean age for sudden death due to hypertrophic cardiomyopathy in the exercise group is younger than that in the nonexercise group. However, it is of interest that this study does not show a difference in the "exercise group" and the "nonexercise" group in sudden death associated with severe atherosclerosis.—G.V. Anderson, M.D.

Concussion in Sports: Guidelines for the Prevention of Catastrophic Outcome

Kelly JP, Nichols JS, Filley CM, Lillehei KO, Rubinstein D, et al (Univ of Colorado, Denver)
JAMA 266:2867–2869, 1991 10–2

Background.—Traumatic brain injuries occur frequently in contact sports. Concussion, a traumatically induced alteration in mental status, not necessarily with loss of consciousness, is too often dismissed as trivial. Repeated concussions can lead to brain atrophy and cumulative neurophysiologic deficits; repeated concussions occurring within a short pe-

Colorado Medical Society Guidelines for the Management of Concussion in Sports*

Grade 1: Confusion Without Amnesia, No Loss of Consciousness
Remove from contest. Examine immediately and every 5 minutes for the development of amnesia or postconcussive symptoms at rest and with exertion. Permit return to contest if amnesia does not appear and no symptoms appear for at least 20 minutes.

Grade 2: Confusion With Amnesia, No Loss of Consciousness
Remove from contest and disallow return. Examine frequently for signs of evolving intracranial pathology. Reexamine the next day. Permit return to practice after 1 full week without symptoms.

Grade 3: Loss of Consciousness
Transport from field to nearest hospital by ambulance (with cervical spine immobilization if indicated). Perform thorough neurological evaluation emergently. Admit to hospital if signs of pathology are detected. If findings are normal, instruct family for overnight observation. Permit return to practice only after 2 full weeks without symptoms.

Prolonged unconsciousness, persistent mental status alterations, worsening postconcussion symptoms, or abnormalities on neurological examination require urgent neurosurgical consultation or transfer to a trauma center.

* Adapted from the Colorado Medical Society, Denver.
(Courtesy of Kelly JP, Nichols JS, Filley CM, et al: JAMA 266:2867-2869, 1991.)

riod can be fatal. The case of a young athlete who died after sustaining repeated concussions is described.

Case Report.—A 17-year-old high school football player sustained a concussion without loss of consciousness in a football game. He complained of headache during the week. A week after his first concussion, he fell unconscious after several impacts in another game. Computed tomography of the head showed diffuse swelling of the brain. Despite resuscitative efforts, the patient died. Autopsy showed massive swelling and vascular congestion of the brain. There were no notable brain hemorrhages, recent or remote anoxic damage, or diffuse axonal injury. A focal axonal swelling in the brain stem was attributed to the original concussion 1 week before death.

Discussion.—Individuals who are symptomatic from a concussion even without loss of consciousness are at risk for the development of diffuse brain swelling after a second impact to the head. Repeated concussions can predispose the brain to vascular congestion from autoregulatory dysfunction. The Colorado Medical Society has developed guidelines that define levels of injury and the appropriate management of these injuries (table). An athlete with grade I concussion with confusion but no loss of consciousness should be examined at regular intervals for the development of amnesia or postconcussive symptoms at rest and with exertion. He may be permitted to return to the game if symptoms do not appear, but the development of amnesia, however, changes the severity of concussion to grade 2 and precludes the athlete's return to the same event. Athletes rendered unconscious or those with persistent mental status alterations, worsening postconcussive symptoms, or abnormalities on neurologic examination require urgent neurosurgical evaluation.

▶ I am always leery of guidelines based on only a few cases. In this report, only 1 illustrative case is presented. Nonetheless, the emergency physician, whether in the emergency department or on the sidelines, should be aware of this publication when giving advice to players, parents, coaches, or others. Until additional data are provided, these guidelines represent a prudent approach to the sports participant sustaining a concussion during contact sports.—J.R. Hedges, M.D.

Anterior Compartment Syndrome of the Thigh in Athletes: Indications for Conservative Treatment

Robinson D, Halperin N (Assaf Harofeh Med Ctr, Zerifin, Israel)

J Trauma 32:183–186, 1992 10–3

Background.—Rarely, anterior compartment syndrome of the thigh results from blunt contusion without an accompanying fracture. Most physicians advocate surgical treatment for this condition. However, wound infection rates are high, and loss of knee range of motion is common. A group of patients treated conservatively was evaluated.

Methods and Outcomes.—Six athletes aged 19 to 28 years were studied prospectively. All had an anterior thigh compartment syndrome immediately after sustaining a blunt contusion to the quadriceps with an accompanying massive hematoma. Fasciotomy was not done, even though sustained pressure rose above 50 mm Hg. The patients' tissue pressure, renal function, and creatinine phosphokinase levels were monitored carefully. Neurologic function remained unaffected. One year later, the athletes had no limitation of joint motion or weakness of the quadriceps.

Conclusions.—Anterior compartment syndrome of the thigh should be treated conservatively when it occurs as an isolated injury in a young athlete without accompanying wound or fracture. Treatment should consist of hospitalization, close monitoring of intracompartmental pressure and neurovascular status, and narcotic analgesics. Corticosteroid use is probably contraindicated. However, when treating patients conservatively, emergency fasciotomy is indicated if a neurologic dysfunction develops.

▶ This article might best be renamed ". . .in **Young** Athletes" because one inclusion criteria for the study was "an age less than 30 years." In addition, this condition may be relatively rare because the authors were able to find only 16 cases previously reported in the literature.

As always, a high index of suspicion is needed to avoid missing the diagnosis. Note that the diagnosis must be based on pressure measurements because (1) the motor function of the femoral nerve is difficult to test clinically in the face of a large extramuscular hematoma and (2) creatinine phosphokinase levels may be within normal levels.

The study underscores a very effective approach to medical care: the concept of "watchful waiting." It is effective, often results in better outcomes, and is by no means a passive process. It is, instead, a process of active waiting through a process of aggressive observation.—E.H. Taliaferro, M.D.

Magnetic Resonance Imaging in the Evaluation of Knee Injuries

Boeve BF, Davidson RA, Staab EV Jr (Univ of Florida, Gainesville)

South J Med 84:1123–1127, 1991 10–4

Background.—The methods for evaluating knee injuries have limitations ranging from patient discomfort and possible morbidity to a wide range of accuracy and expense. Several recent articles have favorably compared the accuracy of MRI with that of arthroscopy. Data from 10 articles on the role of MRI in the diagnosis of meniscal and anterior cruciate ligament tears of the knee were analyzed.

Methods.—Fifteen articles comparing MRI with arthroscopy were selected from MEDLINE and authors' references, and 10 articles were retrieved. Arthroscopy was considered the standard to which MRI was compared. All patients had arthroscopy after MRI. The number of structures evaluated, sensitivity (SN), specificity (SP), positive predictive value (PPV), and negative predictive value (NPV) for tears of the medial meniscus, lateral meniscus, and anterior cruciate ligament were either obtained or calculated from data in the articles.

Results.—In the 10 studies, the medians for measurements of medial meniscus tears were 97% SN, 89% SP, 88% PPV, and 96% NPV. Measurement medians for lateral meniscus tears were 85% SN, 94% SP, 86% PPV, and 95% NPV. Anterior cruciate ligament tear measurement medians were 100% SN, 96% SP, 80% PPV, and 98% NPV. The high NPVs of MRI in the studies, many at 100%, suggest that diagnostic arthroscopy is not necessary in evaluating patients with negative MRI studies. Magnetic resonance imaging also had superior sensitivity in detecting frank posterior horn tears, intrasubstance meniscal tears, and significant incidental findings, and it may be useful in preoperative planning.

Conclusions.—Screening MRI studies can decrease the number of unnecessary diagnostic arthroscopies in patients with clinically suspected meniscal and cruciate ligament tears. Although the cost-effectiveness of MRI utilization has not been calculated, MRI offers a high NPV, noninvasiveness, and a lack of ionizing radiation and has the ability to detect subtle defects and significant incidental findings in the evaluation of knee injuries.

▶ Magnetic resonance imaging studies of the knee can help decrease the need for diagnostic arthroscopy. Diagnostic arthroscopy of the knee is 65% to 95% accurate. This review of 10 articles confirms that MRI has 85% to 100% accuracy in predicting meniscal and anterior cruciate tears.—J. Wasserberger, M.D.

Dislocation of the Knee

Frassica FJ, Sim FH, Staeheli JW, Pairolero PC (Mayo Clinic and Found, Rochester, Minn)

Clin Orthop 263:200-205, 1991 10–5

Introduction.—Knee dislocation is an uncommon but serious injury that can produce disruption of the popliteal vessels as well as the collateral and cruciate ligaments and the posterior joint capsule. Traction injury of the common peroneal nerve is also a possibility. The vascular status of the limb is of prime importance at the time of injury.

Patients.—Twenty patients were seen in an 8-year period with complete knee dislocations. Eight of them had a total of 23 associated injuries. Injuries occurred during athletic activity and motor vehicle accidents as well as during farm work. The mean age was 33 years.

Vascular Injuries.—Ten of the 17 patients seen initially had vascular injuries, and 9 required surgical repair of the popliteal artery. Most often the vessel had avulsed distally. Two patients had thrombosis in the mid-popliteal artery secondary to stretching of the vessel. Intraoperative arteriograms demonstrated both distal thrombosis and anastomotic narrowing in patients seen after popliteal artery reconstruction. Vascular reconstruction succeeded in 8 of the 9 cases.

Ligament Injuries.—Eleven of the 12 patients had satisfactory results after early open repair of the knee ligaments.

Discussion.—All patients suspected of having traumatic knee dislocation should have vascular assessment of the lower extremities, including a Doppler study of the ankle pulses. A younger patient lacking pulses should have immediate femoral arteriography. If the popliteal artery is not normal, it should be explored operatively.

▶ This very serious injury is fortunately exceedingly rare. Unfortunately, when it does occur, serious vascular injury is anything but rare. Indeed, a 1961 study reported that 89% of these patients required amputation. Fortunately, subsequent advances in vascular surgery have lowered the need for amputation.

Beware of the patient who sustained a knee injury with dislocation and spontaneous reduction prior to arrival in the emergency center. The history is not fully obtained until the paramedic run sheet is reviewed and the patient specifically questioned about the occurrence of this event.—E.H. Taliaferro, M.D.

Subject Index

A

B

C

E

F

J

K

L

M

N

O

Q

R

S

U

V

W

Z

Author Index

A

B

C

N

O

P

Q

R

S

T